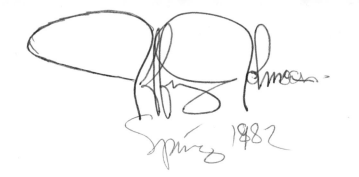

Spring 1882

Trauma Management

Volume I

Abdominal Trauma

Edited by

F. William Blaisdell, M.D.
Department of Surgery
University of California, Davis
Sacramento, California

Donald D. Trunkey, M.D.
Department of Surgery
San Francisco General Hospital
San Francisco, California

1982
Thieme-Stratton Inc. • New York
Georg Thieme Verlag • Stuttgart • New York

Publisher: Thieme-Stratton Inc.
381 Park Avenue South
New York, New York

Illustrations by Marsha Dohrmann
Cover by Leslie H.P. Hurley

TRAUMA MANAGEMENT
VOLUME I: ABDOMINAL TRAUMA

TSI ISBN 0-86577-011-5
GTV ISBN 3-13-598901-1

Last digit is print number   5 4 3 2 1

Contributors

F. William Blaisdell, M.D.
Professor of Surgery
Chairman, Department of Surgery
University of California, Davis
Sacramento Medical Center

John Cello, M.D.
Assistant Professor in Residence
Department of Medicine
University of California, San Francisco
Chief of Gastrointestinal Medicine
San Francisco General Hospital

Norman Christensen, M.D.
Assistant Clinical Professor of Surgery
University of California, San Francisco
Department of Surgery
San Francisco General Hospital

Sebastian Conti, M.D., F.A.C.S.
Associate Clinical Professor
University of California, Davis
Director, Non-invasive Vascular
  Laboratory
Mercy San Juan Hospital

Richard Crass, M.D.
Assistant Professor of Surgery
University of California, San Francisco
Department of Surgery
San Francisco General Hospital

Lawrence Danto, M.D., F.A.C.S.
Associate Clinical Professor
Department of Surgery
University of California, Davis
Sacramento Medical Center

Michael Federle, M.D.
Assistant Professor in Residence
University of California, San Francisco
Department of Radiology
San Francisco General Hospital

Charles Frey, M.D.
Professor and Vice Chairman
Department of Surgery
University of California, Davis
Department of Surgery
Sacramento Medical Center

James Holcroft, M.D.
Associate Professor of Surgery
Director of Trauma Services
Department of Surgery
University of California, Davis
Sacramento Medical Center

Kenneth A. Kudsk, M.D.
Trauma and Burn Research Fellow
University of California, San Francisco
San Francisco General Hospital

Robert C. Lim, Jr., M.D.
Professor of Surgery
University of California, San Francisco
Department of Surgery
San Francisco General Hospital

Jack McAninch, M.D.
Associate Professor of Urology
University of California, San Francisco
Chief, Department of Urology
San Francisco General Hospital

Theodore Schrock, M.D.
Associate Professor of Surgery
University of California, San Francisco
Department of Surgery
San Francisco General Hospital

George F. Sheldon, M.D.
Professor of Surgery
University of California, San Francisco
Department of Surgery
San Francisco General Hospital

Donald D. Trunkey, M.D.
Professor of Surgery
University of California, San Francisco
Chief, Department of Surgery
San Francisco General Hospital

Foreword

As academic surgeons, our interest in trauma developed for multiple reasons. Our discipline, surgery, through the act of operation itself inflicts trauma. Thus the study of trauma provides insight into surgical illness and recovery from operation. The pursuit of trauma involves the need to investigate basic mechanisms of wound healing, immunology, biochemistry and physiology. Trauma is, and will remain, the most secure of all surgical disciplines since the treatment of injury will not be resolved by medical measures as is potentially true of cardiovascular disease, cancer, and biliary and gastrointestinal disorders. Finally, despite increasing specialization, the trauma surgeon must remain a generalist since under emergency circumstances he must be prepared to deal with unexpected problems in any area involving any body cavity.

In the process of developing trauma surgery as a distinct discipline in our university settings, we have acquired colleagues with similar interests. Thus we have accumulated a large clinical experience and a uniform approach to trauma that seems to merit collection in a treatise on trauma rather than remain as a large number of articles scattered throughout the medical literature in journals and in book chapters. We are bringing together from the respective staffs of our two institutions—the University of California, San Francisco at San Francisco General Hospital and the University of California, Davis—a coordinated and united approach to trauma.

In order to make the material more manageable and to permit subsequent revision and expansion of particular areas in which changes are the most rapid, we have elected rather than to incorporate our work into a single volume to organize it into a series of monographs. Our first, *Abdominal Trauma*, should be of the widest general interest and set the tone for the next two monographs on *Cervicothoracic Trauma* and *Initial Management and Resuscitation*. Subsequently we plan monographs on the major specialty areas: orthopedics, neurosurgery, plastic and maxillofacial surgery, burns and eventually the full spectrum of trauma.

The orientation of our trauma monographs will be toward the senior surgical resident and general surgeons who treat trauma in their private practice. We believe our orientation will be both practical and conservative, aimed toward saving the maximum number of lives with minimum morbidity.

After careful consideration of many options we have selected Thieme-Stratton Inc. as our publisher. We believe that this aggressive young publishing company will provide the resources to ensure a high quality series of volumes, which we hope will enhance the libraries of many of our colleagues in surgery.

F. William Blaisdell, M.D.

Donald D. Trunkey, M.D.

Preface

This monograph, *Abdominal Trauma*, is designed as the first of a series of treatises on trauma. It is fitting that *Abdominal Trauma* be the first since the abdomen is the focal point of the evaluation of injury in the multiply injured patient. Abdominal injury is the most subtle of all the injuries to the body, and is the most likely to tax the diagnostic skills of the trauma surgeon. Autopsy studies repeatedly confirm that abdominal injury is the most frequent cause of readily preventable death. Our philosophic approach to trauma, which may seem conservative to some, is to recommend exploratory laparotomy if there is doubt concerning the presence of abdominal injury. There are no statistics available that support the contention that patients die from complications secondary to exploratory laparotomy, whereas it is relatively easy to prove that patients die of delays in the diagnosis of abdominal trauma and that many patients die in sophisticated hospitals of readily treatable injuries without having been subjected to operation at all. We remain surprised at the reluctance of surgeons to explore the abdomen of a traumatized patient and at the same time readily accept a negative exploration rate of 20 to 30 percent for appendicitis as representing good practice.

Although new diagnostic techniques such as peritoneal lavage and CT scanning have provided valuable assistance in making a prompt diagnosis of abdominal injury, there is no substitute for clinical judgment since all ancillary diagnostic methods have inherent false negative rates. That for peritoneal lavage, for example, varies from 1 to 5 percent, but most likely is closer to the higher figure in medical centers that see and treat trauma only occasionally. The tragedy of one preventable death in a previously healthy young person may have permanent impact on the unfortunate surgeon responsible for treatment.

The contributions to this and successive volumes all come from our colleagues with whom we practice, as we believe the value of this work is that it provides a uniform approach to trauma. In the experience of the authors this represents an optimal approach for us as we deal with thousands of trauma victims each year in our combined environments. We believe the guidelines for patient management that we have laid down should be of assistance to those who deal with trauma less frequently as well.

We the editors are grateful to our secretaries who have assisted us with the manuscript preparation by turning out draft after draft. We are indebted to our surgery residents, many of whom have initiated or assisted us with statistical evaluation of our results which have led to numerous papers and manuscripts. Moreover, their suggestions regarding patient management have led to new concepts of patient care and operative management. We are proud of our artist, Marsha Dohrmann, who has been selected to provide consistency for our illustrative material. We in particular are indebted to our long suffering wives and children who have tolerated our emergency commitments so well and in so doing have helped our surgical careers.

Contents

GENERAL ASSESSMENT, RESUSCITATION AND EXPLORATION OF PENETRATING AND BLUNT ABDOMINAL TRAUMA

F. WILLIAM BLAISDELL

INTRODUCTION

Definitive surgical treatment for abdominal injuries for all practical purposes has developed only in this century. Previously, survival was more dependent upon the individual's inherent ability to recuperate rather than on the medical care he received.

Historically, King William, the Conqueror of England, was one of the unfortunate victims of blunt abdominal trauma. In 1087, he was faced with a revolt of his son, Robert, and the treason of his half-brother, Odo. King Philip of France was in open rebellion. William and his army crossed the channel and attacked the French with a viciousness that he had not previously displayed. With a large force, he harried the countryside up to Mantes and fell upon the city in a surprise attack, during which terrible destruction ensued. The city was so completely burned that today it is hard to find traces of eleventh century buildings in the town. As the king rode through the burning streets, his horse, frightened by burning embers, threw the corpulent king against the high pommel of the saddle with such force that he was lethally ruptured. He was taken initially to the Priory of Saint-Gervais where he lived an additional three weeks with great suffering and then died of intra-abdominal sepsis on September 8, 1087. His body was removed to Caen where the final insult occurred. The attendants, who were trying to force his body into the stone coffin, ruptured the abdomen and an incredible stench filled the church. The tomb was destroyed in 1562 by the Calvinists. Only a single thigh bone survived as a remnant

**Table 1–1   CAUSE OF DEATH IN 425 TRAUMA CASES
(SAN FRANCISCO GENERAL AUTOPSY STUDY)**

Type of Injury	Percentage
Head injury	45%
Burns	11%
Heart injury	10.5%
Lung injury	8%
Liver injury	6.5%
Aortic injury	4%
Hemorrhage	4%
Pelvic fracture	2.5%
Miscellaneous	3.0%
Hospital related*	6.5%

*primarily sepsis and respiratory failure

of the king, but this too was lost during the revolutionary riots of 1793. Today a simple stone slab is all that marks the grave of William the Conqueror.

During the nineteenth century, several surgeons attempted laparotomy for gunshot wounds of the abdomen with mixed success. However, mortality for an abdominal wound was 98 percent during the American Civil War. During the Boer War in 1899, there were isolated reports of successful surgical treatment of major abdominal trauma but more patients died after operative intervention than survived.[21]

World War I brought improvements in surgical techniques and perioperative care such that mortality following gunshot wounds to the abdomen dropped to 45 percent. This was further reduced to 25 percent during World War II, to 12 percent during the Korean conflict, and to 8.5 percent in Viet Nam. During the same period, the civilian mortality rate was 55 percent. This has dropped to less than 5 percent today. Much of this resulted from putting into practice lessons learned during the management of military wounds since World War II.[2,7,12,13,15,19,21, 26,28,31]

Autopsy studies of injury show that head and chest trauma are the primary killers in present day society (Table 1-1). Nonetheless, abdominal injuries are responsible for approximately 10 percent of deaths following penetrating and blunt trauma. Isolated major blunt abdominal trauma that results in fatality is relatively rare since pelvic, chest, and head injury are found in association with most abdominally induced fatalities. Penetrating injuries most often cause fatalities secondary to major vascular injury or from septic complications of bowel injury.[16,17,26,34]

PATHOPHYSIOLOGY AND ETIOLOGY

Stab wounds are relatively benign injuries unless a major blood vessel has been lacerated or unless a particularly vital structure has been injured. Rarely do these result in much morbidity. Gunshot wounds, on the other hand, may cause devastating abdominal injury particularly if they are from high-velocity weapons or close-range shotguns (Table 1-2 lists common handguns and weapons with their respective muzzle velocities). [36]

Terminal ballistics, the amount of energy imparted to tissues by the missle, largely determines the injury and killing power (Figure 1-1). Although not all authorities agree, the most widely accepted terminal ballistic theory is the kinetic energy theory. The kinetic energy theory states that kinetic energy released to tissues

Table 1–2 EXAMPLES OF MUZZLE VELOCITY

Weapon		Velocity (ft/sec)
.22	Long rifle	1335
.22	Magnum	2000
.220	Swift	2800
.270	Winchester	3580
.357	Magnum	1550
.38	Colt	730
.44	Magnum	1850
.45	ACP	850

equals mass times velocity squared, divided by two times the gravity, KE $mV^2/2g$. This is thought to provide the best estimate of wounding capacity and it thus follows that modest increases in velocity will result in tremendous increases in the kinetic energy of the missle and resultant killing and wounding power. Simple calculations using this formula demonstrates that a .22 Magnum is capable of eight times the energy release of a .38 revolver. Generally, those weapons capable of generating a missle velocity in excess of 2000 ft/sec are said to be high-velocity.[36]

The amount of energy imparted to the tissue is estimated to be the kinetic energy upon impact minus kinetic energy upon exit. Thus, bullet design becomes important and ideally, a bullet should dissipate all of its energy to the tissue with no residual exit energy. This has led to the development of missiles which disintegrate upon impact, such as soft point and hollow nose bullets. Increased muzzle velocity and disintegrating missles can cause extensive tissue damage creating for example, a

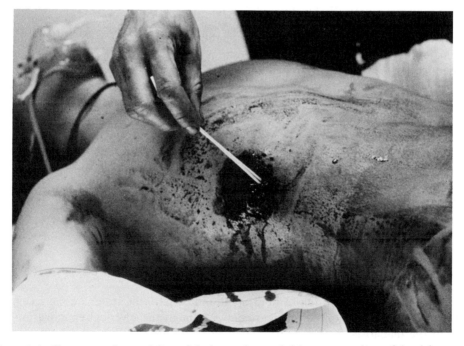

Figure 1–1 Close range shotgun injury of the lower chest and right upper quadrant of the abdomen.

Table 1–3 FREQUENCY OF INJURIES IN TRAFFIC ACCIDENT VICTIMS

	57 Pedestrians	64 Auto Occupants	6 Motorcycle or Bicycle
Head	35 (22)*	43 (30)	6 (6)
Chest	17 (4)	31 (12)	3
Abdomen	14 (2)	24 (10)	–
Spine	4 (2)	4 (1)	–
Upper Extremity	14 (0)	17 (0)	1
Pelvis and lower extremity	40 (16)	27 (2)	2
Genitourinary	5 (0)	4 (1)	–

*The number of times that each injury was the primary cause of death is indicated in parentheses (from Perry and McClellen).

temporary cavity 30 times the size of the entering bullet. This is dependent on ballistics, type of bullet, and the tissue that is transgressed. The damage produced can be worsened by secondary missiles or fragments of disintegrating bone and other tissue.

Close-range shotgun blasts undoubtedly cause the most devastating injuries of any weapon to which civilians are normally exposed. Sherman and Parrish have classified shotgun wounds into three categories: Type I shotgun injuries, sustained at long range (greater than seven yards); Type II shotgun injuries, sustained at close range (three to seven yards); and Type III shotgun injuries, sustained at very close range (less than three yards); illustrated in Figure 1-1.[29] Type I injuries usually present as scatter types and may not even penetrate visceral cavities from distances greater than 40 yards. At 20 yards, penetration is increased and yet expectant management may sometimes be warranted. Type II injuries usually involve damage to deep structures and require more aggressive management. Type III wounds produce massive tissue injury and carry a very high mortality rate (85-90 percent).

Blunt injury can be caused by direct impact, deacceleration, rotary forces, and shear forces. Direct impact may cause significant injury and the severity can be estimated by knowing the force and duration of impact as well as the mass of the patient contact area. Table 1-3 demonstrates the most common sites of injury from motor vehicle accidents. Ejection, steering assembly impact, windshield impact, instrument panel impact, and rear collision account for the majority of these.

Deacceleration injuries are most often associated with high-speed motor vehicle accidents and falls from heights. As the body impacts, the organs continue to move forward at the terminal velocity, tearing vessels and tissues from points of attachment. Rotary forces also tend to cause tearing injuries from a tumbling type of action.

Shear forces have a tendency to produce degloving types of injuries such as are apt to occur when the patient is run over by a large vehicle. As the vehicle passes over the body, the skin and subcutaneous tissues are pushed ahead tearing nutrient blood supply from its muscular sources below. Subsequent extensive soft tissue loss is common following such injury.

ASSESSMENT

The *definitive evaluation* of both blunt and penetrating trauma consists of history, physical, and laboratory assessment. Although the physical examination is a key to the diagnosis of the nature and type of trauma, the *history* should not be neglected (Table 1-4). If not obtainable from the patient, it is often available from

Table 1–4 HISTORY

Mechanism of injury
Time of injury
Status at the scene
   Level of consciousness
   Shock
Complaints
Previous state of health

the ambulance attendants, police, friends, relatives, or bystanders. It is important to obtain information about the mechanism of injury. Was penetrating trauma part of a fight and was there a possibility of blunt trauma as well? Was the injury caused by an auto accident, an auto versus pedestrian accident or a fall? And, in particular, when did the injury occur relative to the patient's admission to the emergency department? This history can be obtained by a nurse or a physician associate while the physical examination is being carried out so that it does not necessarily result in a delay in evaluation. Knowing whether the patient was awake and alert at the scene of the accident and knowing that he is now comatose may well change the priorities of management. What were the patient's complaints at the scene of the accident? What are they now? What was his previous state of health?

Physical examination can be carried out in a relatively short period of time (Table 1-5). One of the areas that is often neglected in the initial physical examination is the backside of the patient. All too often, in a matter of moments, he is tied down by intravenous lines, catheters, and splints. When first seen, the patient can be log-rolled, with someone supporting his head and neck while the back, flanks, buttocks, and posterior aspects of the thigh and neck are inspected. All of this should not take more than a few minutes to accomplish.

The *first priority* overall, in assessment, is the *respiratory system*. If the patient is conscious, he should be asked to take a deep breath. The ability to take deep inspiration without discomfort rules out most thoracic injuries. If the patient is unable to take a deep breath or if he splints with respiration, thoracic wall injury should be assumed. If the patient is comatose and has lost gag, cough, and swallowing reflex, he is at risk for aspiration, and endotracheal intubation should be carried out promptly. If ventilation is rapid and shallow then once again there is presumption of respiratory injury. In all instances in which there is evidence of chest injury, a chest x-ray should be obtained as rapidly as possible and arterial blood gases drawn from the femoral artery and sent for analysis.

Blunt traumatic injuries to the lower six ribs or penetrating trauma through the sixth interspace or below implies the possibility of abdominal injury. Since the

Table 1–5 PHYSICAL EXAMINATION

Back of patient
Ventilation adequacy
Perfusion adequacy
CNS status
Abdominal evaluation
Rectal examination
Extremity evaluation

Repeat PE—any change from above?

diaphragm rises with normal ventilation to the sixth interspace, penetrating trauma at this level may well penetrate the abdominal cavity. Similarly, very little lung tissue lies below the lower six ribs and so, blunt injuries associated with rib fractures may injure an underlying viscus such as liver, spleen, stomach, or kidney.

The *cardiovascular system* should be the *second priority* in assessment. The blood pressure and pulse should be noted. Most patients with discomfort from injury have a rapid pulse. Young patients, by vasoconstricting, can maintain a relatively good blood pressure even though considerable volume has been lost. Assessment of peripheral perfusion, urinary output, and cardiac cerebral function are appropriate to define the level of shock. Warm extremities, good peripheral perfusion, and good urinary output provide assurance that the cardiovascular system is intact.

The *third priority* in assessment is the *central nervous system*. Comatose patients should have their necks splinted until cervical films can be carried out. They should be inspected for evidence of blunt head trauma and for scalp lacerations and the level of consciousness should be noted. A progressive fall in the level of consciousness is the primary indication of increasing intracranial pressure and this dictates the need for early cerebral decompression. An awake, conscious patient obviously has a good margin for safety. If the patient is conscious and moves his head without discomfort, the probability of cervical fracture is minimal. If he is unconscious or reports cervical discomfort, the head and neck should be splinted with sand bags until cervical films can be obtained.

The *fourth priority* is the *abdominal contents - the gastrointestinal and genitourinary systems*. This begins with assessment of the integrity of the chest wall, since the lower six ribs overlie the abdominal cavity. The screening maneuver of asking the patient to take a deep breath is a reliable way of ruling out chest wall injury. If the comatose patient responds to stimuli, gentle pressure over the lower ribs establishes whether or not rib fractures are present. The contour of the abdomen should be noted. The normal fasting abdomen is scaphoid. The abdomen may be relatively flat after a full meal and, of course, the contour of the abdomen of the obese patient may be convex rather than scaphoid. Gentle palpation of the abdomen should be carried out initially by laying the hand on the abdominal wall. This permits assessment of local areas of increased tone which may suggest underlying injury. The presence or absence of penetrating wounds should be noted. Bullet holes and knife wounds should be described and should be marked with a paper clip or radiopaque object so as to permit localization on abdominal film when this is obtained. The bullet wounds should be matched up with the information about the number of shots fired. Two holes may mean either two bullets or a through and through injury. An odd number of holes implies the presence of a foreign body inside the patient and it is mandatory that the bullet be located by x-ray so its exact path can be determined. Failure to locate a foreign body such as a bullet can have serious consequences. When the wounding object is radiopaque, it must be located by x-ray, since major cardiac and vascular injury may lead to embolism of the wounding object to a remote site and early location of the wounding object may be the key to prompt recognition of these potentially lethal injuries.

Deeper palpation should be carried out to elicit guarding, tenderness, and rebound. The flanks should be palpated and the iliac crest and symphysis pubis compressed, to establish the possibility of a pelvic fracture. Inspection of the genitalia should follow. Blood coming from the urethra is diagnostic of urethral injury. If the patient can void, a urine specimen should be obtained promptly. Hematuria requires urinary tract evaluation for renal or bladder injury.

Rectal examination should be carried out. Fullness in the pelvis is diagnostic of retroperitoneal hematoma and pelvic fracture. Blood on the examining glove suggest lower gastrointestinal injury. Pelvic fractures may be associated with perineal lacerations. These compound fractures are extremely serious since they are invariably associated with extensive soft tissue injury and have high mortality.

As *final priority* the *extremities* should be examined. If the patient is awake and can move both lower extremities without discomfort, the probability of fracture is low. Passive motion of the limbs should also be carried out. If the patient is unable to cooperate then pain on motion of the extremity points to a site of probable injury. Instability, of course, is diagnostic of fracture or dislocation. The upper extremity should be examined in a similar fashion, and both upper and lower extremities carefully palpated for pulses, evidence of hematomas, and sites of tenderness which may be associated with fracture or ligamentous injury.

Following the completion of the physical examination, which rarely should take more than a few minutes, the appropriate *laboratory studies*, if not already initiated, should be carried out (Table 1-6). Blood should be sent for typing and crossmatch. Minimal examination should consist of CBC, urinalysis, chest x-ray—upright if possible, and if there is any evidence of abdominal injury, abdominal films consisting of AP and supine and upright or left lateral decubitus films (Table 1-7). Suspected bone injuries should be x-rayed. Hematuria or penetrating trauma that is presumed to pass in the vicinity of the kidneys, ureter, or bladder are indications for radiologic assessment of the urinary tract. This involves urethrograms, cystograms and/or intravenous pyelography (see Chapter 2). It is important to note that disruption of the renal pedicle can occur without the injury being reflected in the urine. The value of an intravenous pyelogram in this instance is that it not only provides information about the renal injury but, even more importantly, it also documents the status of the opposite kidney. If there is a thoracic injury or any question regarding the adequacy of pulmonary function, arterial blood should be drawn for arterial blood gases. If there is evidence of major injury, routine obtaining of an SMA-12 is appropriate. Additional specialized laboratory procedures will be dictated by the specific injuries that are suspected (see subsequent chapters). We have found it useful

Table 1–6 LABORATORY ASSESSMENT

Blood for type and cross match
Hct and WBC
Urinalysis
Arterial blood gases?
Amylase?
SMA–12?
Toxicology?
Blood alcohol?

Table 1–7 X-RAY ASSESSMENT

Chest x-ray—upright if possible
Abdominal film—KUB
Fracture sites
IVP?
CT CNS scan?

to save 10 cc of clotted blood from most patients and send the sample for toxicology, blood alcohol, or other tests, as indicated.

Repeated physical examinations are extremely helpful to the clinician in less obvious cases as are repeated vital signs and laboratory data such as the hematocrit and white count. Serum amylase may assist in diagnosing pancreatic injury.[25] The indications for peritoneal lavage will be discussed in Chapter 3.

Generally, the principle for use of lavage is that if the injury is limited to the abdomen, clinical criteria and not lavage should dictate the need for laparotomy. When there are multiple injuries, and when there is bleeding from other areas so that the hematocrit is an unreliable indication of intraabdominal bleeding, then peritoneal lavage may be an appropriate diagnostic maneuver.[8] It is of particular value when there is an associated head injury or where a history is unobtainable, as when the patient does not respond to examination so that the reliability of the abdominal examination is questionable. Other means of assessing trauma include laparoscopy, sonography, scintillation, and CT scans.[11] These all have serious limitations and will be dealt with in more detail in Chapter 2.

RESUSCITATION

The *first principle* of resuscitation involves *ensuring* an *adequate airway* (Table 1-8). This is more apt to be a problem in a patient with multiple blunt traumatic injuries than with penetrating trauma. When thoracic penetration is present or when there have been rib fractures, there is always the probability that associated lung laceration may be present. When positive pressure ventilation is initiated as part of resuscitation or when anesthesia is induced for the surgical treatment of other injuries, a minor lung laceration can produce lethal tension pneumothorax as air is forced out of the laceration due to increased atmospheric pressure in the airway (Figure 1-2). For this reason, chest tubes are used liberally as part of initial resuscitation, particularly if the unstable condition of the patient contraindicates immediate chext x-ray. In the stable patient, chest tube insertion can await indications based on chest x-ray. However, if the patient with thoracic penetration is going to require immediate abdominal surgery, then prophylactic chest tube insertion may be judicious when there has been thoracic penetration or evidence of rib fractures despite the absence of hemo- or pneumothorax.

Another mechanism for collapse with introduction of mechanical ventilation is air embolism. This results when air enters a pulmonary vessel with resultant coronary air embolism.[32] This is most apt to occur in the presence of shock when pulmonary vascular pressures are low. One indication for endotracheal intubation is altered consciousness with loss of gag, cough, and swallowing reflexes so that the patient is at risk for aspiration; major maxillofacial injury that produces bleeding into the upper airway is another. Whenever the patient has altered ventilation as manifested

Table 1–8   PRIORITIES OF MANAGEMENT

1. Airway
2. Cardiovascular
3. Central nervous system
4. Gastrointestinal and genitourinary
5. Orthopedic and plastic

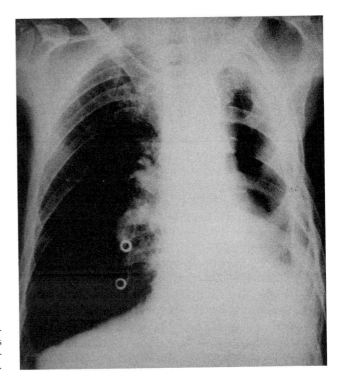

Figure 1–2 Right tension pneumothorax. The mediastinum is shifted to the left with compromise of function of the good lung.

by difficulty taking a deep breath, rapid respirations (over 30-35 per minute), and evidence of abnormalities of arterial blood gases, such as the PO2 level below 60 in a previously healthy patient or a PCO2 level below 30 or above 50, intubation is indicated.

The *second priority* is resuscitation of the *cardiovascular system*. If the patient demonstrates blood loss as manifested by the previously described signs of shock, frequent assessment of skin perfusion and temperature is appropriate. A urinary catheter should be inserted for monitoring urinary output. If there is any evidence of significant blood loss, access to the vascular system via cutdown is essential. If evidence of shock is minimal, this can be accomplished using a cutdown on an accessible antecubital vein. A 5 mm diameter plastic catheter threaded up the basilic vein to an intra-thoracic position facilitates rapid administration of volume or central venous pressure assessment techniques. This and the appearance of neck veins are always important aspects of initial triage. Distended neck veins or a high CVP in the presence of shock means tension pneumothorax, or pericardial injury or tamponade. Once these possibilities are recognized, immediate appropriate steps to identify and deal with the pathology are essential. These can consist of chest tube placement or pericardiocentesis (Figure 1-3).

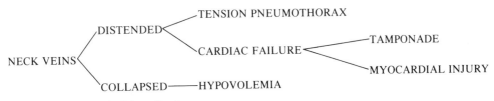

Figure 1–3 Neck Vein Triage Shock.

If the patient presents in shock, upper and lower extremity cutdowns should both be utilized. The saphenous vein at the ankle or at the saphenofemoral junction in the groin permits the introduction of the entire cross-section of intravenous tubing (8 mm diameter) in the average male patient. With saphenous and antecubital line in place, almost any patient who survived long enough to reach the Emergency Room can be successfully resuscitated, albeit briefly. Our resuscitation fluid of choice is Ringer's lactate or acetate. Two liters of fluid can be administered in two to five minutes in the average adult. If the patient responds and shock is alleviated, time is available for definitive evaluation.

If the patient does not respond or responds briefly to fluid infusion, urgent operation becomes part of the resuscitation.[23] Chest x-ray is the only diagnostic study necessary. This will tell the surgeon what body cavity to open first. If there is no blood in either hemithorax, the abdomen is the source of problems. The patient should be taken immediately to the operating room, the most appropriate body cavity opened and tamponade of the bleeding site carried out while fluid resuscitation is continued. We do not use plasma, albumin, or dextran as part of initial resuscitation, and whole blood is reserved for administration in the operating room; all initial resuscitation is carried out with balanced salt solution, even to the point of seeing the hematocrit fall below 20. The reason for this is that with adequate volume, a patient can maintain oxygenation of tissues despite a low hemoglobin. If bleeding is active, transfusing blood results in depletion of blood reserves through the loss of blood into a body cavity or externally so that once control of bleeding is obtained there may not be sufficient reserves of blood to restore the hematocrit to the optimal level of about 30.

The *third priority* is the *central nervous system* so that once the respiratory and cardiovascular systems have been stabilized, definitive evaluation can be carried out to determine if there are injuries which compromise the brain or spinal cord. If the patient does not respond to painful stimuli or voice commands and the cardiovascular function is good, severe intracranial damage is presumed. Administration of 1 to 2 units of mannitol or endotracheal intubation with hyperventilation will usually permit medical decompression of increased intracranial pressure so that time can be bought for obtaining definitive diagnostic procedures such as the CT scan. When the abdominal or thoracic injuries are extremely urgent, time may not permit obtaining definitive assessment of the neurological system. In these circumstances, the neurosurgeons may wish to place burr holes while thoracotomy or laparotomy is going on so that temporary decompression can be obtained. Later the patient can be taken for definitive scanning studies followed by reoperation as indicated to control intracranial bleeding and to evacuate intracerebral hematomas.

The *fourth priority* for resuscitation is the *gastrointestinal* and *genitourinary systems*. Generally, laparotomy should be carried out within six to eight hours, during the "golden period" of wounding. It is during this period of time that contamination such as that due to perforation of the intestine remains on the peritoneal surface so that local irrigation and debridement can be carried out and much of the risk of infection eliminated. After that so-called "golden period", the bacteria invade tissue so that the wound is not easily cleaned. It is for this reason that we do not observe stab wounds since we feel that prompt operation permits early recognition of injury and can avoid many of the infectious complications in the abdominal cavity and in the wounds and incisions.

The *final priority, orthopedic* and *maxillofacial injuries* and *plastic procedures* can await definitive evaluation and treatment of the other injuries. Generally, compound wounds should be treated within the "golden period" of wounding, that is, within six to eight hours. Since these injuries usually do not immediately threaten life, wound protection with or without organic iodide dressings should be utilized while more serious injuries are definitively treated.

INDICATIONS FOR OPERATION

In many respects, the diagnosis of *penetrating trauma* of the chest and abdomen is far easier than that of blunt trauma. The reason, of course, relates to the fact that the injury is obvious and the prediction of possible underlying injuries is relatively easy. As a general rule, wounding from knives and similar penetrating objects such as glass is relatively benign compared to gunshot wounds, which generally carry four times the mortality.

Because the major volume of the abdominal cavity is composed of hollow viscus, penetrating trauma, particularly stab wounds, is statistically most apt to produce a hollow viscus injury (Table 1-9).[1,4,10,18,19,24,28,25]

Assessment of the possibility of hollow viscus injury involves evaluation for peritonitis or retroperitoneal sepsis. A full bowel, when injured, readily evacuates into the peritoneal cavity and signs of injury are obvious. When an empty bowel is injured or when the site of penetration of the bowel involves its retroperitoneal portion, egress of bowel contents may be negligible initially, and therefore, findings minimal. Increasing abdominal tenderness demands exploration. An elevated white count or fever appearing several hours following the injury are keys to early diagnosis.

The likelihood of a major vascular injury is far higher on a percentage basis with penetrating as opposed to blunt abdominal injury in those patients who survive to reach the hospital. If a patient presents in shock a short time after the injury, the probability of major vascular injury should be assumed and appropriate resuscitation initiated.

Table 1-9 PENETRATING TRAUMA
(RELATIVE INCIDENCE OF ORGAN INJURY)

Organ	Percentage
Small bowel	30
Mesentery and Omentum	18
Liver	16
Colon	9
Diaphragm	8
Stomach	7
Spleen	6
Kidney	5
Major Vascular	4
Pancreas	3
Duodenum	2
Bladder	1
Ureter	1
Biliary	1

Collected Series

Although we recognize there is controversy regarding treatment of penetrating injuries to the abdomen, we believe in the general principle that most penetrating trauma should be explored immediately. When a hollow viscus has been injured, delay in treatment results in progression of intraperitoneal or retroperitoneal contamination to the point of invasive infection and a high incidence of septic complications.[9,24,30]

All gunshot wounds which penetrate the lower chest or the abdominal wall are explored. The incidence of major intraabdominal injury exceeds 90 percent in most series.

Patients with abdominal stab wounds or stab wounds of the chest wall at the level of the sixth intercostal space or below who have clinical evidence of intraabdominal injury undergo immediate laparotomy.[5] In the absence of findings, "selective mandatory exploration" for the management of penetrating stab wounds has been our policy. This involves immediate laparotomy or observation depending upon the location of the injury. Because we have found a 90 percent association with intra-abdominal penetration from stab wounds of the abdominal wall anterior to the posterior axillary line, all anterior stab wounds are explored. If there is any question of the depth of the injury, the wound may be explored under local anesthesia in the emergency room. Fascial penetration is an indication for laparotomy. Since we have found that wounds posterior to the posterior axillary line have a low incidence of peritoneal penetration, injuries to the back and flank may be observed expectantly if no physical, laboratory, or x-ray findings are present which suggest intra-abdominal injury. Injuries to the abdominal wall or lower intercostal spaces between the anterior axillary line and the posterior axillary line are selectively managed. However, because retroperitoneal injury to the colon is possible, laparotomy is used liberally in the presence of minimal abdominal findings.

This policy was subjected to review.[27] Between January 1975 and December 1976, 757 patients underwent exploratory laparotomy at San Francisco General Hospital for blunt and penetrating abdominal trauma. Only 12 of the 159 patients with gunshot wounds of the abdomen did not have a major visceral injury. Most of these missed the peritoneal cavity since penetration of the abdomen by gunshot wounds necessitated repair or drainage of an abdominal viscus in 99.3 percent of the records analyzed. This reconfirmed our belief that all patients with gunshot wounds suspected of entering the peritoneal cavity should be treated by mandatory laparotomy.

Of the 367 patients with stab wounds of the abdomen, 106 had insignificant or absent intra-abdominal injury. The main determinant of the need for laparotomy in the patients with negative findings at exploration had been possible peritoneal penetration. Signs of peritoneal irritation were present in 38 patients or 40 percent of those who had a negative exploration. However, in 21 of these there had been no peritoneal penetration. A total of 18 patients in this group with negative findings had laparotomy based on clinical suspicion of penetration alone in the absence of clinical, laboratory, or x-ray abnormalities.

Nineteen complications occurred in the 118 patients whose laparotomy was negative following penetrating trauma from gunshot wounds and stab wounds. Most of the complications were minor and did not prolong hospitalization, the mean hospital stay being six days. Hospitalization was prolonged in two patients who had serious complications. One patient had a pulmonary embolus and remained in the hospital for fourteen days. Another patient with a wound infection was hospitalized on two occasions for 28 days. In the remainder, the complications of atelectasis and minor wound infection did not result in prolongation of the hospitalization. There were no deaths in this group with negative findings at laparotomy. Thus, we believe that a policy of exploration of stab wounds is appropriate. The rate of 20 percent for negative findings at laparotomy is considered acceptable for another potentially lethal illness, appendicitis, and we believe that the potential lethality of penetrating wounds is reduced to a bare minimum by this policy of prompt exploration. Since retroperitoneal and diaphragmatic injuries, for example, are frequently asymptomatic, peritoneal lavage often is negative in this group as well. Not only can immediate complications occur from diaphragm injuries, but delayed complications can and do result and can compromise the patient years later. Although the production of adhesions which can result in delayed complications of bowel obstruction can theoretically occur following a negative exploration, this has been most unusual in our experience; only one such patient has been encountered during the period of review for this series.

Blunt abdominal trauma is far more subtle than penetrating trauma. The degree of injury is difficult to establish and findings even with serious injury may be minimal. In blunt abdominal trauma, the organs most likely to be injured are solid organs such as the liver, spleen, kidney, pancreas, and mesentery (Table 1-10).[1,3,6,7,12,20,22,33,35]

A hollow viscus is much less commonly injured by blunt trauma and the diagnosis of hollow viscus injury when it occurs is not particularly difficult. The reason for this relates to the fact that an empty hollow viscus is relatively invulnerable to injury. The commonest hollow viscus injury is to the small bowel; this is ruptured by trapping a loop against the vertebral colon and this bursting type of injury is associated with severe peritoneal signs. The incidence of intestinal injury of this type has increased with the use of seat belts.

The next most common hollow viscus to be injured is the full bladder, and lower abdominal tenderness in association with hematuria and/or pelvic fractures strongly suggests the possibility of bladder rupture. The duodenum and stomach are less commonly involved with blunt trauma.

Since a primary manifestation of solid organ injury is bleeding, assessment of the patient with blunt trauma includes monitoring the patient for evidence of hem-

Table 1–10   BLUNT TRAUMA
(RELATIVE INCIDENCE OF ORGAN INJURY)

Organ	Percentage
Spleen	25
Liver	15
Retroperitoneal hematoma	13
Kidney	12
Small Bowel	9
Bladder	6
Mesentery	5
Large Bowel	4
Pancreas	3
Urethra	2
Diaphragm	2
Vascular	2
Stomach	1
Duodenum	1

Collected Series

Table 1–11   LEVELS OF SHOCK
(CLINICAL CLASSIFICATION OF HEMORRHAGIC SHOCK)

Mild Shock (up to 20% blood volume loss)
  Pathophysiology: decreased perfusion of nonvital organs and tissues (skin, fat, skeletal muscle, and bone).

  Manifestations: pale, cool skin. Patient complains of feeling cold. Urine is concentrated.

Moderate Shock (20–40% blood volume loss)
  Pathophysiology: decreased perfusion of vital organs (liver, gut, kidneys).

  Manifestations: oliguria to anuria and slight to significant drop in blood pressure.

Severe Shock: (40% or more blood volume loss)
  Pathophysiology: decreased perfusion of heart and brain.

  Manifestations: restlessness, agitation, coma, cardiac irregularities, ECG, abnormalities, and cardiac arrest.

orrhage (Table 1-11). This includes careful assessment of peripheral perfusion and urine output along with blood pressure, pulse, and hematocrit. The first manifestations of acute volume loss is peripheral vasoconstriction; the patient appears pale, the extremities are cool and he complains of feeling cold. Under such circumstances, shock should be assumed regardless of the blood pressure and a catheter should be inserted into the bladder for monitoring the urinary output. Urinary output in excess of 0.5 cc/kg/hr suggests that renal perfusion is adequate and shock, if present, is minimal and limited to non-vital structures such as skin and subcutaneous tissue. Manifestations of severe shock are impaired cerebral and coronary perfusion. These are manifest in the heart as EKG abnormalities such as arrhythmias or myocardial ischemia and may progress to myocardial arrest. The initial manifestations of inadequate cerebral perfusion, or inadequate supplies of oxygen or glucose to the brain for that matter, are restlessness or agitation. If such a patient has evidence of peripheral vasoconstriction, severe shock should be assumed and treatment initiated promptly using large bore cutdowns. Bladder catheterization should be carried out and urine output monitored. As shock progresses, coma may ensue.

Ordinarily, blood in the belly is irritating and intraperitoneal bleeding is associated with definite peritoneal signs. This produces a secondary ileus with overt abdominal distention. However, on occasion, the blood is bland and minimal peritoneal irritation results. The abdomen can accommodate most of the blood volume with a change in girth of only four to five centimeters. When blood in the abdominal cavity does not produce peritoneal irritation, there is little associated ileus and distention may not be particularly impressive, even through several liters of blood have been lost into the abdominal cavity.

An unexplained fall in the hematocrit together with evidence of cardiovascular instability means bleeding into the abdomen unless some other source has been established and this provides an indication for laparotomy.

INITIAL SURGICAL APPROACH

Preoperative antibiotics are useful adjuncts in the management of massive abdominal injuries. Broad spectrum antibiotic coverage such as penicillin and an aminoglycocide are particularly useful in all patients suspected of having colon or small bowel injuries as would be likely following penetrating trauma. Antibiotics are not necessarily indicated for blunt trauma since solid viscus injury is the most likely complication and these are clean injuries.

A team approach is often appropriate in the patient with multiple injuries and may include simultaneous decompression of the space-occupying intracranial lesion by neurosurgeons while the general surgeons explore the abdomen. In the patient with massive abdominal injuries and associated widened mediastinum, exploration of the abdomen with repair of injuries is indicated first. Following laparotomy, an aortagram can be carried out and thoracic aortic rupture, if present, treated. If the patient has associated major vascular injuries to the extremities, control of these must be obtained prior to abdominal exploration. If the patient remains unstable, exploratory laparotomy should be carried out before definitive treatment of the peripheral vascular injuries.

When dealing with trauma, the possibility that any body cavity may be opened exists and drains or chest tubes may be required expeditiously. Therefore, the patient should be prepared with iodide paint from clavicles to groin and table line to table line. He should be draped so exposure of any of this area is possible quickly without contaminating the fields when shock is present. Prepping should not involve more than a few minutes and is preferably carried out prior to induction of anesthesia so that should deterioration occur, immediate laparotomy or thoracotomy can be carried out. For rapid access and wide exposure, the midline abdominal incision is the incision of choice. Only rarely will transverse or oblique incisions be appropriate for trauma. Surgeons should always be prepared to extend the midline incision up to the sternun as a sternal splitting incision or into the right or left chest if necessary. The chest should, therefore, be prepped along with the abdomen.

When the presence of abdominal injury is questionable or the site of pathology uncertain, it is usually appropriate to start with an upper midline incision extending from just below the xiphoid to just above the umbilicus. The incision can be centered on the umbilicus if the injury is presumed to be in the lower abdomen. Most of the complicated problems, however, will lie in the upper abdomen, hence, the decision for xiphoid to umbilical exploratory incision. When intra-abdominal pathology is encountered, the incision should be rapidly extended below the umbilicus all the way to the pubis if the injuries appear major. If the abdomen is filled with bright red blood, this is highly indicative of an arterial injury. The patient should be eviscerated, each corner of the abdomen rapidly inspected and packs placed temporarily to control any bleeding encountered. All quadrants of the abdomen and the mesentery should be inspected on the first pass. This can be done within a minute or two so that the most major source of hemorrhage can be located and dealt with first. Minor injuries and minor sources of hemorrhage should not distract the surgeon from dealing with major ongoing hemorrhage. Venous bleeding may not be obvious unless looked for since it is low pressure and may not be as dramatic or as evident as the arterial hemorrhage. Almost all venous bleeding can be controlled by the judicious application of packs permitting time for restoration of volume. This is also true of many arterial injuries and if the injury can be controlled by pack or direct pressure this should be done while volume is restored. The reason for not entering the injury directly is that the vascular system may suddenly decompress; massive amounts of blood volume lost in a previously hypovolemic patient leads to a high probability of cardiac arrest.

If the injury appears to be arterial and in the upper abdomen, the possibility of injury to the visceral portion of the aorta or one of its major upper abdominal branches should be considered and proximal control must be ensured. If there is hematoma extending into the level of the diaphragm, the left chest should be opened and the aorta encircled. If there is no hematoma at the level of the aortic hiatus, dissection can be carried down around the aorta by severing the cursa of the diaphragm as they wrap around the aorta and an occluding clamp placed temporarily at this region (see Chapter 12).

As soon as bleeding has been identified and controlled, the next priority is preventing gross contamination from hollow viscus injury, particularly in the colon. When bowel injuries are encountered as part of routine exploration, time should not be taken to suture them initially. Instead they should be temporarily approximated with the application of a Babcock or Allis forceps or an occluding clamp such as a Kocher or intestinal clamp if the disruption is major.

Once the gross injuries have been identified and controlled, there is time for definitive exploration. This should be carried out systematically and deliberately. This is best accomplished utilizing a generous incision carried below the umbilicus which permits evisceration of the entire small bowel. The small bowel mesentery should be spread out on the abdominal wall and inspected in entirety first on one side and then the other. The transverse colon and omentum should be retracted upward and the base of the mesocolon inspected. The small bowel can then be run from the Ligament of Trietz to the ileocecal valve. The right colon, transverse colon, descending colon, sigmoid, and rectum are examined and palpated in order. When there is presumption of injury of ascending or descending colon or hepatic or splenic flexure, these should be mobilized by severing lateral attachments and bringing the bowel upward into the wound to permit inspection of all sides of the large bowel.

The left upper quadrant should then be examined completely. The presence of clot localizes the probable source of bleeding and if present in the left subphrenic area strongly suggests injury to the spleen or left lobe of the liver. Careful palpation and inspection of the spleen should be done using the left hand to exert gentle traction while first the hilar area, then the outer convex surface are inspected. If no clot and no overt injury to the spleen is seen, the left upper quadrant should be completely evacuated of blood and the pack left in place temporarily to monitor bleeding. The left lobe of the liver, then the anterior wall of the stomach should be inspected. If there has been any evidence of trauma to the upper abdomen, the lesser sac should be explored. This is best done by severing the attachment of the omentum to the transverse colon so as not to devascularize the omentum or the greater curvature of the stomach. Once the lesser sac is found through the omentocolic junction, the attachment of the omentum to the colon can usually be rapidly and bloodlessly developed until the entire posterior wall of the stomach and body and tail of the pancreas can be inspected. Hematomas around the body and tail of the pancreas require further mobilization and careful palpation of the pancreas since a small hematoma will fill out the contour of a completely disrupted pancreas. If there is any loss of integrity of the pancreas, this organ should be completely mobilized by severing the lateral attachment of the spleen and mobilizing the spleen and the tail of the pancreas and greater curvature of the stomach upwards and into the midline of the wound. This is facilitated by completely dividing the attachments of the omentum to the splenic flexure of the transverse colon so this can be mobilized upwards. Following inspection of the left upper quadrant, the right upper quadrant should be examined. The liver should be carefully palpated on both surfaces and inspected as far as possible. The presence of clot usually points to the the site of probable injury, whereas nonclotting blood accumulating in the upper quadrants of the abdomen usually will have come from some other region of the abdomen.

The duodenal sweep should be inspected. If there is hematoma about this region or overlying the duodenum, a Kocher maneuver should be carried out and definitive palpation of the head of the pancreas and inspection of the posterior surface of both duodenum and pancreas carried out. The retroperitoneum on both sides should be inspected through the root of the mesentery. The presence of hematomas in the flank does not necessarily require exploration of the kidney (see Chapter 11).[14] Following exploration of the upper abdomen, the lower abdomen should be inspected. Hematomas in the pelvis generally result from pelvic fractures and should be left intact (see Chapter 4). Penetrating injuries which pass in the vicinity of the ureter dictate exploration of the ureter. This is carried out on the right by mobilizing the right colon lateral attachments and sweeping this upwards as described in a subsequent chapter.

Following completion of the exploration and surgery, the abdominal incision is closed in layers. We favor a running closure using synthetic collagen suture for the peritoneum, and an interrupted, heavy absorbable or non-absorbable suture for the fascia, although a continuous closure with heavy (#1) synthetic collagen suture is now being used with increasing frequency. Antibiotics, if indicated, are continued for two or three days postoperatively.

REFERENCES

1. Andersen CB, Ballinger WF: Abdominal Injuries From the Management of Trauma. W.B. Saunders, Philadelphia, 1975, p. 431.
2. Bailey H: Surgery in Modern Warfare, Vol. II, 3rd. ed, Williams & Wilkins, Baltimore, 1944.
3. Bolton PM, Wood CB, Quartey-Papafio JB, Blumgart LH: Blunt abdominal injury: A review of 59 consecutive cases undergoing surgery. Br J Surg 60; 657-663, 1973.
4. Buchsbaum HJ: Diagnosis and managemnt of abdominal gunshot wounds during pregnancy. J Trauma, 15:425-430, 1975.
5. Bull JC, Mathewson CF: Exploratory laparotomy in patients with penetrating wounds of the abdomen. Am J Surg 116:223, 1968.
6. Davis JJ, Cohn I, Nance FC: Diagnosis and management of blunt abdominal trauma. Ann Surg 183:672-678, 1976.
7. DiVincenti FC, et al: Blunt abdominal trauma. J Trauma, 8:1004, 1968.
8. Fisher RP, Beverlin BC, Engrav LH, Benjamin CI, Perry JF Jr: Diagnostic peritoneal lavage. Am J Surg 136:701704, 1978.
9. Forde KA, Ganepola GAP: Is mandatory exploration for penetrating abdominal trauma extinct? The morbidity and mortality of negative exploration in a large municipal hospital. J Trauma 14:764-766, 1974.
10. Freeark RJ: Penetrating wounds of the abdomen. NEJM 291:185-188, 1974.
11. Gazzaniga AB, Stanton WW, Bartlett RH: Laparoscopy in the diagnosis of blunt and penetrating injuries to the abdomen. Am J Surg 131:315-318, 1976.
12. Griswald RA, Cellier HS: Blunt abdominal trauma. Abst Surg 112:209, 1961.
13. Heaton LD, et al: Military surgical practices in the US Army in Vietnam. Curr Probl Surg, Nov. 1966.
14. Holcroft JW, Trunkey DD, Minagi H, Korobkin MT, Lim RC: Renal trauma and retroperitoneal hematomas—indications for exploration. J Trauma 15:1045-1052, Dec. 1975.
15. Hopsen WB, et al: Stab wounds of the abdomen. Amer Surg 32:213, 1966.
16. Hossack DW: Investigation of 400 people killed in road accidents with special reference to blood alcohol levels. Med J Aust 2:255-258, 1972.
17. Hossack DW: The pattern of injuries received by 500 drivers and passengers killed in road accidents. Med J Aust 2:193-195, 1972.
18. Jordan GL, Beall AC: Diagnosis and management of abdominal trauma. Curr Probl Surg Nov. 1971.
19. Kazarian KK, et al: Stab wounds of the abdomen, an analysis of 500 patients. Arch Surg 102:465, 1971.

20. Longmire WP Jr, McArthur MS: Occult injuries of the liver, bile duct, and pancreas after blunt abdominal trauma. Am J Surg 125:661-666, 1973.
21. Loria FL: Historical aspects of abdominal injuries. Charles C. Thomas, Springfield, Ill., 1968.
22. Lucas CE, Ledgerwood AM: Factors influencing outcome after blunt duodenal injury. J Trauma 15: 839-846, 1975.
23. Mattox KL, Allen MK, Feliciano DV: Laparotomy in the Emergency Department. JACEP 8:180-183, 1979.
24. Nance FC, Wennar MH, Johnson LW, Ingram JC, Cohn I Jr: Surgical judgment in the management of penetrating wounds of the abdomen: Experience with 2212 patients. Ann Surg 179:639-646, 1974.
25. Olsen WR: The serum amylase in blunt abdominal trauma. J Trauma 13:200-204, 1973.
26. Perry JF Jr, McClellan RJ: Autopsy findings in 127 patients following fatal traffic accidents. Surg Gynecol Obstet 119:586-590, 1964.
27. Petersen SR, Sheldon GF: Morbidity of a negative finding at laparotomy in abdominal trauma. Surg Gynecol Obstet 148:23-26, 1979.
28. Pridgen JE, et al: Penetrating wounds of the abdomen: Analysis of 776 operative cases. Ann Surg 165:901, 1967.
29. Sherman RT, Parrish RA: Management of shotgun injuries. J Trauma 3:76, 1963.
30. Stein A, Lisoos I: Selective management of penetrating wounds of the abdomen. J Trauma 8: 1014, 1968.
31. Surgery in World War II, General Surgery, Office of the Surgeon General, Department of the Army, Washington D.C., 1955.
32. Thomas AN: Air embolism following penetrating lung injuries. J Thor C-V Surg 66:533, 1973.
33. Trollope ML, Stalnaker RL, McElhaney JH, Frey CF: The mechanisms of injury in blunt abdominal trauma. J Trauma 13:962-970, 1973.
34. Trunkey DD, Lim RC Jr: Analysis of 425 consecutive trauma fatalities: An autopsy study. J Am Coll Emerg Phys, 368, Nov-Dec. 1974.
35. Walt AJ, Wilson RF: Management of trauma: Pitfalls and Practice. Lea and Febiger, Philadelphia 1975, p. 348.
36. Wilson JM: Shotgun ballistics and shotgun injuries. West J Med 129:149-155, 1978.

Chapter Two

SPECIAL DIAGNOSTIC PROCEDURES

DONALD D. TRUNKEY, MICHAEL FEDERLE, and
JOHN CELLO

INTRODUCTION

Severely injured patients will usually declare themselves within a few minutes as to whether or not special diagnostic procedures can be carried out. If the patient arrives in an unstable condition and remains so despite resuscitation, there is only one diagnostic procedure that will be of use: a chest x-ray. Any other diagnostic procedure will delay operation, which has now become part of the resuscitation. Conversely, patients may arrive in a stable condition or stabilize secondary to the resuscitation. In these instances special diagnostic procedures are often of great value in developing priorities for management and treatment.

HISTORY

Special diagnostic procedures are of recent vintage, most developed within the past century. Prior to that, clinicians relied almost exclusively on history and physical examination for diagnosis. Sushruta was one of the first to use tasting of urine to diagnose diabetes.[1] He also noted that the sweetness of the discharge could be inferred from its ability to attract flies and ants. Pare, in his book *The Methods of Treating Wounds Made by Arquebueses and Other Firearms*, describes how he would have the patient assume the same position as when the injury occurred in order to determine the course of the projectile through the body. Whether or not this diagnostic technique influenced outcome is not clear in his manuscript.

The importance of diagnosis was well recognized by the early trauma surgeons, as pointed out by Brunshwig.[2] In his *Duties of the Surgeon* he comments;

The surgeon should also know anatomy and be aware that there is a connection and a separation of the members of the body so that he knows where he should cut or cauterize so that he will not incur fatal injury through cutting and cauterization, and so that he will not tear or wrench a member of the body. He should also understand how he can repair something of that nature, he should know whether someone was shot with an arrow or a gunshot or whether the iron is still in the body, or a part of the bullet or a stone, whether he should cut this out or draw it out with plasters or whether he should soften the spot with softening poultices or how you can bring every member back into its correct form and appearance.

It was not, however, until the publication by Wilhelm Conrad Roentgen's *A New Kind of Ray* in 1895 that special techniques have permitted diagnostic procedures never before anticipated.

COMMON DIAGNOSTIC PROCEDURES IN TRAUMA

Before progressing to more special types of diagnostic procedures, we shall describe the more commonly done procedures, their indications, and their limitations.

Probably the most common diagnostic procedure is examination of the peripheral blood, including red cells, hemoglobin, white blood count, and differential blood count. One of the variables of oxygen transport is the amount and function of available hemoglobin. This, in turn, is dependent on the amount of hemoglobin present in whole blood, expressed in grams of hemoglobin per deciliter of whole blood; the proportion of whole blood that red cells contribute, expressed as the hematocrit, or percentage of red cells in whole blood; and the absolute number of red cells in whole blood, usually expressed as a number (in millions) per cubic milliliter of blood. Of these three variables, the most often used in trauma is the hematocrit. This is usually performed on venous or capillary blood by the "micro" technique. Its limitations in the acute situation have been appropriately pointed out and are primarily due to the slowness in equilibration and to its dependence upon the resuscitation itself. Carey and his co-workers showed that in severe hemorrhage the hematocrit equilibrated faster than previous investigations had shown.[3,4] This is in part due to plasma refill, but it also probably reflects initial resuscitation with balanced salt solution. More important than a single determination is the information gathered from serial hematocrits performed over time. The hematocrit will fall 3 to 4 points for each 500 ml blood loss, the exact amount related to the size of the patient. A falling hematocrit is probably indicative of sequestration of blood, usually at hidden sites such as the peritoneal cavity, retroperitoneum, pelvis, and long bone fracture sites.

Peripheral blood contains approximately 4,000 to 10,000 white cells per microliter (ul). Total white count can be determined by lysing red cells and counting the nucleated white cells directly in a counting chamber or by automated techniques, the most popular of which is the Coulter counter. More important than the total white count is the differential white count, which gives the proportions of different cell types that comprise the total number of white cells. Of primary importance in the patient who has sustained trauma is the "shift to the left," which reflects an absolute increase in the number of neutrophiles and, in particular, of the more immature forms. Conditions causing neutrophilia (greater than 8000 PMN's ul) are shown in Table 2-1. Serial white count determinations are again of more value in the trauma patient than a single determination. This may give the clinician early clues that there is an inflammatory response, usually in the peritoneal cavity, that is causing early mobilization of neutrophiles.

Routine urinalysis in the acutely injured patient is usually limited to the presence or absence of red cells in the urine and using a reagent strip method such as Bililabstix, Hemastix, (Ames Company, Alcarte, Indiana). This plastic strip has 6 impregnated reagent areas which allow simultaneous testing for urinary pH, protein, glucose, ketone bodies, bilirubin, and occult blood. This reagent strip method is quite accurate

Table 2–1   CAUSES OF NEUTROPHILIA

1. Infections
    Pyogenic bacteria
    Abscess
    Septicemia
2. Acute inflammation or necrosis
    Infarction
    Collagen disease
    Acute hemolysis
3. Neoplasms
4. Intoxication
    Drugs
    Chemicals
5. Acute hemorrhage

and very simple to use. An additional test includes measuring the specific gravity, usually with a urinometer.

If the patient has a history of crushing injury or severe burns, evaluation of the urine should include measurement for hemoglobin and myoglobin. If the reagent strip test is positive, three conditions are possible. The positive test may represent red blood cells, which case is easily eliminated by microscopic examination for the presence of either hemoglobin or myoglobin within the urine. Hemoglobinuria occurs when all haptoglobin, a serum mucoprotein, has been completely bound by the hemoglobin present in the blood stream. A positive reagent strip test in the absence of red cells as determined by microscopic examination therefore implies the presence of either hemoglobin or myoglobin. Myoglobin can be differentiated from hemoglobin by the following three characteristics: (1) myoglobin is soluble in 80 percent ammonium sulphate while hemoglobin is not, (2) myoglobin has one half the electrophoretic mobility of hemoglobin, and (3) myoglobin can be differentiated from hemoglobin by immunochemical methods. The simplest way of differentiating myoglobinuria from hemoglobinuria in the acute situation is to add an 80 percent solution of ammonium sulphate to an aliquot of urine. This will precipitate the hemoglobin, leaving undenatured myoglobin in the supernatant. If the supernatant tests positive with reagent strips, myoglobinuria is probably present.

Other laboratory blood tests that should be considered but not done routinely on trauma patients include serum electrolytes (sodium, potassium, chloride), blood urea nitrogen, glucose, creatinine, amylase, and liver function tests. After the first intravenous line has been inserted, approximately 40 cc of whole blood should rapidly be obtained. Ten cc should be sent immediately for type and cross-match and the remainder is kept for the above tests and performed when indicated either by history or subsequent events. Ten cc of blood are also kept aside for toxicology and blood alcohol determinations, which are done when history warrants it.

Amylase is an enzyme secreted by both the pancreas and salivary glands and splits starch into its component sugars. Damage to either the glandular cells or the ductal systems may cause amylase to enter the blood stream. It was first reported as a diagnostic aid in pancreatic injury by Naffziger and McCorkle in 1942.[6] Amylase activity is measured by one of two methods, both depending on its ability to digest a starch solution. In the Somogyi method the sugars are measured colorimetrically and normal values are 40 to 140 units/dl. The second method utilizes a starch dye substrate and the amount of dye is measured. This gives lower values with the upper limits of normal being 25 units/dl.

It has been our experience that the serum amylase is a relatively poor indicator of pancreatic injury. We are in total agreement with the findings of Olson, who concluded that patients with levels of 300 Somogyi units/dl which remain persistently elevated or increase are the patients most likely to have pancreatic injury.

The third most common blood test done in the acutely injured patient is arterial blood gas determination including oxygen level (pO2), blood CO2 level (PCO2) and blood pH. The arterial pO2 is indicative of the amount of oxygen passing from inspired air into the blood. It is influenced by respiratory capacity, pulmonary perfusing surfaces, distribution of pulmonary blood flow, and the adequacy of pulmonary and systemic circulation. The pCO2 is a more accurate measure of ventilation, since carbon dioxide diffuses more readily across alveolar surfaces than does oxygen. Blood pH values accurately reflect the body's acid base balance, but will not as a single value tell the clinician whether it is due to metabolic or respiratory causes. In the severely traumatized patient, the pH is most commonly below 7.4 and reflects a metabolic acidosis secondary to the accumulation of hydrogen ion and lactic acid. This may be altered by compensatory respiratory akalosis if the patient is spontaneously ventilating and by the resuscitation procedure itself, which is often done with balanced salt soulution containing variable amounts of bicarbonate ion. Isolated measurements may give the clinician some index as to ventilatory status or perfusion, but it is far better to determine serial measurements over time which give more information.

Arterial blood should be obtained anaerobically, into a heparinized container, from the femoral, radial or other accessible artery and determination should be performed within 15 minutes. Results should be corrected to body temperature.

SPECIAL DIAGNOSTIC PROCEDURES

Imaging Procedures

Conventional radiography, radionuclide scanning, ultrasonography, angiography, and computed tomography are diagnostic modalities that may be employed for early diagnosis and accurate evaluation of suspected internal abdominal injuries. Various factors must be considered in selecting which to use in any given clinical situation, including the cost, safety, and availability of the procedure, the accuracy of the results, and the experience and expertise of the radiologist performing and interpreting the examination.

The type and extent of injury usually dictates the nature of the radiologic evaluation. Life-threatening injuries accompanied by unstable vital signs will permit only the most cursory radiologic evaluation. In less urgent circumstances, clinical and laboratory findings indicate the most appropriate imaging modality. Referring physicians should be requested to supply information as to the mechanism of injury, presence of ecchymoses or focal tenderness, and relevant laboratory data such as falling hematocrit or hematuria. Rib, spine, or pelvic fractures on the preliminary radiograph can suggest the need for a close scrutiny of adjacent viscera and direct the choice of further diagnostic examinations.

Plain Radiographs And Contrast Studies

The major contribution of abdominal plain films in the diagnosis of abdominal trauma is the detection of intraperitoneal fluid (blood). Although other findings, such as free air and alteration of visceral contours, are of importance, the frequency with which they are seen does not approach that of intraperitoneal fluid. The classic signs of free intraperitoneal fluid (i.e., separation and floating of bowel loops and diffuse haziness over the abdomen) are not pertinent to this discussion, since massive quantities of fluid are required to produce them. Of major importance in the recognition of intraperitoneal fluid are (1) separation of the ascending and descending colon from the adjacent properitoneal fat (flank stripe sign) (2) loss of definition of the hepatic angle (hepatic angle sign) and (3) the presence of homogeneous shadows of water density in and adjacent to the pouch of Douglas (''dog ear'' sign).

In the normal state, there is a pericolonic gutter formed on each side of the abdomen by reflections of peritoneum over the vertical colon segments and lateral abdominal wall. Intraperitoneal fat ordinarily occupies the space between the colon and the peritoneum. Just outside the peritoneum and medial to the three layers of abdominal musculature is a zone of properitoneal fat. The flank stripe is the radiolucent zone comprised of intra- and properitoneal fat. The medial border of the

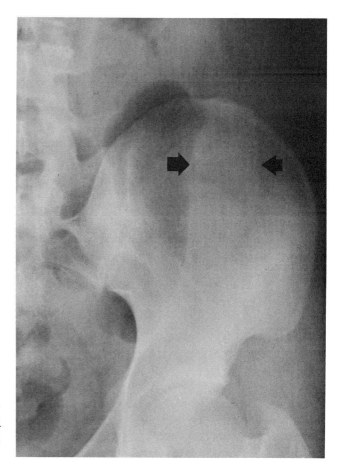

Figure 2–1 Flank stripe sign. Descending colon is displaced from properitoneal fat by water band of water density blood (arrows) in pericolic gutter.

flank stripe in normal cases is usually poorly defined as an undulating curve. With accumulation of fluid in the pericolonic gutter, a water density band with a sharp lateral margin formed by the peritoneum separates the properitoneal fat zone from the lateral margin of the colon (Figure 2-1).[8-10] Some diagnostic pitfalls may be encountered. Fluid-filled small bowel lying lateral to the colon may cause a false positive flank stripe sign, particularly on the left side. If the colon is not visualized, owing to either contraction or intraluminal fluid, the flank stripe sign is unreliable.

The inferior and right lateral margins of the liver (hepatic angle) are commonly identified on routine films of the abdomen. This finding is dependent upon the liver (and parietal peritoneum) being closely applied to the extraperitoneal fat laterally and the greater omentum and pericolic fat inferiorly. Intraperitoneal fluid interposed between the lower edge of the liver and the omental fat obscures the hepatic angle (Figure 2-2).[11] Unfortunately, the hepatic angle may also be obscured by overlying colon, respiratory motion or retroperitoneal hematoma.

The pelvis is the most dependent part of the peritoneal cavity in the supine position and may constitute one-third of its total volume. As such, large amounts of blood may accumulate in the pelvis following injury, although small amounts of blood may not be detectable on plain radiographs. Classic radiographic findings with larger accumulations of blood are due to the homogeneous density of the liquid blood displacing the gas, stool, and fluid-filled loops of bowel.

Blood in the peripelvic space extending cephalad to the bladder may suggest the projecting ears of a dog - "dog ear" signs, although rounded, pear-shaped, and other configurations may be assumed (Figure 2-3).[12] Fluid-filled loops of bowel within

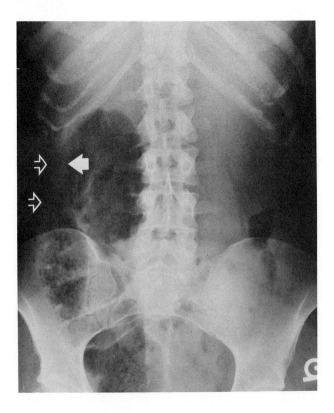

Figure 2–2 Hepatic angle and flank stripe sign. Ascending colon displaced from abdominal wall by band of water density blood (arrows). The blood also obliterates the inferior-lateral margins of the liver (hepatic angle sign). Positive flank stripe also present on left side. Liver and spleen laceration found at surgery.

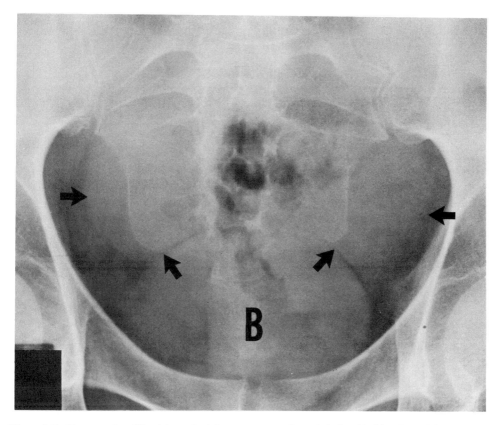

Figure 2–3 Dog ear sign. Blood in peripelvic spaces extends cephalad to bladder (B) and is separated from it by perivesical fat.

the pelvis are a frequent source of potential error. Retroperitoneal hematoma, bladder diverticula, and uterine or ovarian masses may also resemble fluid collections.

Cadaver experiments have demonstrated that 800 cc of intra-abdominal fluid was the minimum amount that could be detected roentgenologically.[13] Intra-abdominal injuries which cause relatively little bleeding constitute the principle source of error on plain films. Because of this, a negative plain film is of little value.

Orally administered contrast media can be useful in diagnosing injuries of the upper gastrointestinal tract. Its fixed retroperitoneal position directly over the spine renders the duodenum the portion of the bowel most susceptible to injury. Laceration of the duodenum allows bowel contents, blood, and gas to enter the anterior pararenal space. Gas bubbles may be detected surrounding the duodenum or outlining the top of the right kidney or ascending colon (Figure 2-4). [14]

In the absence of gas on plain films, a clinical suspicion of duodenal perforation calls for immediate evaluation of bowel integrity by water soluble contrast media given orally or by nasogastric tube. Extravasation of contrast media indicates the site and extent of duodenal laceration.

Blunt trauma may also result in intramural hematoma of the duodenum. If laceration has been excluded, barium studies should be performed and are usually diagnostic. Intramural hemorrhage widens the mucosal folds, producing a pattern

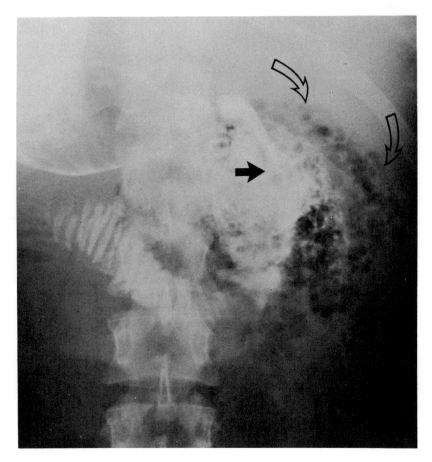

Figure 2–4 Ruptured duodenum. Multiple gas bubbles surround top of kidney (curved arrows) and extend down retroperitoneum. Oral aqueous contrast material extravasates from duodenum at site of rupture (straight arrow).

of "accordion pleating," "picket fence,"or "coiled spring" appearance. More extensive hemorrhage into the submucosa may occlude the lumen.[15]

Blunt trauma rarely results in significant injury to the colon. Tearing of the rectum has been associated with buttock laceration and sacrococcygeal fractures. A more common cause of injury is unusual sexual practices, accomplished by insertion of foreign bodies or a fist which may lacerate the rectosigmoid colon intra- or extraperitoneally. Digital and proctoscopic examination is the perferred method of diagnosis of such injuries. In equivocal cases a water-soluble contrast enema may confirm the presence and site of perforation (Figure 2-5).

The mainstay of diagnosis of renal injuries is excretory urography (intravenous pyelography). This study should be performed with a large dose of concentrated contrast media (100 cc of 60 percent urographic contrast) and should be accompanied by nephrotomography whenever there is any doubt about the integrity of the kidneys. About 75 to 85 percent of renal injuries are minor, consisting of contusions and minor cortical lacerations. Urography is usually adequate to confirm the absence of more serious injury. Major or catastrophic injuries comprise 15 to 25 percent of cases and urographic findings in this group are frequently nonspecific. Complete nonfunction of a kidney may indicate renal pedicle injury, although this sign is occasionally seen

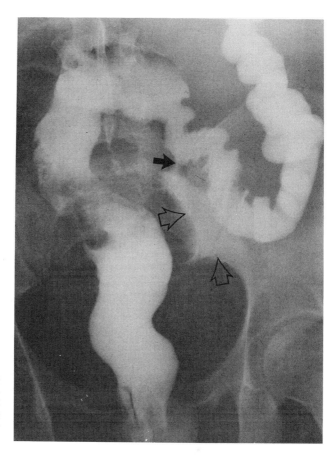

Figure 2–5 Lacerated sigmoid colon. Wall of colon lacerated (straight arrow) by insertion of fist of homosexual partner. Collection of extravasated contrast in peritoneal cavity (open arrows).

with relatively minor injuries. Extravasation of opacified urine indicates injury extending into the collecting system, generally considered a sign of major trauma. Unfortunately, this sign may be absent even in the presence of complete renal fracture, usually owing to a failure of the traumatized kidney to concentrate and excrete the contrast media adequately. In acute trauma, excretory urography with nephrotomography accurately depicts the extent of renal injury in about 70 to 85 percent of cases, leaving a large number of patients (particularly those with more severe injuries) in whom the diagnosis is uncertain.[16-18] In such cases, other important information may be provided by radionuclide scintigraphy, angiography, or computed tomography.

Ultrasonography

There has been very limited experience with sonography in the evaluation of acute abdominal trauma. Splenic injuries have not been detected with high sensitivity or specificity due to the difficulty in distinguishing hematoma from the underlying splenic parenchyma which can have a similar low-level echogenicity.[19-20] Occasionally, subcapsular hematomas of the spleen or liver are visualized as sonolucent bands located peripherally around the involved organ (Figures 2-6, 2-7). Scattered and variable internal echoes may also be seen within the hematoma in association with clot formation. The focal nature of the sonolucency and its failure to change in

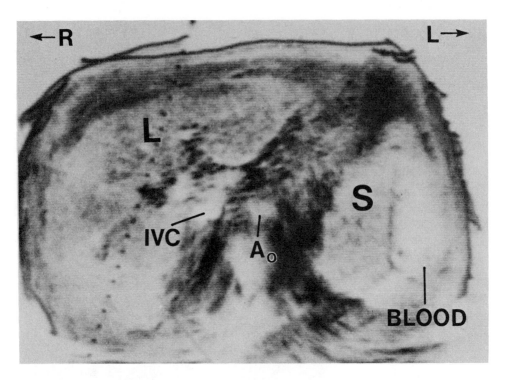

Figure 2–6 Transverse ultrasonogram of upper abdomen demonstrating subcapsular hematoma of the spleen (S). The blood appears as a peripheral sonolucent band. L–liver, IVC–inferior vena cava, Ao–aorta (Courtesy Faye C. Laing, M.D., San Francisco General Hospital).

decubitus position allow subcapsular hematomas to be differentiated from free peritoneal blood or ascites.

In renal trauma, sonography can delineate the extent of extrarenal hematoma (assuming technically adequate scans), but provides only limited information about the nature of underlying parenchymal injuries.[21-22] Sonography provides morphologic information only and does not evaluate the function of the kidney.

Sonography has major technical limitations in the setting of acute trauma. Intestinal ileus, which frequently accompanies trauma, effectively shields much of the abdomen and retroperitoneum from evaluation, since the ultrasound beam cannot penetrate gas. The left upper quadrant is a particularly difficult region to scan adequately because of the gasfilled stomach. Complete evaluation of organs usually requires scanning in multiple oblique, prone or upright positions, often difficult or impossible to achieve with the acutely injured patient. The presence of open wounds, rib fractures, dressings, tubes, and so forth, all limit the ultrasound examination.

Radionuclide Scintiscanning

In the setting of acute trauma, radionuclide studies are essentially limited to liver-spleen or kidney examinations. Minor splenic and hepatic ruptures (subcapsular hematomas) may be manifested by flattening of the lateral organ contour and displacement from the lateral abdominal wall (Figures 2-8, 2-9).[23-25] Collections of blood

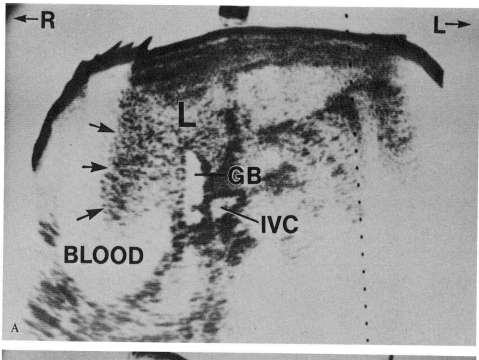

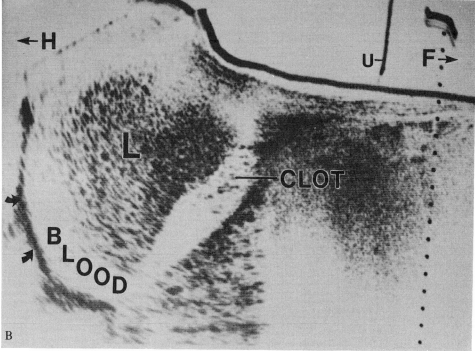

Figure 2–7 *A*, Transverse ultrasonogram in patient with subcapsular hematoma of liver (L). Edge of liver is flattened (arrows) by peripheral sonolucent collection of blood. GB–gallbladder, IVC–inferior vena cava. *B*, Longitudinal scan. Focal collection of blood separates liver from diaphragm (curved arrows). Echogenic material representing clot can be seen within the hematoma. H–head of patient, F–feet, U–umbilicus.

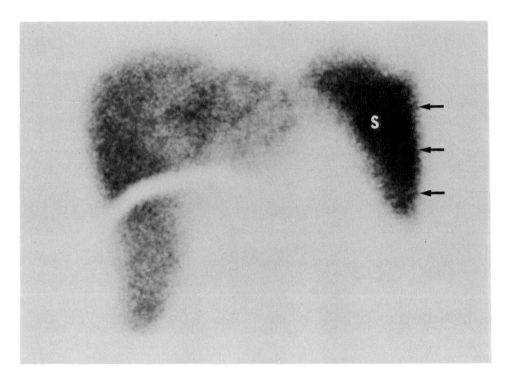

Figure 2–8 Sulfur colloid liver–spleen scintiscan. Lateral margin of spleen (S) is flattened (arrows) by subcapsular hematoma.

within the parenchyma and the attendant compression of surrounding tissue are detected as focal areas of nonfunction ("photopenic areas"). The area of involvement seen on the scintiphoto may appear larger than the volume of the hematomas, because the surrounding compressed tissue is often hypofunctioning.

In our experience, radionuclide studies have been of most value in detecting larger parenchymal injuries. It is frequently difficult to detect slight flattening of contour or displacement from the abdominal wall. The "cold defect" on a liver spleen scintiscan is also a nonspecific finding that can be seen with abscesses, cysts, tumors, and infarctions.

Radionuclide studies should include multiple oblique views and should be interpreted with consideration of the variety of shapes and sizes which the normal spleen and liver may assume. Congenital clefts in these organs, large renal or gallbladder indentations, and other variations are causes of false-positive interpretations. Equivocal results occur in about 10 percent of cases, usually requiring confirmation by other studies such as angiography or computed tomography. [23-25]

Newer radiopharmaceuticals, such as Tc99m glucohepatonate, have improved the quality of renal scans in trauma. Bolus injection of the agent is followed by rapid-sequence images to assess renal vascular integrity. Delayed static images may reveal focal photopenic areas indicative of parenchymal injury. Radionuclide studies have the advantage of being fairly simple and non-invasive and provide important information about the function and vascular supply of the kidney. Disadvantages include the necessity for multiple oblique views and the relatively poor anatomic detail provided. Extrarenal hematomas and injuries to other organs are not revealed. [26-28]

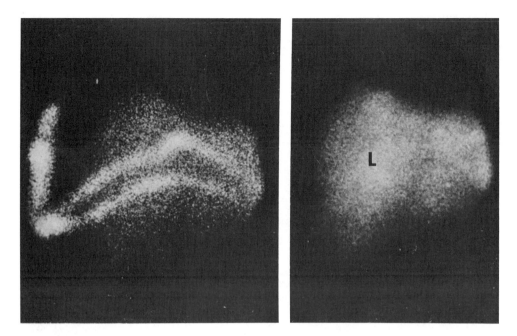

Figure 2–9 Subcapsular hematoma of liver. Liver (L) appears normal but is displaced from lateral abdominal wall (indicated by radioactive marker).

Arteriography

Arteriography can be useful in both blunt and penetrating trauma, and in the past has been recommended as the procedure of choice when plain films and radio-nuclide studies were not definitive. The angiographic findings of splenic or hepatic laceration include extravasation of contrast medium into the tear, early venous filling, displacement of intrasplenic branches due to hematoma, and mottled accumulation of contrast medium during the capillary phase (Figure 2-10). [29,30] Subcapsular hematomas (minor lacerations) may be detected by displacement of a flattened paren-chymal contour from the lateral abdominal wall (Figure 2-11). False-positive results are encountered owing to congenital variations in the size and shape of these organs, and hematomas located along the upper pole are difficult to detect. Angiography may detect arterio-venous fistulas, false aneurysms, or arterio-biliary fistulas, es-pecially with penetrating trauma. These conditions are sometimes self-limited, but if there is clinical suspicion of ongoing vascular injury, arteriography is the radi-ographic procedure of choice.

Renal parenchymal injuries are accurately depicted by angiography, and some authors have recommended its use in virtually all cases of renal trauma.[31] More commonly, it is reserved for cases in which excretory urography suggests a major renal injury, or in which there is clinical evidence of major injury in spite of an

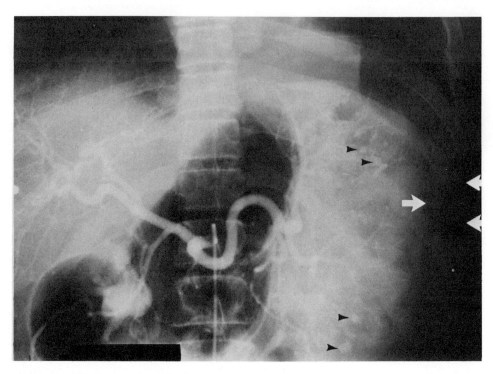

Figure 2–10 Splenic laceration—arteriogram. Multiple sites of intraparenchymal extravasation of contrast material (arrowheads). Perisplenic blood displaces spleen from lateral abdominal wall (arrows).

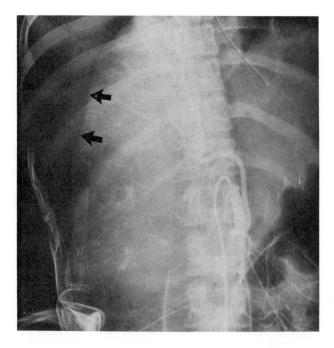

Figure 2–11 Subcapsular hepatic hematoma-arteriogram. Liver surface is flattened (arrows) and displaced from lateral abdominal wall.

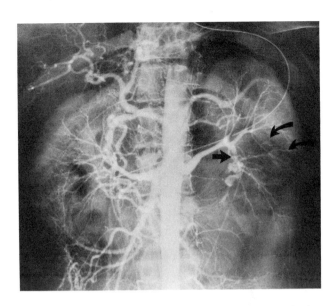

Figure 2–12 Renal fracture arteriogram. Lower pole of kidney fails to opacify (curved arrows). Artery to lower pole is avulsed and extravasates contrast material (straight arrow).

unremarkable or equivocal urogram. Angiography can help distinguish minor injuries such as contusions or small cortical lacerations from major injuries, such as renal fracture (Figure 2-12). Renal pedicle injuries, usually arterial occlusions, and arteriovenous fistulas and false aneurysms are best diagnosed by arteriography. Extrarenal hematomas are manifested by displacement of the capsular artery. It may be difficult to distinguish subcapsular from perirenal hematomas or to accurately judge the extent of the hematoma.

One serious limitation shared by both radionuclide studies and angiography is their "organ specificity". A specific radiopharmaceutical is selected to image either the liver and spleen or the kidney. Such studies cannot evaluate other parenchymal injuries, or retroperitoneal or intraperitoneal bleeding. Similarly, the need to selectively catheterize multiple visceral arteries sequentially limits angiography, as this is time consuming and may increase morbidity in the badly traumatized patient. The rapid evaluation of possible associated injuries is of more than theoretical importance, since there are multiple major thoraco-abdominal injuries in as many as 10 percent of cases coming to surgery. [32]

Computed Tomography

Perhaps the single greatest advance in the radiographic evaluation of abdominal trauma is the recent application of computed tomography (CT). Reports of large series are now appearing in the literature as modern CT scanners become available at major trauma centers.[33-34] Unlike plain radiography, nuclide scans, and angiography, CT appears to be not only specific for a wide variety of traumatic lesions but also very sensitive. CT appears capable of detecting any substantial amount of intraperitoneal or retroperitoneal blood, and is much more sensitive in this regard than other studies.

Splenic injuries are detected by CT with a sensitivity and specificity of about 93 percent.[35] Subcapsular hematoma (minor laceration) appears as a lenticular low density fluid collection which flattens the underlying splenic contour (Figure 2-13).[36]

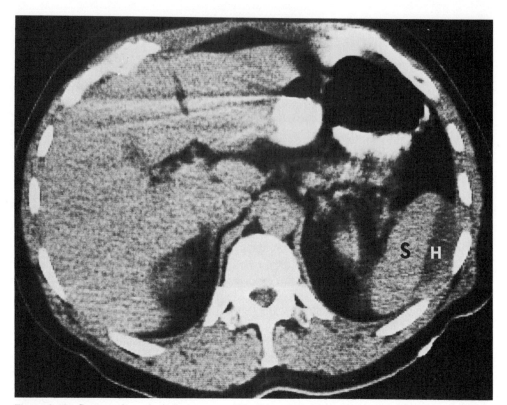

Figure 2-13 Supcapsular splenic hematoma—CT. (Reproduced by permission of Radiology. See reference #26.) Low density lenticular hematoma (H) flattens lateral margin of spleen (S).

More extensive lacerations are seen as clefts through the splenic parenchyma with perisplenic hematoma and intraperitoneal blood detected in almost all cases (Figure 2-14).[37]

Hepatic hematomas and lacerations are similar to the splenic counterpart in appearance (Figure 2-15).[33] Complications of hepatic trauma such as arterio-venous or biliary fistulas, infected hematomas, and bile pseudocysts are detected on CT (Figure 2-16). In cases of suspected vascular injury, we obtain CT scans after an intravenous bolus of contrast media in order to visualize hepatic arteries and veins. Cholangiographic contrast media can be used similarly.

Pancreatic injuries, both traumatic and nontraumatic, have been extensively studied by CT. Pancreatitis is manifested by swelling of the gland and spread of inflammation into peripancreatic tissues. Associated hemorrhage and injuries to adjacent organs such as the duodenum can also be detected. Pancreatic phlegmon, pseudocyst, and abscess may result from trauma, and all are easily detected by CT.[33] Pancreatic abscesses contain gas in about one-third of cases.[38,39] In the absence of this finding, it may be difficult to distinguish infected from non-infected fluid collections. We employ CT or ultrasound-guided percutaneous thin-needle aspiration in suspicious cases.

Retroperitoneal hemorrhage is fairly common after blunt or penetrating trauma and clinically may simulate intra-abdominal pathology. CT is ideally suited to its detection and can simultaneously rule out accompanying abdominal trauma (Figure 2-17).[40]

When major renal trauma is suspected on the basis of excretory urography or

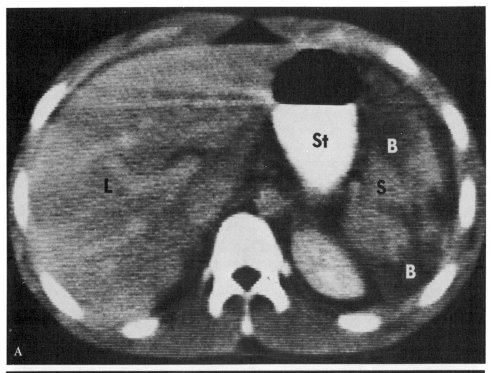

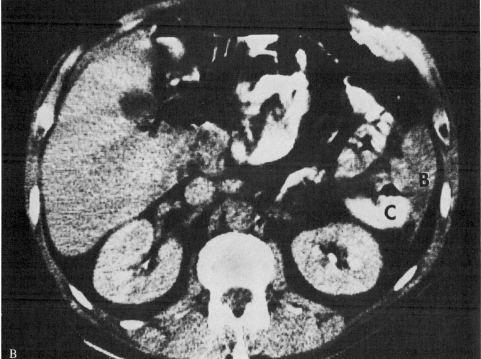

Figure 2–14 Splenic laceration—CT. *A*, Spleen (S) divided my multiple fracture planes. Perisplenic blood clot (B). St–stomach; L–liver. *B*, Blood (B) in pericolonic gutter displaces descending colon (C) from properitoneal fat. This is the CT equivalent of the ''flank stripe'' sign (Reproduced by permission of Radiology, reference #26.)

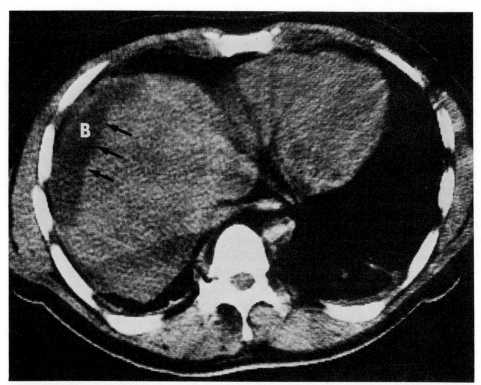

Figure 2–15 Subcapsular hematoma of liver—CT. Lenticular blood collection (B) flattens lateral margin of liver (arrows).

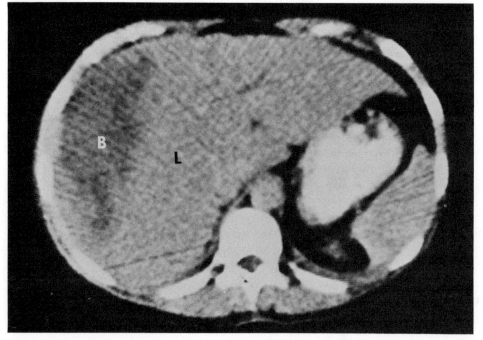

Figure 2–16 Intrahepatic and subcapsular hepatic hematoma. Mottled low-density blood collection (B) in and adjacent to liver (L), which developed secondary to percutaneous liver biopsy. (Reproduced by permission of Radiology, reference #26.)

clinical evaluation, CT is very valuable.[33,41,42] Contusions, incomplete lacerations, complete lacerations and fractures have characteristic appearances and are readily diagnosed (Figure 2-18). CT is much more sensitive than urography to the detection of extravasated urine, an important sign of extension of injury into the collecting system.[41] CT is the best modality for determining the type and extent of extrarenal hematomas. In addition to superior anatomic detail, CT offers functional information; areas of vascular injury and non-perfusion fail to enhance following intravenous contrast media administration.

CT studies offer major advantages over other imaging modalities in evaluation of patients with abdominal trauma. This single non-invasive study, requiring no repositioning of the patient, is completed in about half an hour. CT simultaneously evaluates all intra-abdominal and retroperitoneal structures for injury and provides superior anatomic detail. The confidence with which the scan is interpreted allows one to plan therapy without resorting to further radiologic or other diagnostic procedures (such as peritoneal lavage). With personal experience amounting to more than 200 cases, we are unaware of any in which management of the patient was inappropriately guided by the CT scan.

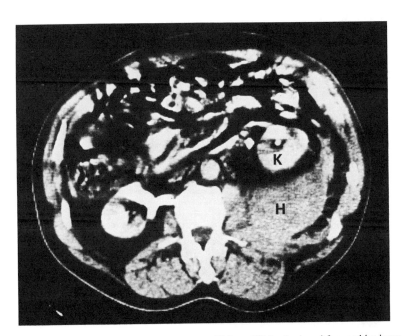

Figure 2–17 Retroperitoneal hemorrhage. Kidney (K) is displaced forward by large retroperitoneal hemorrhage (H). Minor trauma in patient on coumadin therapy.

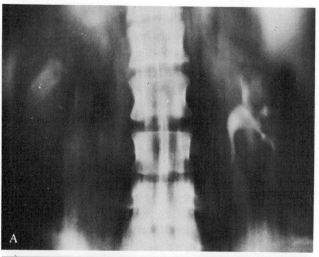

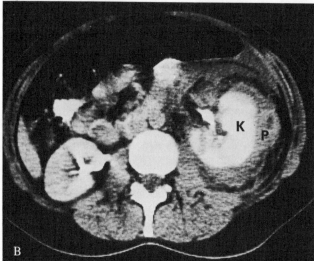

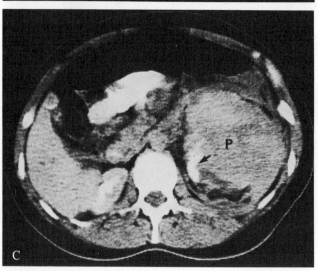

Figure 2–18 Renal fracture. *A*, Excretory urogram with nephrotomography. Decreased function of left kidney. No extravasation of opacified urine. Nonspecific findings. *B*, CT scan. Kidney (K) is rotated and displaced by a perirenal collection of fluid (P). *C*, At this level no functioning renal parenchyma. Arrow indicates extravasation of opacified urine implying laceration into renal collecting system. Large perirenal collection (P) of blood and urine. At surgery, complete fracture of kidney found at this level.

Endoscopy

Endoscopy has limited indications in the acutely injured patient. We include this section primarily because of its use in the post-injury state and in anticipation of increased utilization in the future.

The introduction of flexible, fiberoptic endoscopes with improved optics and high-powered, cold light sources has exposed a large percentage of the gastrointestinal tract to thorough visual examination. These newer instruments, with lengths up to 1.8 meters, have allowed thorough evaluation of the upper gastrointestinal tract down to the proximal jejunum. Endoscopic evaluation of the upper gastrointestinal tract is unparalleled in its diagnostic accuracy when performed by a competent clinician with excellent equipment and in a well prepared patient.[43,44]

Fiberoptic endoscopy is, however, contraindicated in the unstable patient who is in shock following a massive hemorrhagic event or the patient who is in a state of severe cardiopulmonary collapse. Thorough endoscopic examination of unstable patients must await hemodynamic, cardiac, and pulmonary resuscitation. Endoscopic evaluation is also contraindicated in a patient who is totally uncooperative for the physical examination, unless appropriate analgesia and anesthesia can be arranged. In patients with severe, caustic burns of the esophagus, flexible fiberoptic endoscopy should stop at the margin of severe deep circumferential ulceration. In patients with lesser degrees of caustic damage to the esophageal mucosa, thin flexible fiberoptic endoscopes can be passed safely beyond the esophageal burns to examine the stomach and duodenum.

Adequate patient preparation is essential for both patient safety and adequacy of examination. All patients with evidence of recent upper gastrointestinal tract bleeding must be thoroughly lavaged with a large-bore Ewald tube prior to endoscopy. Failure to vigorously lavage the stomach of retained blood and food will render a large portion of the upper gastrointestinal tract invisible to even the most experienced observers. In patients who are totally uncooperative or who are exsanguinating from the upper gastrointestinal tract, consideration should be given to elective endotracheal intubation for airway protection and neuromuscular blockade with analgesia to ensure safety for both patient and endoscopist. When conducted in a well prepared patient, with adequate equipment, the trained endoscopist should be able to identify bleeding lesions with greater than 90 percent accuracy. Routine examination of the third and fourth portions of the duodenum are not possible with standard 1-m adult flexible fiberoptic endoscopes. Enteroscopes, 1.8 m in length, are essential for this purpose. Fortunately, the vast majority of significant pathology will be found proximal to the inferior duodenal angle.

Routine attention to standard coagulation parameters must be observed. Foreign body extraction is possible with flexible fiberoptic endoscopy. The size of objects which can be safely removed is limited by the small size of extracting forceps. A number of grasping forceps are available, however, for removing foreign bodies. Variceal hemorrhage can be controlled using the flexible fiberoptic endoscope with the injection of sclerosing agents, such as sodium morrhuate, into the varices.[45] The exact insertion of small injection needles is possible, given the extremely precise focus at the distal tip of the endoscope. Specific bleeding lesions such as arteriovenous malformations and ulcerations may be coagulated using either electrofulguration or the more recently designed laser photocoagulation systems.[46,47] The place of such coagulation therapy in individuals with significant upper gastrointestinal tract bleeding has yet to be thoroughly evaluated; however, in some centers careful electrocoagulation by laser coagulation in high-risk patients has avoided the necessity of emergency surgical therapy.

Colonoscopy

Colonoscopy has two distinct differences when compared to upper gastrointestinal tract endoscopy in the evaluation of acutely ill patients. First, the tortuosity and length of the colon make routine thorough examination a more difficult procedure than upper GI endoscopy. Second, even vigorous lavage of the colon in patients without dietary or laxative preparation is unlikely to produce a clear field for thorough evaluation. Colonscopy is contraindicated for patients with cardiopulmonary collapse as well as for uncooperative patients.

The lack of adequate preparation of the colon renders the examination less helpful in evaluating lower gastrointestinal pathology than is the endoscopy in evaluating patients with upper gastrointestinal tract symptomatology or signs. [48] In patients vigorously bleeding from the lower gastrointestinal tract or unprepared for colonoscopic examination, the view is obscured and the likelihood of demonstrating substantial helpful endoscopic findings is low. On occasion, colonoscopic evaluation, as well as upper endoscopic evaluation of acutely ill patients can be delayed until just prior to or during the course of an exploratory laparotomy. The colonoscope can be guided with the assistance of the operating team to thoroughly evaluate areas of large or small bowel. However, since adequate evaluation of the bowel by endoscopy requires the use of air insufflation of the bowel, a markedly dilated distended bowel may result from intra-operative endoscopic evaluation of the upper or lower gastrointestinal tract.

Endoscopic Retrograde Cholangiopancreatography

The ERCP evaluation of patients with acute abdominal pain or catastrophic disease involving the pancreas or biliary tree is possible even in the most acutely ill patient. In unstable patients with cardiopulmonary collapse, however, and in uncooperative patients, once again, the examination must be delayed until stabilization and adequate analgesia and cooperation can be assured. Since a side-viewing endoscope is required for ERCP, patients with known large esophageal diverticula or esophageal obstruction must be examined with a great degree of caution, since the endoscope is passed blindly through the esophagus into the stomach. Patients undergoing ERCP must be able to lie prone on the fluoroscopy table to ensure high quality radiographic visualization of the pancreas or biliary tree. The examination requires high quality fluoroscopy with image intensification to ensure the safe yet adequate distention of the necessary duct. The evaluation of the pancreaticobiliary system must, therefore, be performed in fluoroscopy suites and not in the operating room or intensive care centers unequipped for such techniques. Cannulation of the pancreatic or biliary ducts is made difficult by previous gastric surgery, especially the Billroth-II anastomosis. Nonetheless, with a little more caution and expertise,

ERCP is possible even in these patients with previous gastric surgery. In patients with acute abdominal catastrophes, adequate distention of the second portion of the duodenum to allow for selective cannulation of the papilla may be difficult. Moreover, in patients with retroperitoneal trauma, hemorrhage, or pancreatitis, proper distention of the duodenum may likewise be difficult and visualization of the papilla for cannulation impossible. In addition to the endoscopic and radiographic evaluation of pancreatic or biliary pathology, endoscopic sphincterotomy, using electrofulguration, allows for non-operative common duct stone removal in the poor surgical candidate.[49]

Laparoscopy

Laparoscopic evaluation of the peritoneal cavity is possible using either local or general anesthesia. This technique is particularly helpful in patients with suspected or demonstrable focal hepatic mass lesions incompletely evaluated by either non-invasive diagnostic imaging techniques such as CT or ultrasonography or through standard percutaneous liver biopsy techniques. Laparoscopy with single or double puncture techniques allows for precise biopsy of focal left hepatic lobar, anterior right hepatic lobar lesions.[50-51] In addition to selective biopsy of hepatic mass lesions, peritoneal disease can be accurately diagnosed through a combination of aspiration cytology of peritoneal fluid or selective biopsy of focal peritoneal implants. Laparoscopy is, however, contraindicated in the unstable patient with cardiopulmonary disease or in the totally uncooperative patient. In these latter patients, the examination can be conducted under general anesthesia. The laparoscopic examination of the abdomen using local anesthesia with insufflation of air, carbon dioxide, or nitrous oxide is ideally suited for stable, cooperative patients. In most cases, the laparoscope is inserted in the midline sub-umbilically. The thorough visualization of the anterior peritoneal surface and liver will be obscured by previous surgical procedures around this area. In some centers, the laparoscopy trocars are routinely introduced in other portions of the abdomen to gain access to the free peritoneal cavity in patients with midline surgical scars. Adequate attention must be paid to coagulation factors. A depressed platelet count or elevated prothrombin time, partial thromboplastin time, or bleeding time should be considered absolute contraindications to the performance of the laparoscopy unless replacement therapy is undertaken. Although the anterior and superior aspects of both lobes of the liver, the entire anterior peritoneal surface, and the omentum can be examined laparoscopically, a large portion of the abdomen is invisible to laparoscopy, especially retroperitoneal structures.

REFERENCES

1. Kaviraj Kunja Lal (ed.): The Sushruta Samhita, Vol. 1. Bhishagratna, 3 volumes Calcutta, Wilkins Press, 1907.
2. Zimmerman L, Veith I: Great Ideas in the History of Surgery, 2nd ed. New York, Dover Publications, 1967.
3. Hemorrhagic Shock—Current Problems in Surgery, Chicago, Yearbook Medical Publishers, 1971.
4. Moore FD: The effects of hemorrhage on body composition, N Eng J Med 273:567, 1965.
5. Widmann FK: Clinical Interpretation of Laboratory Tests, 8th ed. FA Davis, Philadelphia, 1979.
6. Naffziger HC, McCorkle HJ: The recognition and management of acute trauma to the pancreas with particular reference to the use of the serum amylase test. Ann Surg 118:594, 1943.

7. Olsen WR: The serum amylase in blunt abdominal trauma. J Trauma 13:200, 1973.
8. Cimmino CV: Ruptured spleen: Some refinements in its roentgenologic diagnosis. Radiology 2:57, 1964.
9. Frimann-Dahl J: Roentgen Examinations in Acute Abdominal Disease. 2nd ed., Springfield, Charles C Thomas, 1960.
10. Budin E, Jacobson G: Roentgenographic diagnosis of small amounts of intraperitoneal fluid. Am J Roentgen 99:62-70, 1967.
11. Margulies M, Stoane L: Hepatic angle in roentgen evaluation of peritoneal fluid. Radiology 88:51-54, 1967.
12. McCort JJ: Radiographic Examination in Blunt Abdominal Trauma. Philadelphia, WB Saunders, 1966.
13. Keefe EJ, Gagliardi RA, Pfister RC: The roentgenographic evaluation of ascites. Am J Roentgen 101:388389, 1967.
14. Ting YM, Reuter SR: Hollow viscus injury in blunt abdominal trauma. Am J Roentgen 119:408-412, 1973.
15. Mahboubi S, Kaufmann HJ: Intramural duodenal hematoma in children: The role of the radiologist in its conservative management. Gastrointest Radiol 1:167-171, 1976.
16. Richter MW, et al: Radiology of genitourinary trauma. Radiol Clin No Am 11:593-631, 1973.
17. Mahoney SA, Persky L: Intravenous drip nephrotomography as an adjunct in the evaluation of renal injury. J Urol 99:573-576, 1968.
18. Cass AS: Immediate radiological evaluation and early surgical management of genitourinary injuries from external trauma. J Urol 122:772-774, 1979.
19. Wilson RL, Rogers WF, Shaub MS: Splenic Subcapsular hematoma—ultrasonic diagnosis. West J Med 128: 68, 1978.
20. Asher Wm, et al.: Echographic evaluation of splenic injury after blunt trauma. Radiology 118:411-415, 1976.
21. Kay CJ, Rosenfield At, Armm M: Gray-scale ultrasonography in the evaluation of renal trauma. Radiology 134:461-466, 1980.
22. Conrad MR, et al.: Sonography of the Page kidney. J Urol 116:293-296, 1976.
23. Nebesar RA, Rabinov KR, Potsaid MS: Radionuclide imaging of the spleen in suspected splenic injury. Radiology 110:609-614, 1979.
24. Lutzker L, et al.: The role of radionuclide imaging in spleen trauma. Radiology 110:419-425, 1974.
25. Evans GW, et al.: Scintigraphy in traumatic lesions of liver and spleen. JAMA 222: 665-667, 1972.
26. Woodruff JH Jr, et al.: Radiologic aspects of renal trauma with the emphasis on arteriography and renal isotope scanning. J Urol 97:184-188, 1967.
27. Kazmin MH, Swanson LE, Cockett AT: Renal scan: the test of choice in renal trauma. J Urol 97:189-195, 1967.
28. Freedman GS: Radionuclide imaging of the injured patient. Radiol Clin N Am 11:461-477, 1973.
29. Redman HC, Reuter SR, Bookstein JJ: Angiography in abdominal trauma. Ann Surg 169:57-66, 1969.
30. Berk RW, Wholey MH, Stockdale RL: The angiographic diagnosis of splenic and hepatic trauma. J Can Assoc Radiol 21:230-234, 1970.
31. Lang EK: Arteriography in the assessment of renal trauma. The impact of arteriographic diagnosis on preservation of renal function and parenchyma. J Trauma 15:553-566, 1975.
32. Stivelman RL, Glaubtiz JP, Crangston RS: Laceration of the spleen due to nonpenetrating trauma. One hundred cases. Am J Surg 106: 888-891, 1963.
33. Federle MP, et al.: Evaluation of abdominal trauma by computed tomography. Radiology 138:637-644, 1981.
34. Berger PE, Kuhn JP: CT of blunt abdominal trauma in childhood. Am J Roentgen 136:105-110, 1981.
35. Jeffrey RJ Jr, et al.: CT of splenic trauma. Radiology (in press).
36. Korobkin M, et al.: Computed tomography of subcapsular splenic hematoma. Clinical and experimental studies. Radiology 129:441-445, 1978.
37. Mall JC, Kaiser JA: CT diagnosis of splenic laceration. Am J Roentgen 134:265-269, 1980.
38. Federle MP, et al.: Computed tomography of pancreatic abscesses. Am J Roentgen 136:879-882, 1981.
39. Mendez G Jr, Isikoff MB: Significance of intrapancreatic gas demonstrated by CT: A review of nine cases. Am J Roentgen 132:59-62, 1979.
40. Sagel SS, et al.: Detection of retroperitoneal hemorrhage by computed tomography. Am J Roentgen 129:403407, 1977.
41. Federle MP, et al.: The role of computed tomography in renal trauma. Radiology (in press).
42. Schaner EG, Balow JE, Doppman JL: Computed tomography in the diagnosis of subcapsular and perirenal hematoma. Am J Roentgen 129:83-88, 1977.
43. Katon, RM, Smith FW: Panendoscopy in the early diagnosis of acute upper gastrointestinal bleeding. Gastroenterology 65:728-734, 1973.
44. Cello JP, Thoeni RF: Gastrointestinal hemorrhagecomparative values of double-contrast upper gastrointestinal radiography and endoscopy. JAMA 243:685688, 1980.

45. Clark AW, et al.: Prospective controlled trial of injection sclerotherapy in patients with cirrhosis and recent variceal hemorrhage. Lancet III:552-554, 1980.
46. Volpicelli NA, et al.: Endoscopic electrocoagulation—an alternative to operative therapy in bleeding peptic ulcer disease. Arch Surg 113:483-486, 1978.
47. Silverstein FE, et al.: Endoscopic laser treatment. Gastroenterology 73:481-486, 1977.
48. Thanik KD, Cheu WY, Abbott J: Vascular dysplasia of the cecum as a repeated source of hemorrhage — role of colonoscopy in diagnosis. Gastrointest Endoscopy 23:167-169, 1977.
49. Liguory C, Loriga P: Endoscopic sphincterotomy analysis of 155 cases. Am J Surg 136:609-613, 1978.
50. Balfour TW: Laparoscopy in liver disease. Lancet 612-613, 1976.
51. McCallum RW, Berci G: Laparoscopy in hepatic disease. Gastrointest Endoscopy 23:20-24, 1976.

Chapter Three

PARACENTESIS AND DIAGNOSTIC PERITONEAL LAVAGE

LAWRENCE A. DANTO

Diagnostic procedures should be limited to those examinations which have proven effective. . . . One should not jeopardize the care of the seriously injured patient by obtaining examinations of low yield.[9]

"Often the most difficult surgical decision is when not to operate." (Author)

DEVELOPMENT

The origin of paracentesis as a diagnostic technique goes back at least to 1906 when Saloman, in Berlin, reported placing a ureteral catheter through a trochar needle into the peritoneal cavity to evaluate the fluid produced by various acute intra-abdominal conditions.[45] He predicted expanded use of the study in the future, but this concept was slow to be accepted.

Two decades later, in 1926, Neuhof and Cohen reported the first comprehensive study using needle paracentesis as an aid in the diagnosis of various acute abdominal conditions including trauma, pancreatitis, and peritonitis of differing causes.[31] They were also the first to realize that needle paracentesis could miss significant amounts of hemoperitoneum.

Fifteen years passed before Steinberg, in 1941, reported the first completed and organized analysis of peritoneal fluid in various abnormal and normal conditions.[48] In 1950, Keith and others added to this by reporting the analysis of peritoneal amylase values in acute pancreatic conditions.[25]

In 1959, Williams and Zollinger reported a 79 percent accuracy with needle paracentesis in diagnosing intraperitoneal injury in trauma patients.[55] This was the first comprehensive study using paracentesis in trauma patients. They concluded that needle paracentesis was the best procedure for diagnosing intraperitoneal and pancreatic injuries, but that x-ray studies were best for urinary tract injuries. They also pointed out that needle paracentesis was significant only when positive.

A year later, in 1960, Giacobine and Siler showed that the accuracy of needle paracentesis is directly related to the amount of fluid in the peritoneal cavity.[17] The

45

low rate of positive results with small amounts of fluid were shown by I[131]studies to be due to pooling of fluid in the pelvis, paravertebral gutters, and subphrenic spaces where it was hard to reach with a needle. With 200 cc of fluid the accuracy was 16 percent while with 500 cc of fluid the accuracy rose to 78 percent. Again, while a positive needle paracentesis was likely to be associated with injury, a negative study had no clinical significance.

They also showed that while visceral penetration by the paracentesis needle might be a frequent occurrence (39 percent experimentally and 4 percent clinically), the bowel has a remarkable ability to seal itself and leakage requires high (over 200 mm Hg) intralumenal pressures, rarely found in vivo, even in the presence of bowel obstruction. They concluded that needle paracentesis, when positive, facilitated diagnosis of intra-abdominal injury before clinical signs and symptoms developed when morbidity and mortality can be expected to be low. However, relatively large amounts of peritoneal fluid are required for a significant degree of accuracy.

In 1965, however, Root and colleagues reported a new paracentesis technique utilizing a disposable catheter with multiple side holes.[41] This allowed sampling from the pelvis, where Giacobine and Siler showed that blood is most likely to accumulate.[17] If paracentesis was negative, then peritoneal saline lavage was performed. This allowed dilution and dissemination of any abnormal fluids and automatically provided enough volume for a high degree of accuracy early in the course of triage. In this way, lavage increased further the probability of retrieving a clinically significant sample.

Their initial evaluation of 28 blunt abdominal trauma patients proved to be very accurate. Sixteen of 16 patients were correctly diagnosed as having significant intraperitoneal injury. Not only was their technique accurate in proving injury before the symptoms developed, but it was also accurate in ruling out injury; a distinct advantage over conventional paracentesis. Soon other reports appeared supporting the accuracy of paracentesis and lavage over needle paracentesis alone. [3,19,23]

Veith and others, in 1967, reported the lavage findings in a variety of acute abdominal conditions: inflammatory and vascular, as well as traumatic.[54]

Subsequently, reports have shown that paracentesis and diagnostic peritoneal lavage can be safely used in children and during pregnancy.[10,39,43] It has also been used with a high degree of success in penetrating torso injuries.[8,28,30,51,53]

As the use of paracentesis and diagnostic peritoneal lavage expanded over the next few years, it became apparent that lavage was so sensitive that even minor intraperitoneal injuries were detected. In one study, a false positive rate of 20 percent was reported.[32] In the early 1970's, various techniques were devised to quantitate the lavage results to accurately differentiate significant from insignificant injuries. Various methods have been described. Each, in spite of their differences, has lessened the incidence of the false positive and false negative study.[4,7,13,32,33,34,38]

RATIONALE

The diagnosis of intraperitoneal injury, especially when associated with altered consciousness and/or multiple extra-abdominal injuries, has always been difficult. Added difficulties are encountered in children and pregnant women. These remain the classic indications for lavage and are generally agreed to by all.

Clinical signs of visceral injury are notoriously nonspecific, frequently minimal or absent even when life-threatening injury is present. As a result, life-threatening injury can easily be overlooked. This is true for both blunt and penetrating abdominal injuries. It is also true that some patients will show signs and symptoms of intraperitoneal injury when none has occurred. The overall *inaccuracy* of the initial physical evaluation in trauma patients with regard to the presence or absence of intra-abdominal injury has been reported to be from 16 to 45 percent.[2,4,8,9,13,15,32,34,35,36,43,46,51,53,55]

Even documented peritoneal penetration may not be associated with visceral injury in as much as 40 + percent of cases. Other laboratory values and organ imaging techniques are of surprisingly selective and limited value. In addition, these studies are often time consuming, thus leading to unnecessary delay.[1,8,9,27,36,47,53,55]

Because of a certain, albeit limited, morbidity and mortality associated with the negative celiotomy, the policy of selective or expectant observation became popular.[46] Patients without obvious signs and symptoms of intra-abdominal injury were serially and frequently re-evaluated. If and when positive signs and symptoms developed, they underwent exploration. However, expectant observation once again led to morbidity and mortality in these patients. This factor was due to the delay encountered in making a positive diagnosis in about 25 percent of patients being selectively observed.[6,16] Numerous studies have documented the fact that delay in diagnosis is associated with increased morbidity and decreased survival. These same studies show that rapid triage is associated with decreased morbidity and increased survival, including less blood loss, fewer transfusions, and shorter recovery periods. Delay has been encountered in as much as 50 percent of fatal cases and has been felt responsible for as much as 16 percent of these deaths. With combined head injury, unsuspected intraperitoneal injury has been found responsible for 20 to 40 percent of deaths. Finally, over 40 percent of selectively observed patients have been found to have what was considered a prolonged recovery.[4,5,13,25,29,36,39,43,55,56]

The use of catheter paracentesis and diagnostic peritoneal lavage as originally described by Root in 1965 is now recognized as a means of facilitating rapid diagnosis in problem cases. It can be performed anywhere, quickly, and with little equipment. It has the highest degree of accuracy of any test for the diagnosis of intra-abdominal injury. A review of the literature shows its use in an accumulated 9588 reported patients with both blunt and penetrating torso injuries; in pregnancy and childhood as well.[1,4,5,8,10,12,13,15,19, 22,23,30,33,34,35,38,39,41,43,47,50,51,53]

Special mention should be made of the importance of diagnostic peritoneal lavage in other surgical problems. It allows retrieval of representative fluid early in the course of disease when recovery can be expected to be optimal. It is so sensitive that various studies have shown it is often the only reliable indication for operation or observation. It is diagnostic peritoneal lavage that has given the study the high degree of accuracy so widely reported, and as mentioned, this also has given the study significance, not only when it is positive but also when it is negative.[8,9,15,27,28,30,32,33,53]

Finally, a word about who should do paracentesis and diagnostic peritoneal lavage. In general, the surgeon who will perform the celiotomy or observe the patient (as indicated) should perform the paracentesis and diagnostic peritoneal lavage. This is for two reasons: first, this person should be able to perform the procedure with the least morbidity and will best be able to handle any complications, though rare, that might arise; second, it is always good practice for a surgeon to establish his own indications for operation or observation.

However, on occasion, paracentesis and diagnostic peritoneal lavage can be performed by a triaging physician who is faced with sending a multiple trauma patient to a trauma center and needs to know the abdominal status so the patient is not transported with uncontrolled intra-abdominal hemorrhage. Even here, it would be best for a surgeon to consult and perform the study.

INDICATIONS

The indications for paracentesis and lavage as reported in the literature have been varied. Some authors believe the study is indicated in all acute abdominal conditions for which operation might be indicated. They feel that paracentesis and lavage is so superior to all other methods of evaluation that it should always be used. Others are much more reserved. We feel that its greatest value is facilitating rapid diagnosis in patients with altered consciousness, in the patient with thoracic injury—particularly when there are fractures of the lower six ribs—and in the multiply-injured patient in whom blood loss is difficult to assess. Along with these indications, there are other indications which will vary with the nature of the patient, the experience of the surgeon, and the hospital resources available. For simplicity, the relative indications are included in our Emergency Room Protocol (Table 3–1).[1,14,21,31,35,38,39,40,41,47]

Table 3–1 INDICATIONS
PARACENTESIS AND DIAGNOSTIC PERITONEAL LAVAGE

Blunt Torso Trauma

1. Celiotomy if:
   A. Involuntary guarding
   B. Distended/distending abdomen
   C. Unexplained deterioration of vital signs
   D. Blood in gastrointestinal tract
   E. X-ray abdomen (optional)—free air

2. If A–D are negative, equivocal, there are multiple injuries, an unexplained falling hematocrit, or altered consciousness with the possibility of abdominal injury.

A. Paracentesis	Positive	Celiotomy
	Negative	
B. Lavage	Positive	Celiotomy
	Negative	Observe
Equivocal	Observe and re-evaluate	
	Organ imaging	
	RBC, WBC, and amylase on lavagate	

Unconsciousness/Altered Consciousness and Small Children

1. X-ray abdomen (optional)
2. Paracentesis and lavage as above

Penetrating Torso Trauma

1. Celiotomy if:
   A. Evisceration
   B. Distended/distending abdomen
   C. Deteriorating vital sings
   D. Blood in GI or GU tract
   E. Fascial penetration anterior to posterior axillary line.

2. If A–E are negative, paracentesis and lavage, as above.

No patient should be observed in the hospital with the possibility of significant torso trauma without a negative paracentesis and diagnostic peritoneal lavage.

Our protocol recognizes certain clinical signs which, though not pathognomonic of intra-abdominal injury, are highly suggestive and would be intellectually and emotionally difficult not to act upon even if paracentesis and diagnostic peritoneal lavage were negative. It has been used successsfully since 1972. This protocol is not meant to be an absolute or rigid "cook book" list. The use of paracentesis and diagnostic peritoneal lavage is not meant to eliminate the use of other special studies when necessary, and conditions permit. Though paracentesis with diagnostic peritoneal lavage is the most sensitive test available for hemoperitoneum or pyoperitoneum, it is nonspecific. On occasion, organ imaging is of value.

CONTRAINDICATIONS

As with the indications, the contraindications for paracentesis with diagnostic peritoneal lavage, as reported in the literature, have considerable variation. Some authors ignore the subject altogether; some state there are no contraindications; others present a rather detailed list of contraindications, including positive clinical signs, multiple previous abdominal operations, distended bowel, supected localized acute inflammatory process, abdominal mass, childhood, and pregnancy. Still others, ourselves included, advise a moderate approach. We believe there are not absolute contraindications other than obvious signs of intra-abdominal injury. However, the relative contraindications include scars from previous types of surgery in which there would be anticipated numerous adhesions, abdominal distension, or suspected abdominal masses. In any situation where the traditional percutaneous stab technique is felt to be compromised the minilap technique can be used. Although somewhat more complicated and time consuming, it avoids completely the few intraperitoneal complications that can occur when the stab technique is improperly used.[1,8,32,34,41,44,49,54]

TECHNIQUE

The technique for paracentesis and diagnostic peritoneal lavage is quite simple. There are a few precautions and first it should be practiced, if possible, in the morgue. However, the procedure is easy to master and, once it is learned, can be performed anywhere, quickly, with little equipment, and with minimal interruption in patient care.

One precaution concerns x-rays. If x-rays are to be obtained to evaluate the abdominal cavity for free air, they should be obtained first, as paracentesis may introduce room air into the abdominal cavity. If the abdomen is distended an. tympanitic (with a functioning NG tube in place) celiotomy is indicated without "routine" x-rays or paracentesis. If the abdomen is not distended, the yield from x-rays is so low that lavage need not be delayed.

The most optimal and safest technique has been made posasible by the Lazarus-Nelson Peritoneal Lavage technique which utilizes a needle and stylet technique.*

---

* Commercial tray—Lazarus-Nelson Peritoneal Lavage Tray produced by Kormed.

Table 3–2   OUTLINE OF TECHNIQUE

1. Prepare skin and anesthetize site with local anesthetic containing epinephrine.
2. Make stab wound with #11 blade; through fascia if possible.
3. Insert stylet and catheter, removing stylet as peritoneum is penetrated, and advance catheter towards pelvis.
4. Aspirate with 20 cc syringe—if 20 cc of blood, paracentesis is positive.
5. If paracentesis is negative, lavage with Ringer's lactate or normal saline.

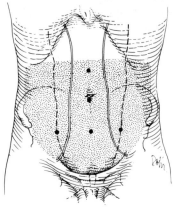

Figure 3–1 Sites used for paracentesis. Primary sites are in the midline below the umbilicus and in the lower portion of the umbilicus itself.

The technique is especially safe in inexperienced hands. The largest sharp object introduced into the peritoneal cavity is an 18 gauge needle. As previously stated, this should not cause morbidity even if the bowel is penetrated[17] in contrast to the large disposable commercial catheters which have caused the various injuries reported in the literature.

The site selected is usually in the midline somewhere in the middle third between the umbilicus and symphysis pubis (Figure 3-1). The site can be located higher in smaller patients and lower in larger patients so the catheter tip will reach into the pelvic depths. A site other than the midline can be used depending on scars from previous celiotomies and masses. The rectus sheath should be avoided.

The bladder should be ensured empty; usually with a Foley catheter. If a suprapubic approach is used, such as in pregnancy, the stomach should first be decompressed with a nasogastric tube. Lazarus and Nelson consider the gravid uterus a contraindication for peritoneal lavage but we and others[43] disagree.

Antiseptic is painted on the skin. Shaving is not necessary. The site is infiltrated with a local anesthetic containing epinephrine. The epinephrine will help prevent false positive results from bleeding along the catheter tract (skin, subcutaneous tissue, and fascia should be infiltrated). This is appropriate even in unconscious patients.

The skin is then incised transversely with a #11 blade. The incision is carried through subcutaneous tissue and the linea alba is palpated with the tip of the blade and incised 2-3 mm blindly. No significant bleeding should be encountered. Local pressure is then applied as needed to suppress capillary leaking.

An 18 gauge needle is then introduced through the incision and directed slightly inferiorly to engage the fascial incision. The needle is then advanced through the fascia and peritoneum with a slight popping sensation. If possible voluntary abdominal wall tension will aid in the performance of this maneuver (Figure 3-2A).

The floppy end of a guide wire is then passed through the needle into the peritoneal cavity (Figure 3-2B). The wire should fall easily into the abdomen towards

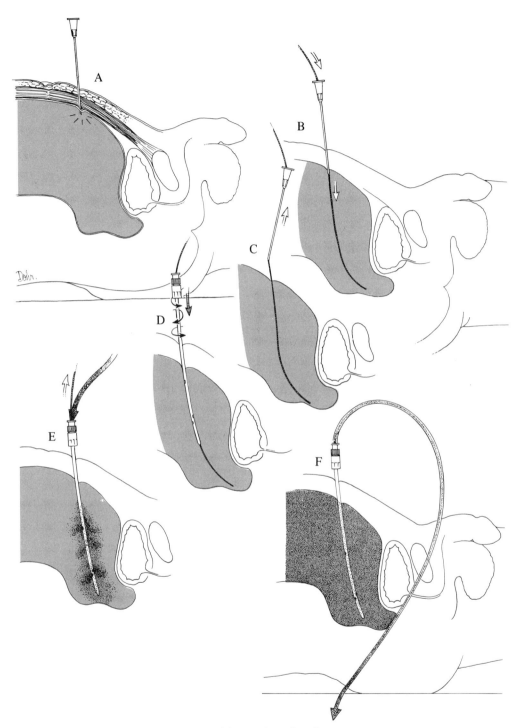

Figure 3–2 *A*, Top left—needle is inserted into peritoneal cavity
B, Flexible guide wire is passed through needle
C, Needle is withdrawn leaving guide wire in place
D, Teflon catheter is advanced over the wire
E, The wire is withdrawn and salt solution infused through catheter
F, Seal on intravenous solution is broken and fluid allowed to drain into infusion container

the pelvis. If it does not then it should be removed and the needle advanced or changed to ensure that the tip is in the free abdominal cavity and the wire passed again until free placement is achieved. After approximately half the wire is in the abdomen the needle is removed (Figure 3-2C).

A tight fitting teflon catheter is now placed over the wire and into the peritoneal cavity with a twisting motion applied just above the skin level to aid facial penetration (Figure 3-2D).

The wire must protrude from the end of the catheter and be held while the catheter is advanced. When the catheter is fully introduced, the guide wire is removed.

The abdominal cavity is then aspirated with a 10 cc syringe. If free return of 10 cc or more of blood can be achieved the study is considered positive and celiotomy is required. If aspiration is otherwise negative then the peritoneal cavity is lavaged (by connecting IV tubing to the catheter) with lactated Ringer's solution or normal saline to the amount of about 20 ml/kg in small people and a liter in adults (Figure 3-2E). If possible, the patient is shifted or rolled from side to side to increase mixing. The bottle is then placed on the floor (or below abdominal level) and the fluid is allowed to return (Figure 3-2F). Most IV tubing contains a one-way valve. If present, it should be removed and the tubing re-inserted into the bottle or allowed to drain into an open container. Wiggling or twisting the catheter or applying abdominal pressure may aid flow when it is hesitant.

It is not necessary to remove all of the fluid. When about 10 to 20 percent has returned a representative sample can be relied upon, readings and specimens taken, and the procedure terminated.

Table 3–3   TRADITIONAL INTERPRETATION*

Positive:	Free aspiration of blood/grossly bloody fluid
	over 100,000 RBC/mm$_3$ over 500 WBC/mm$_3$ over 175u amylase/100 ml
Intermediate:	small amount of blood (fills catheter)
	50,000–100,000 RBC/mm$_3$ 100–500 WBC/mm$_3$ 75–175u amylase/100 ml

*Adapted from Root et al.[42]

Table3–4   QUANTITATIVE PERITONEAL LAVAGE*

Positive:	Free blood or bloody fluid; Newsprint unreadable
Negative:	Clear fluid
Intermediate:	Pink fluid but newsprint readable (about 20% of lavages).
Unstable	Celiotomy
Stable	Observe and re-evaluate Organ imaging RBC, WBC, and amylase on lavagate (as in Table 3–3)

Adapted from Olsen et al.[33]

ALTERNATIVES

There are alternative methods which should be kept in mind. The original method that many articles have reported is the percutaneous thrust using one of the disposable peritoneal dialysis catheters with multiple perforations and an intra-lumenal stylet (Figure 3-3). This is not as controlled a technique as that reported above but in experienced hands is very safe.

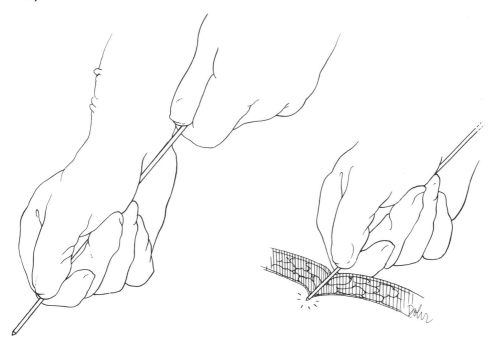

Figure 3–3 The obturator should be grasped as shown to preclude uncontrolled or inadvertent excessively deep penetration. One hand acts as the guard while the other applies the force necessary to push the trocar through the abdominal wall.

In infants and small children a 14 or 16 gauge of appropriate length angiocath can be used. Side holes are cut in the tip of the catheter with the stylet left in place (Figure 3-4).

Finally, the minilap technique (Figure 3-5) can be used whenever a blind procedure might be considered unwise (such as when there are anticipated adhesions at the procedure site, pregnancy, the presence of abdominal masses, or any other uncertainty on the part of the operator). Although inherently safer than the percutaneous thrust, this open technique is more time consuming, requires more equipment and assistance, and has more minor wound complications. It has been largely replaced by the Lazarus-Nelson technique.

In all techniques, the optimal location for the catheter is deep in the pelvis.

INTERPRETATION

A reliable interpretation can be expected unless the abdominal cavity is unusually compartmentalized or obliterated by adhesions from multiple operations or episodes of peritonitis. This is unusual.

Paracentesis is considered positive if there is aspiration of 20 cc or more of non-clotting blood (10 cc or more in children).

The interpretation of diagnostic peritoneal lavage took some time to evolve. Diagnostic peritoneal lavage is so sensitive that it can detect even minor, clinically insignificant injuries; the results must, therefore, be quantitated. The original approach is to perform various laboratory determinations on the lavage fluid (RBC, WBC, and amylase) (Table 3-3). This is accurate but time consuming.[7,33,41,42,54].

In 1972, Olsen described a method of bedside quantitative determination which retained the high degree of accuracy yet required no special equipment and could be instantly performed in the majority of cases. This is the method which is preferred (Table 3-4).[33]

Diagnostic peritoneal lavage is considered positive if the lavage fluid is observed leaving through a Foley catheter or chest tube.[16]

As the lavage fluid leaves the abdomen, it is usually pink or clear and becomes pink. Assessment should not be made on the initial lavage return. After 10 to 20 percent of the fluid has returned, representative specimens can be taken and reliably assessed. It is not necessary to retrieve all of the fluid. If the fluid is grossly bloody,

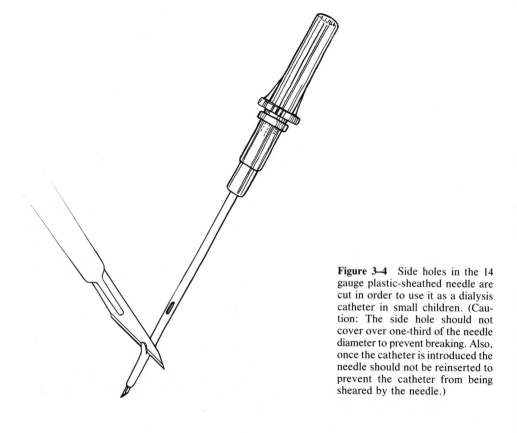

Figure 3-4 Side holes in the 14 gauge plastic-sheathed needle are cut in order to use it as a dialysis catheter in small children. (Caution: The side hole should not cover over one-third of the needle diameter to prevent breaking. Also, once the catheter is introduced the needle should not be reinserted to prevent the catheter from being sheared by the needle.)

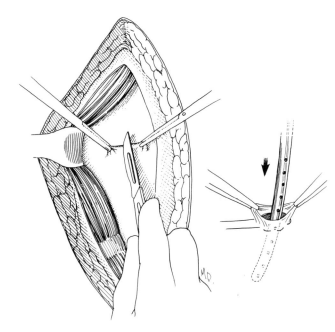

Figure 3–5. The minilap technique. The anterior rectus sheath is entered lateral to the midline, and the rectus msucle is retracted laterally. After opening the posterior sheath and cleaning the preperitoneal fat off the peritoneum, the peritoneum is carefully clamped lateral to the midline and tented up between two hemostats.

Four hemostats keep the peritoneum tented up. The dialysis catheter is gently inserted, and a pursestring suture is placed under direct vision.

lavage is positive. If the fluid is pink to red, newsprint or something similar is placed behind the tubing. If the newsprint cannot be read through the tubing, the lavage is positive. If the newsprint can be read but the fluid is pink, the lavage is termed intermediate. If the fluid is clear, the lavage is negative and the patient is observed.

The patient with the intermediate lavage can be handled selectively. If the patient is unstable, celiotomy is indicated. If the patient is stable, RBC, WBC, and amylase determinations should be done; alternatively, the patient should be observed and periodically re-evaluated (even the paracentesis catheter can be left in and lavage repeated later on). Organ imaging studies can be instituted meanwhile to actively search for specific injuries. If follow-up examination and all studies are negative, observation can be continued. If RBC, WBC, and amylase determinations are done on the intermediate lavage fluid, two hours is usually required after injury for a reliable cellular peritoneal response.[42] For this reason, laboratory tests are usually not carried out on the lavage fluid.

In Olsen's series only about 20 percent of lavaged patients fall into this intermediate group.[33] Nonetheless, the identification and management of this intermediate group helps give diagnostic peritoneal lavage its extremely high degree of accuracy. In the majority of cases, however, an accurate plan of action can be chosen on the initial patient contact without using special studies.

RESULTS

The results of triage with paracentesis with diagnostic peritoneal lavage have been uniformly excellent. As mentioned earlier, a review of 23 papers published since Root's initial report in 1965 shows a total of 9588 documented patients (both blunt and penetrating injuries); 4053 of these had a positive test and 5535 had a negative test. A positive test was 97 percent accurate. Restated, this is a 3 percent false positive or negative celiotomy rate. A negative test was 98.7 percent accurate for a false negative rate of 1.3 percent. Whereas most authors report some false positive results, over half reported no false negative results; further emphasizing the accuracy of a negative test. The overall accuracy of paracentesis and diagnostic peritoneal lavage in these patients was 98 percent.

False positive results are usually related to bleeding from the catheter insertion site or from an omental or mesentery laceration produced by the catheter. Other causes include a large retroperitoneal hematoma associated with a pelvic fracture or a minor intraperitoneal injury. This all points to the high degree of sensitivity of the test. This margin of error towards the side of overdiagnosis provides a reassuring safety factor.

False negative studies, though unusual, can be due to faulty catheter placement or some other technical problem (such as compartmentalization by adhesions). Occasionally a retroperitoneal injury of significance (kidney, pancreas, duodenum, colon) when present by itself can be missed. Also, a ruptured diaphragm or bladder can be missed. Rarely, a significant injury which is not associated with bleeding may be encountered. Paracentesis and diagnostic peritoneal lavage may have been performed so early that the results are negative due to lack of development of an appropriate peritoneal inflammatory response. These false negative lavages, however, are most often questionably negative or intermediate.

All authors reporting the use of paracentesis and diagnostic peritoneal lavage repeatedly point to the large number of clinically negative patients who were discovered early by paracentesis and diagnostic peritoneal lavage to have significant intraperitoneal injury. Conversely, they show that even clinical signs traditionally associated with "obvious" intraperitoneal injury (such as abdominal rigidity, absent bowel sounds, falling hematocrit, and leukocytosis) are far less accurate indications than paracentesis and diagnostic peritoneal lavage. Many patients with these signs have been spared unnecessary operation and safely observed. Even in patients with penetrating injuries—both stab wounds and gunshot wounds—paracentesis and diagnostic peritoneal lavage can be used and relied upon as an accurate method of triage.[8,28,30,51,53]

COMPLICATIONS

Complications of paracentesis are uncommon. Of the 23 studies previously summarized, 21 reported no complications. Of a total of 9385 patients reported in these studies, there were 127 complications for an overall complication rate of 1.4 percent. There were 83 minor complications consisting of wound problems, rectus sheath hematomas, rectus sheath lavage, or retroperitoneal bladder penetration. Most were wound hematomas and infections occurring in patients undergoing open placement of the lavage catheter by the minilap technique. They required no special therapy and did not contribute significantly to morbidity.[1,4,5,8,10,12,13,15,19,21,22,23,33,34,38,39,41,43,47,50,51]

There were 44 major complications for a significant complication rate of 0.5 percent. These included mostly trochar penetrations of the stomach, small bowel, colon, mesentery, and occasionally a venous injury or rupture of an ovarian cyst. Although these injuries usually require surgical correction, in one large series of

1465 patients the complication was the sole reason for operation in only 2 of the 15 patients with complications.[13] Most required celiotomy for an intra-abdominal injury. There has been no long term morbidity associated with these complications and no complication-related deaths have been reported.

One final word about complications. They are virtually always due to errors in technique caused by either operator inexperience or failure to follow the precautions described in the section on technique. Several authors mention that their few complications occurred early in their experience and, subsequently none were encountered.[20,23,33,54]

REFERENCES

1. Ahmad W, Polk HC Jr: Blunt abdominal trauma: A prospective study with selective peritoneal lavage Arch Surg 111:489-492, 1976.
2. Baker RJ: Newer techniques in evaluation of injured patients. Surg Clin N Am 55:31-42, 1975.
3. Baker WNW, Mackie DB, Newcombe JF: Diagnostic paracentesis in the acute abdomen. Br Med J 3:146-149, 1967.
4. Bivins BA, Jona JZ, Belin RP: Diagnostic peritoneal lavage in pediatric trauma. J Trauma 16:739-742, 1976.
5. Bivins BA, Sachatello CR, Daugherty ME, Ernst CB, Griffin WO Jr: Diagnostic peritoneal lavage is superior to clinical evaluation in blunt abdominal trauma. Am Surg 44:637-641, 1978.
6. Bull JC, Mathewson C Jr: Exploratory laparotomy in patients with penetrating wounds of the abdomen. Am J Surg 116:223-228, 1968.
7. Caffee HH, Benfield JR: Is peritoneal lavage for the diagnosis of hemoperitoneum safe? Arch Surg 103:4-7, 1971.
8. Danto LA, Thomas CW, Gornbein S, Wolfman EF Jr: Penetrating torso injuries: The role of paracentesis and lavage. Am Surg 43:164-170, 1977.
9. Davis JJ, Cohn I Jr., Nance FC: Diagnosis and management of blunt abdominal trauma. Ann Surg 183:672-678, 1976.
10. Drew R, Perry JF Jr, Fischer RP: The expediency of peritoneal lavage for blunt abdominal trauma in children. Surg Gynecol Obstet 145:885-888, 1977.
11. DuPriest RW Jr, Khaneja SC, Rodriguez A, Cowley RA: A technique for open diagnostic peritoneal lavage. Surg Gynecol Obstet 147:241-243, 1978.
12. DuPriest RW Jr, Rodriguez A, Khaneja SC, Soderstrom CA, Maekawa KA, Ayella RJ, Cowley RA: Open diagnostic peritoneal lavage in blunt trauma victims. Surg Gynecol Obstet 148:890-894, 1979.
13. Engrav LH, Benjamin CI, Strate RG, perry JR Jr: Diagnostic peritoneal lavage in blunt abdominal trauma. J Trauma 15:854-859, 1975.
14. Fallazadeh H, Mays ET: Disruption of the diaphragm by blunt abdominal trauma. Am Surg 41:337-341, 1975.
15. Fischer RP, Beverlin BC, Engrav LH, Benjamin CI, Perry JF Jr: Diagnostic peritoneal lavage: Fourteen years and 2586 patients later. Am J Surg 136:701-704, 1978.
16. Forde KA, Ganepola GA: Is mandatory exploration for penetrating abdominal trauma extinct? The morbidity and mortality of negative exploration in a large municipal hospital. J Trauma 14:764, 1974.
17. Giacobine JW, Siler VE: Evaluation of diagnostic abdominal paracentesis with experimental and clinical studies. Surg Gynecol Obstet 110:676-686, 1960.
18. Generelly P, Moore TA, LeMay JT: Delayed splenic rupture: Diagnosis by culdocentesis. JACEP 6:369371, 1977.
19. Gumbert JL, Froderman SE, Mercho JP: Diagnostic peritoneal lavage in blunt abdominal trauma. Ann Surg 165:70-72, 1967.
20. Hickman TC: Abdominal paracentesis. Surg Clin N Am 49:1409-1412, 1969.
21. Hornyak SW, Shaftan GW: Value of "Inconclusive Lavage" in abdominal trauma management. J Trauma 19:329-333, 1979.
22. Jacob ET, Cantor E: Descriminate diagnostic peritoneal lavage in blunt abdominal injuries: Accuracy and hazards. Am Surg 45:11-14, 1979.
23. Jahadi MR: Diagnostic peritoneal lavage. J Trauma 12:936-938, 1972.
24. Jergens ME: Peritoneal lavage. Am J Surg 133: 365-369, 1977.
25. Keith LM, Zollinger RM, McCleery RS: Peritoneal fluid amylase determinations as an aid in diagnosis of acute pancreatitis. Arch Surg 61:930-936, 1950.
26. Kirkpatrick JR, Walt AJ: The high cost of gunshot and stab wounds. J Surg Res 14:260-264, 1973.

27. Lowe RJ, Boyd DR, Folk FA, Baker RJ: The negative laparotomy for abdominal trauma. J Trauma 12:853-861, 1972.
28. Lucas CE: The role of peritoneal lavage for penetrating abdominal wounds. J Trauma 17:649-650, 1977.
29. Maynard AL, Oropeza G: Mandatory operations for penetrating wounds of the abdomen. Am J Surg 115:307-312, 1968.
30. McAlvanah MJ, Shaftan GW: Selective conservatism in penetrating abdominal wounds: A continuing reappraisal. J Trauma 18:206-212, 1978.
31. Neuhof H, Cohen I: Abdominal puncture in the diagnosis of acute intraperitoneal disease. Ann Surg 83:454462, 1926.
32. Olsen WR, Hildreth DH: Abdominal paracentesis and peritoneal lavage in blunt abdominal trauma. J Trauma 11:824-829, 1971.
33. Olsen WR, Redman HC, Hildreth DH: Quantitative peritoneal lavage in blunt abdominal trauma. Arch Surg 104:536-543, 1972.
34. Pacey J, Forward AD, Preto AF: Peritoneal tap and lavage in patients with blunt abdominal trauma: Their contribution to surgical decisions. CMAJ 105:365-370, 1971.
35. Parvin S, Smith DE, Asher WM, Virgilio RW: Effectiveness of peritoneal lavage in blunt abdominal trauma. Ann Surg 181:255-261, 1975.
36. Perry JR Jr: A five year survey of 152 acute abdominal injuries. J Trauma 5:53-61, 1965.
37. Perry JR Jr: Initial hospital management of the injured patient. Curr Prob Surg, 1970.
38. Perry JF Jr, Strate RG: Diagnostic peritoneal lavage in blunt abdominal trauma: Indications and results. Surgery 71:898-901, 1972.
39. Powell RW, Smith DE, Zarins CK, Parvin S, Virgilio RW: Peritoneal lavage in children with blunt abdominal trauma. J Pediat Surg 11:973-977, 1976.
40. Prout WG: An evaluation of diagnostic paracentesis in the acute abdomen. Br J Surg 55:583-587, 1968.
41. Root HD, Hauser CW, McKinley CR, LaFave JW, Mendiola RP: Diagnostic peritoneal lavage. Surgery 57:633637, 1965.
42. Root HD, Keizer RI, Perry JF Jr: The clinical and experimental aspects of peritoneal response to injury. Arch Surg 95:531, 1967.
43. Rothenberger DA, Quattlebaum FW, Zabel J, Fischer RP: Diagnostic peritoneal lavage for blunt trauma in pregnant women. Am J Obstet 129:479-481, 1977.
44. Sachatello CR, Bivins B: Technic for peritoneal dialysis and diagnostic peritoneal lavage. Am J Surg 131:637-640, 1976.
45. Saloman H: Diagnostiche puncktion des bauches. Berl Klin Wchnschr 43:45, 1906.
46. Shaftan GW: Indications for operation in abdominal trauma. Am J Surg 99:657-664, 1960.
47. Sloop RD: The dominant role of paracentesis technics in the early diagnosis of blunt abdominal trauma. Am J Surg 136:145-150, 1978.
48. Steinberg B: Peritoneal exudate: A guide for the diagnosis and prognosis of peritoneal conditions. JAMA 116:572-578, 1941.
49. Stephens GL, Amis RE: Polyethylene tube technique of diagnostic paracentesis. J Trauma 5:805-811, 1965.
50. Thal ER, Shires GT: Peritoneal lavage in blunt abdominal trauma. Am J Surg 125:64-69, 1973.
51. Thal ER: Evaluations of peritoneal lavage and local exploration in lower chest and abdominal stab wounds. J Trauma 17:642-648, 1977.
52. Thavendran A, Vijayaragavan A, Rasaretnam R: Selective surgery for abdominal stab wounds. Br J Surg 62: 750-752, 1975.
53. Thompson JS, Moore EE, Moore SVD, Moore JB, Galloway AC: The evolution of abdominal stab wound management. J Trauma 20:478-484, 1980.
54. Veith FJ, Webber WB, Karl RC, Deysine M: Peritoneal lavage in acute abdominal disease: Normal findings and evaluation in 100 patients. Ann Surg 166:290-295, 1967.
55. Williams RD, Zollinger RM: Diagnosis and prognostic factors in abdominal trauma. Am J Surg 97:575-581, 1959.
56. Yurko AA, Williams RD: Needle paracentesis in blunt abdominal trauma: A critical analysis. J Trauma 6:194-200, 1966.

Chapter Four

ABDOMINAL WALL
AND PELVIS

F. WILLIAM BLAISDELL

INTRODUCTION

Injuries which are limited to the abdominal wall and pelvis are often taken lightly but the significance of what initially appears to be a trivial injury may be great. This is because underlying injuries may be masked. Moreover, major pelvic fractures are associated with a considerable degree of soft tissue injury, and this is associated with disproportionately high incidence of secondary complications.

The first recorded survival of a major abdominal wall injury appears in Xenophon's history of the Anabasis. The Greek generals went to the Persian camp to assure Tissaphernes that the Greeks were not plotting to kill him. What followed was one of history's most daring acts of treachery. The Persians turned on the Greek generals and killed all but Nicarcus, the Arcadian, who escaped and warned the other Greeks. He "came there with a wound in his stomach and holding his intestine. He told them everything which happened." Nicarcus somehow survived this wound, possibly with the aid of one of the eight doctors assigned to the Greek soldiers who may have bandaged and attended the injury.

The incidence of abdominal wall injury independent of other injuries is not well documented. In the experience at San Francisco General Hospital, approximately 50 percent of stab wounds of the abdomen were not associated with significant intra-abdominal injury.[17] Therefore, it would be our estimate that there are approximately twice as many abdominal wall injuries as there are viscus injuries reported in association with stab wounds. In our experience, 92 percent of gunshot wounds are associated with significant intraperitoneal injury and therefore in only a minor number of gunshot wounds are the injuries limited to the abdominal wall, yet certain types of shotgun blasts of the abdominal wall can be devastating.[17]

Blunt trauma may produce contusion of the abdominal wall in the absence of significant abdominal injury but the abdominal wall is so resiliant that most abdominal wall injuries of any significance are associated with intraperitoneal injury. One exception is perhaps related to the rectus muscle where the largest vessels of the abdominal wall, the superior and the inferior epigastric artery meet, and with severe contusions of this muscle, significant hemorrhage may occur which produces disability or may simulate intra-abdominal injury.[5,27] Another injury which can be associated with severe complications is avulsion injury. In this instance, the wheels of the car passing over the abdomen may produce a shearing force which separates skin and underlying subcutaneous tissue from the fascia (Figure 4-1).[12]

59

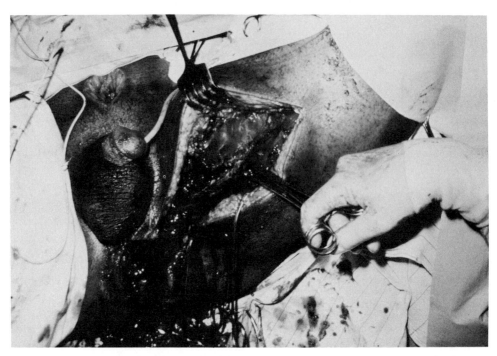

Figure 4–1   Compound pelvic fracture—extensive undermining. Perineal and thigh lacerations are demonstrated.

Significant pelvic injuries rarely result from penetrating trauma.[13] Almost all injuries are due to blunt trauma, the most frequent cause being the crushing types of injury most often associated with motor vehicle accidents.[7,26] At San Francisco General Hospital, 173 patients were noted to have pelvic injuries in one three-year-period, during which time some 4500 injuries were seen and managed.[26] Thus, the incidence was approximately three percent of our injuries. This translates into an incidence between five and ten percent of all blunt injuries. Mortality rates vary from minimal with minor fractures up to 50 percent with certain compound fractures (Table 4-1).[3,4,8,10,15,20,26]

The injuries to the chest wall involving the lower six ribs should also be considered abdominal injuries because the mass of underlying lung is minimal and major abdominal structures, including liver, spleen, and both kidneys, lie subadjacent. In our experience, one in five, or 20 percent, of all fractures to the ninth and tenth ribs on the left side are associated with splenic rupture and it is probable that a corresponding incidence of secondary liver damage occurs in association with rib fractures

Table 4–1   MORTALITY OF PELVIC FRACTURES

	Classes I and II	Class III
Trunkey et al.	14% (89 patients)	4.4% (89 patients)
Conolly et al.	26% (109 patients)	2.2% (91 patients)
Flint et al. (later group)	21% (28 patients)	–
Rothenberger	16.5% (242 patients)	7.2% (347 patients)

on the right side of the abdomen. It is our contention (see Chapter 7) that many minor liver injuries are not recognized clinically and have no significance, whereas for all practical purposes, there is never a minor splenic injury. Therefore, the incidence of major splenic injury associated with left rib fractures appears to correspond or to be actually higher in incidence than corresponding right rib fractures associated with injuries to the liver. The greater mass of the liver, however, more than compensates for its decreased vulnerability to injury so that the incidence of clinically significant injury appears similar.

The significance of pelvic injury relates to associated extensive soft tissue injury and the possibility of injury to urethra and bladder, and more rarely, the rectum. The pelvis is most often fractured by direct compression. The exception is the compound fracture of the pelvis in which there is a perineal tear in association with an unstable fracture of the pelvis. This results from a shearing force in which the leg is literally partially torn from the body (Figure 4-1). This type of injury is an abduction type of injury most commonly associated with motorcycle accidents. Mortality from this injury exceeds 50 percent because of problems of hemorrhage and extensive soft tissue damage and predisposition to secondary infection.

ANATOMY

The anatomy of the lower six ribs and overlying musculature is not particularly complex and does not require definition in this text except to indicate that posteriorly the right kidney overlies the tenth, eleventh, and twelth ribs. On the left side, the left kidney lies over the ninth, tenth, eleventh, and twelth ribs. The spleen centers on the posteior axillary line with the normal spleen overlying the ninth and tenth ribs. The liver can be found under any of the ribs, 6 through 11, depending upon the respiratory cycle.

The abdominal wall, over approximately 40 percent of its surface, consists of three muscle groups; the transversus abdominis, internal oblique, and external oblique. The muscular aponeurosis of these muscles surround the anterior longitudinally placed rectus muscle, the external oblique always passing in front, the internal oblique dividing and passing both back and front in the upper two-thirds of the abdomen and completely in front of the rectus muscle in the lower one-third of the abdomen, the lower edge of this being the semicircular line. The transversus abdominis and its inserting fascia passes posterior to the rectus muscle throughout its extent. The direction of the external oblique musculature parallels the inguinal ligament, and the internal oblique in the upper two-thirds of the abdomen passes obliquely in the opposite direction, paralleling the costal margin at the level of the iliac crest. However, the internal oblique passes transversely and, below the iliac crest, passes obliquely downward as its fibers insert with those of the transversus abdominis on the pubic tubercle. The transversus abdominis, as its name indicates, takes origin from the lumbosacral fascia with the other two muscles and passes transversely across the abdomen over most of its extent, although below the anterior superior spine of the ilium its fibers curve downward to insert on the pubic tubercle with those of the internal oblique as the conjoined tendon. An areolar plane separates these three muscles and the preperitoneal fat, and in the lower abdomen, the transversalis fascia separates the transversus abdominis from the underlying peritoneum.

The rectus muscle passes downward from its origin on the costal cartilages of the lower anterior ribs and sternum and inserts on the symphysis pubis and the pubic tubercle. It is composed of multiple segments corresponding to the vertebrae. These segments in the upper abdomen are marked by fibrous bands, "inscriptions," which are adherent to the anterior fascia but are free posteriorly so there is an areolar plane deep to the muscle and anterior to the deep fascia through which blood can dissect. The only major vessels of the abdominal wall, the superior and inferior epigastric arteries, run through the posterior aspect of the rectus muscle. The superior epigastric artery is a continuation of the internal mammary artery above, which becomes the former as the vessel passes through the mammary foramen of the diaphragm. It enters the center of the body of the rectus muscle and passes downward to meet the inferior epigastric artery coming up from below. The inferior epigastric artery takes origin from the external iliac artery at the inguinal ligament, curves upward in a plane between the peritoneum and transversalis fascia in the preperitoneal fat, on an oblique course toward the umbilicus joining the rectus muscle to anastomose with the superior epigastric artery. The rectus muscles are in close proximity in the lower abdomen, the separation between the right and left rectus muscle is often difficult for the surgeon to find below the umbilicus. Above the umbilicus, the rectus muscles progressively diverge from one another and at the level of xiphoid are normally separated by a distance of approximately 1 cm by a facial line, the linea alba. The linea alba is composed of anterior and posterior fascial layers which encircle the rectus muscle and join in the midline as an avascular fascial layer. The umbilicus constitutes a full thickness scar involving the peritoneum, fascia, and overlying skin. This contains the remnant of the obliterated umbilical vein which passes upwards under the linea alba in a fold of peritoneum as the ligamentus teres. Along the lateral margin of the rectus muscle is the semilunar line, an avascular area which is composed of the interweaving fascia of the more lateral flat muscles as they converge to surround the rectal muscle.

Posterior to the posterior axillary line, the lumbodorsal fascia, the fascia of the insertion of the anterior flat muscles of the abdomen covers the quadratus lumborum muscle which runs between the twelfth rib above and the iliac crest below. The latissimus dorsi muscle takes origin from the iliac crest and the sacral fascia and passes obliquely upward along the back, its anterior edge forming the posterior axillary line. The thick extensor muscles of the back fill in te gutter between the spinous process of vertebrae and its transverse processes of the angles of the ribs.

The innervation of the abdominal wall muscles is by the segmental intercostal nerves 8 through 12 (Figure 4-2). The tenth intercostal nerve passes through the corresponding thoracic vertebral foramen and circles the abdomen in nearly a transverse direction supplying the musculature opposite the umbilicus and the sensory nerves to the overlying skin. The ninth nerve lies just above the parallels and the tenth nerve in its course and, anterior to the anterior axillary line, curves obliquely upward to reach the rectus muscle. The eight thoracic nerve innervates the abdomen below the costal margin and therefore, anterior to the anterior axillary line, passes obliquely upward paralleling the costal margin to reach the rectus muscle. The course of T-11 is obliquely downward to innervate the lower abdomen and rectus muscle. T-12 innervates the suprainguinal and suprapubic region of the lower abdomen before ending in the rectus muscle. When lateral incisions are made in the abdominal wall, the course of these nerves should be recognized and optimal location of incisions should be parallel to the direction of the abdominal wall nerves.

The parietal peritoneum underlies the muscles and fascia of the abdominal wall,

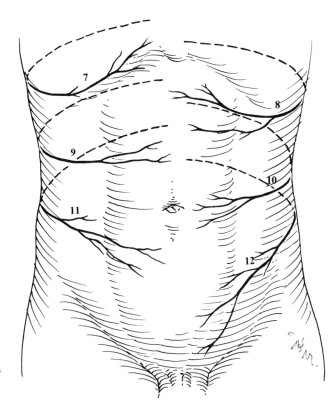

Figure 4–2 Anatomy of the nerves of the abdominal wall.

separated from them by a variable degree of preperitoneal fat. The peritoneum underlying the abdominal wall is richly innervated by somatic nerves, whereas that lining the pelvis and that surrounding the viscera has little or no innervation. That covering the peripheral portion of the diaphragm is innervated by the local intercostal nerves, whereas the peritoneum overlying the central tendon of the diaphragm is innervated from C5. Pain in the instance of central tendon irritation is referred to the shoulder (Kehr's sign). A midline longitudinal abdominal wall incision that permits entry and exposure of all corners of the abdomen is the standard incision used for exploratory laparotomy in the trauma cases. This has the advantage of avoiding all critical anatomy, both blood vessels and nerves. The abdominal cavity can generally be likened to a barrel and the incision of the linea alba corresponds to the removal of a stave of a barrel permitting access to all segments of the interior. A transverse incision, unless very generous, limits exposure to upper or lower portion of the abdomen depending upon its location. A midline incision is rapid and quick to make, a transverse incision requires longer. However, transverse incisions have a major advantage over longitudinal incisions as the stresses on the abdominal wall are such that they tend to close transverse incisions and disrupt longitudinal incisions (Figure 4-3). The rectus abdominal muscle is the one longitudinal muscle in the abdominal wall, but its effective force is negligible compared to the lateral flat muscles. The vector of forces of these muscles which pass obliquely upward, obliquely downward, and transverse is in a transverse direction. Therefore, a transverse wound which is left open will tend to close as abdominal muscles tense, whereas a longitudinal wound will tend to gape. This is a consideration primarily when incisions are planned to drain or explore infected or heavily contaminated

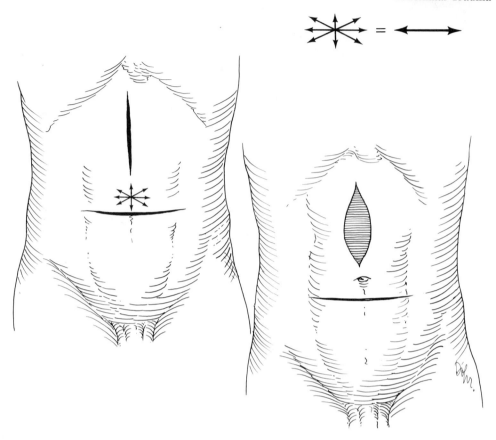

Figure 4–3 *A,* Vectors of forces acting upon wounds of the abdominal wall. *B,* The effective force of these vectors is in a transverse direction tending to result in gaping at longitudinal wounds while closing transverse wounds.

areas. Under these circumstances, when there is a possibility of secondary wound disruption, transverse rather than longitudinal incisions may be optimal.

The pelvis constitutes the bony box which protects the lower abdomen. As a result of this protection, the underlying peritoneum requires minimal innervation compared to the parietal peritoneum of the upper abdomen. Characteristically, a patient with pelvic irritation is unable to localize the source of irritation and may feel little, if any discomfort with trauma of the pelvic peritoneum. The bony ring of the pelvis is composed of the sacrum posteriorly, a large wing or ilium posteriolaterally, the pubis anteriorly, and the ischium inferiorly, the three bones joining in the acetabulum. The superior and inferior ramus of the pubis pass around the obturator foramen and join at the symphysis pubis. Injuries anterior to the acetabulum that disrupt the bony ring are stable fractures since the weight is transmitted through the acetabulum to the sacrum and vertebral column and if this and the posterior structures are intact and the sacroiliac joint stable, the patient can bear weight without compromise of healing and with minimal discomfort. Fractures involving the acetabulum and posterior elements including the sacroiliac joint are unstable and must be treated in non-weight bearing fashion until a bony union or integrity of ligamentous structures has developed. Blows to the anterior abdominal wall may result in fractures of the superior or inferior ramus of the pubis or the symphysis and, as indicated previously, may be associated with injury to the underlying bladder or urethra. The mass of soft tissue overlying the anterior components of the pelvis is minimal, therefore, these injuries generally have a good prognosis and have a relatively low incidence of secondary complications, once bladder and urethral injury have been ruled out.

In contrast, the posterior elements of the pelvis are strong stable structures and violent trauma is required to produce disruption. Therefore, when posterior elements of the pelvis are injured, the associated soft tissue injury is often considerable. Moreover, major blood vessels, the common iliac arteries, overlie the sacroiliac joint; the internal iliac arteries, and veins spread fan-wise over the pelvis to supply adjacent abdominal organs. These may be disrupted by posterior element injuries that produce major bleeding and pelvic hematomas (see Chapter 14 on retroperitoneal hematoma). The rectum occupies the hollow of the pelvis and the perineum and levator sling closes the pelvic outlet. Injuries which tend to avulse or abduct the thigh violently may produce tear of the rectum and/or muscles and ligaments of the pelvic outlet; this is almost inevitably associated with perineal laceration. The presence of a perineal laceration in association with pelvic fracture indicates that this serious avulsion-type compound fracture is present.

ASSESSMENT

The assessment of injuries to the lower six ribs is relatively easy. An excellent screening maneuver is to ask the patient to take a deep breath and cough. The ability to do both of these without discomfort indicates that there has been no compromise in the integrity of the lower six ribs, since fractures of the ribs are almost inevitably associated with pleural injury and severe pain with ventilation. In an uncooperative patient, compression of the lower rib cage can be utilized. If acute discomfort is elicited, rib fracture is likely, whereas minimal discomfort usually rules out the possibility of significant chest wall injury. If chest wall injury is documented by the above maneuvers then the individual ribs can be palpated and the extent of the injuries noted. X-ray is frequently misleading and underdiagnoses the severity of chest wall injury, since many rib fractures cannot be seen and separation of costal cartilages cannot be diagnosed on any film.

Trauma to the abdominal wall is often evident on inspection. There may be abrasions, ecchymosis, or splinting as the patient breathes. In the normally nourished patient, a rectus hematoma is often evident as a mass which usually increases in prominence as the patient tenses his abdominal wall. Lacerations of the thorax or abdominal wall are evident on inspection also. Palpation of the abdomen following blunt injury is generally associated with tenderness and the patient unable to splint or tighten the muscles without aggravating the discomfort. Ultrasound has proven recently to be capable of assisting in the diagnosis of the injury.[27] Since injuries sufficient to produce abdominal wall injury most often are associated with underlying injury, it may be both difficult and unnecessary to differentiate injury of the overlying abdominal wall from that in the abdomen. Signs of peritoneal irritation should always be interpreted as irritation coming from within the abdominal cavity since, statistically, this is overwhelmingly the most likely probability. The probing of penetrating wounds is of little value unless the probing results in the dropping of the instrument into the abdominal cavity, since the abdominal wall muscles change with the position of the patient. Therefore, the probing object may not reveal the true depth of the injury because deeper muscle layers of the abdominal wall may change an inch or more in relationship to the injury to the outermost muscle layer. Therefore, once a penetrating wound has passed through fascia, penetration of the full thickness of the abdominal wall must be assumed.

Occasionally, contusion of the lateral portion of the abdominal wall may be associated with relatively large hematomas. However, this is unusual because of the lack of large blood vessels in most of the abdominal wall. As indicated previously, the exception is the rectus muscle which contains the epigastric vessels. Because of the presence of inscriptions which prevent the hematoma's spreading longitudinally within the substance of the muscle, the rectus hematoma may appear as a specific mass. In patients with thick subcutaneous layers, this may be difficult to differentiate from an abdominal mass. If tenderness and peritoneal irritation exist, abdominal exploration may well be indicated to rule out intraperitoneal injury as this, in the last analysis, is the only way to differentiate between abdominal wall injury and intraperitoneal injury, particularly when peritoneal irritation exists.

Avulsion injuries inevitably are associated with irregular lacerations which usually extend down to fascia. Usually there is considerable ecchymosis. Exploration of the laceration will reveal extensive undermining of the skin and subcutaneous tissue.

Examination of the pelvis is initiated by leaning on the iliac crest. If this can be done without eliciting discomfort, injury to the posterior elements of the pelvis are unlikely. Movement of the hips without eliciting discomfort tends to rule out acetabular injury. If compression over the symphysis pubis elicits no tenderness, then significant injuries to the pelvis are generally ruled out. The elicitation of tenderness on any of the preceding maneuvers requires pelvic x-rays for definitive evaluation. This, of course, should be done as well whenever there is evidence of injury to the lower abdomen, back, or hips. Separation of the symphysis pubis and widening of the sacroiliac joint are subtle manifestations that may require radiologic interpretation but most fractures and pelvic separations are obvious even to the radiologic neophyte (Figure 4-4).

We have utilized the following classification of pelvic injuries to assist us with prognosis (Table 4-2). Class I injuries are comminuted, unstable fractures of the pelvic ring in which there has been injury to three or more structures of the pelvic ring (Figure 4-5).

Class II injuries are unstable fractures which are often referred to as diametric fractures, as originally described by Malgaigne in 1847. A diametric fracture is any fracture in which the fractures extend through the pubic rami or pubic symphysis anteriorly and through either the sacrum, sacroiliac joint, or ilium posteriorly so that there is potential or actual cranial displacement of the hemipelvis (Figure 4-6). Class II-a is the diametric fracture with displacement. Class II-b is a diametric fracture without displacement. Class II-c is the "open book" or sprung pelvis, in which, because of anterior disruption, the pelvis is open like a book hinging on intact posterior structures, but necessarily with some disruption of these. The classic injury is separation of the pubic symphysis accompanied by separation of the sacroiliac joint. The "open book" injury can also occur with pubic rami fractures and sacroiliac joint separation. When pelvic fractures are associated with a perineal or other overlying laceration, a compound fracture of the pelvis is present. This is most commonly associated with Class II-c injuries.

Because of the instability of these Class II fractures, persistent hemorrhage is

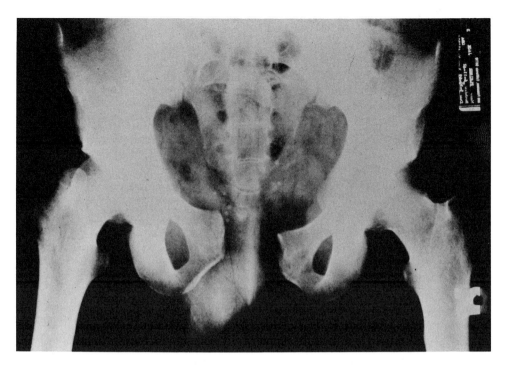

Figure 4–4 "Open book" pelvic fracture due to separation of the pubic symphisis and fracture at the superior and interior left pubic rami.

Table 4–2   CLASSIFICATION OF PELVIC FRACTURES

I.	Comminuted (crush) injuries:
	A. Three or more major components involved (rami, ilium, acetabulum, sacrum)
	B. Often unstable
	C. Usually are combinations of II—A, B, C, D
II.	Unstable (Require immobilization or traction to reduce hemorrhage or maintain position of weight bearing portions of pelvis)
	A. Diametric fractures with cranial displacement of hemiplevis (Froman and Stein, 1967; Malgaigne, 1847)
	B. Diametric fractures, undisplaced
	C. Open-book (sprung) pelvis
	D. Acetabular fractures
III.	Stable (immobilization usually unnecessary except for symptomatic relief)
	A. Isolated fractures
	B. Fractures of the pubic rami

often a problem. To reduce hemorrhage, these fractures usually require a pelvic sling or external fixation or other reduction to hold it stable. Class II-d fractures are fractures of the acetabulum that can be either displaced or undisplaced. The displaced fractures usually are accompanied by a simple dislocation of the femoral head.[6] Posterior dislocation of the femoral head with fracture of the acetabulum is also included. These fractures usually require longitudinal and horizontal traction in order to reduce the fracture and to maintain adequate position of the acetabular fragments.

Class III fractures are stable fractures that can be divided into two types: the isolated fractures (type a) and fractures of the pubic rami (type b) (Figure 4-7). An example of an isolated fracture is an avulsion fracture of the iliac wing. With the exception of the comminuted fractures of the iliac wing, these usually present no problem from the standpoint of either hemorrhage or the need for immobilization.

PRE-OPERATIVE PREPARATION AND INDICATIONS FOR OPERATION

Operation is not necessarily required for blunt in juries of the abdominal wall unless underlying injury is suspected, unless there is a major devitalizing injury, or unless an extremely large hematoma such as a rectus hematoma exists. Blood loss associated with injuries to the pelvis can be from one or two units all the way to loss of the blood volume several times over, so these injuries should not be taken lightly. [1,7,21] Rothenberger, for example, found that of patients with pelvic fractures admitted in shock, 63 percent had major associated vascular injury.[21]

Pelvic fractures themselves do not require operation; the association of underlying injury is relatively frequent and this will dictate the need for surgical treatment. Peritoneal lavage can be used in assessing pelvic injury, but is often positive in the absence of significant injury, since retroperitoneal hematoma is often associated with extravasation of small amounts of blood that will render the lavage positive. [11] If bladder and urethra are intact and the injury is not compound, operation is not necessarily indicated. When the pelvic injury is unstable, and bleeding is continuous, some form of stabilization of the injury with external fixation is indicated and will usually result in control of hemorrhage. (Definitive treatment of bleeding is described in the chapter on retroperitoneal hematoma.) When transportation of major pelvic injuries is required, the mast suit has been utilized. [2] This tends to stabilize unstable fractures and the counter pressure of the suit may slow venous bleeding.[2,8]

Type III-c compound fractures of the pelvis will require operation for control of bleeding.[20] This can be attempted by local exploration of the perineal laceration and inevitably will require an associated colostomy; this to prevent contamination of the laceration and the pelvic hematoma, even if the rectum is intact. Persistent, ongoing bleeding associated with pelvic fractures is an indication for some type of

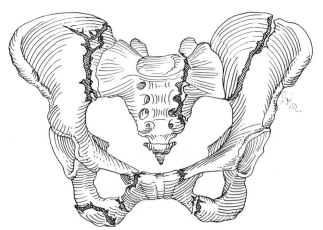

Figure 4–5 Class I injuries—comminuted, unstable fractures.

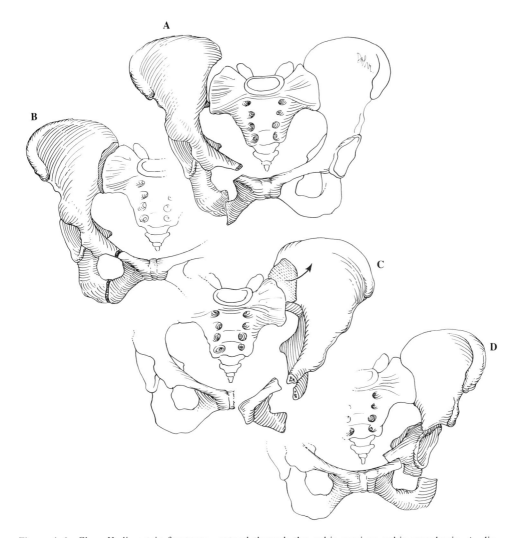

Figure 4–6 Class II diametric fractures—extend through the pubic rami or pubic symphysis. *A*, displacement; *B*, undisplaced; *C*, open hook; *D*, acetabular.

vascular control. The alternatives available are arteriographic embolism and exploratory laparotomy. The absolute indication for angiographic localization and definitive treatment of the bleeding point is blood loss that is persistent and exceeds 6 units. If the bleeding point can be localized by angiography, embolization is the treatment of choice. If not, a direct surgical approach with internal iliac artery ligation or definitive clamping of the bleeding point is indicated (see Chapter 14).[7,8,9,14,15,16,18,19,22,23,25,26]

Preparation of the patient for surgical treatment of the abdominal wall or pelvic injury involves assessment of blood volume loss with appropriate replacement. Sufficient crystalloid should be administered to maintain a brisk urine output and blood should be administered only if the heatocrit falls below 30. Since associated injuries

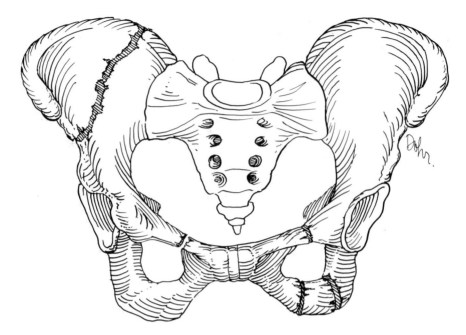

Figure 4–7. Class III fractures—two types of stable fratures.

are frequent, a complete careful examination of the patient is indicated. The presence of blood in the urine requires urinary tract evaluation and urethrograms and cystograms performed as described in Chapter 11.

Abdominal wall trauma may require surgery to rule out intra-abdominal injury, to drain large hematomas, or to repair gross disruption. A stab wound that is in the anterior abdominal wall and is one cm or more in transverse diameter, if anterior to the anterior axillary line, should have the fascial and peritoneal defect closed, if only to prevent subsequent evisceration or hernia. Penetrating injuries always carry the possibility of hollow viscus injury and should be treated with preoperative antibiotics. Avulsion injuries are usually followed by skin necrosis and infection of the elevated flap. If trauma to the subcutaneous tissue is extensive, removal of devitalized fat from the skin flap is often indicated with the skin reapplied to the abdominal wall as a full thickness graft. Shotgun and high velocity tangential injuries of the abdominal wall require debridement of all dead and devitalized tissue. [24]

DEFINITIVE TREATMENT

Multiple rib fractures do not, as a rule, require operative treatment; however, if a flail segment is present that results in compromised ventilation, the early institution of endotracheal intubation and mechanical ventilation will permit pain relief, since pain medication can be administered without fear of compromise of ventilation and adequacy of ventilation can be ensured. Injection of isolated rib fractures with a long-acting local anesthetic may provide considerable symptomatic relief and per-

Table 4–3 INDICATIONS FOR CONTINUOUS MECHANICAL VENTILATION

I. Ventilatory (mechanical) failure
    A. Respirations $\geq$ 35 to 40/min
    B. Inadequate alveolar ventilation with $PaCO_2 \geq 48$ torr
    C. Vital capacity $\leq$ 10 to 15 ml/kg body weight
    D. Maximal inspiratory force $\leq$ − 25 cm H_2O
II. Pulmonary (parenchymal) failure
    A. Alveolar-arterial oxygen gradient $(A - aDO_2)$ $\geq$ 300 torr
       ($FiO_2 = 1$)
    B. Right to left shunt fraction (Q_s/Q_t) $\geq$ 15 to 20 percent
    C. Wasted ventilation (V_d/V_t) $\geq$ 0.6
    D. Compliance less than 30 ml/cm H_2O

mit the patient to cough, deep breathe, and clear secretions. Operative treatment of rib fractures is indicated only when there are severe compound injuries, major flail segments, or underlying intra thoracic injury.

Penetrating abdominal wall injuries such as stab wounds of one cm or larger are best treated by laparotomy with closure of peritoneum and fascia from inside the abdomen, despite the absence of intraperitoneal injury. Even though the external fascial defect is closed, it is possible for a knuckle of bowel to herniate into the deeper layer of the abdominal wall.

Abdominal wall hematomas rarely require operation, although a large rectus hematoma may be treated operatively with resultant less morbidity overall than conservative management. This permits ligation of the injured epigastric artery and evacuation of the hematoma. If exploratory laparotomy is indicated, either the stand-ard midline incision is utilized and the rectus sheath opened, or the hematoma decompressed using paramedian incision which provides direct access to the injured muscle.

Shotgun injuries and other high velocity injuries which produce devitalization of the abdominal wall should be explored and all overtly necrotic tissue debrided.[24] If this involves full thickness of the abdominal wall, some type of plastic procedure or prosthesis may be appropriate to prevent evisceration of abdominal contents. It may be possible to mobilize skin flaps to close a fascial defect. Marlex mesh can be sutured circumferentially to viable fascia and later covered with split thick skin grafts. In desperate circumstances, particularly when there are associated injuries, the abdominal wound can be packed with antibiotic dressings containing organic iodide and evisceration prevented with an abdominal binder.

Avulsion type injuries should be explored and the degree of undermining de-termined. If the flaps raised exceed a hand's breadth, the flap is best elevated, defatted, and all underlying devitalized tissue removed.[12] The skin can then be put back as a full thickness graft, the wound allowed to develop vascularity and then covered with split thick skin grafts.

Unstable pelvic fractures, dislocation of the hip with acetabular fragmentation or sacroiliac migration may require the insertion of a Steinmann pin in the distal femur for traction or operative reduction and fixation with external fixation devices. Pelvic bleeding will be described under the section on pelvic hematoma.

Compound pelvic injuries are essentially degloving type injuries in which skeletal muscle is literally stripped from the pelvis. As a result, there is usually severe external hemorrhage. This requires pelvic stabilization and sigmoid diverting colos-tomy. Vigorous pelvic bleeding can be treated by ligation of the bleeding point, if it can be seen through the perineal wound, or by packing, if the pack controls the bleeding. If these techniques are not successful, arteriographic embolization or internal iliac artery ligation can be done, preferably after identifying the bleeding point by arteriography. This will depend a great deal on the magnitude of the hematoma present in the pelvis at the time a diverting colostomy is carried out. It is usually advisable not to enter the hematoma since, while arterial bleeding usually can be controlled with ligation of the internal iliac artery, venous bleeding is decompressed thereby and is very difficult to control once the retroperitoneum has been opened. This is because bleeding occurs from both proximal and distal segments and multiple disruptions of great veins are common. Venous injury in the pelvis cannot be devascularized by arterial ligation despite misconceptions to the contrary (see Chapter 14).

When a colostomy is indicated for associated rectal injury or in the instance in which a compound pelvic fracture alone is present, colostomy can be carried out using a small midline laparotomy incision, if no intraperitoneal hemorrhage is encountered and no abdominal injury was suspected prior to laparotomy. A sigmoid loop can be mobilized into the lower abdominal wound, divided proximally and brought out the middle of the left lower quadrant as an end sigmoid colostomy. The colostomy opening can either be matured after the laparotomy incision is closed by suturing the bowel mucosa to skin or be brought out so that there is no tension. In this latter instance, the colostomy clamp is left in place and petroleum jelly gauze placed about the colostomy stoma. In both instances, fixation of the mesentery of the bowel to the peritoneum and fascia is helpful, so that should there be any tension on the colostomy with the development of a subsequent ileus, the bowel will not retract back into the abdominal cavity. The distal end of the bowel is brought out through the lower portion of the incision as a mucous fistula or through a separate stab wound in the abdominal wall, well away from the end colostomy, so as to permit the application of a colostomy appliance. A large bore rectal tube can be inserted below, and the mucous fistula irrigated above, with the patient in the lithotomy position so that through-and-through irrigation of the rectal segment can be carried out. When the irrigation is clear, one gram of Neomycin and 500 mg of Erythromycin base should be left in the segment. The perineal laceration should be irrigated vigorously with sterile saline followed by antibiotic irrigation.

POSTOPERATIVE CARE

Penetrating injuries to the abdominal wall should be treated with preoperative antibiotics continuing for 24 hours in the postoperative period if there has been injury to an underlying hollow viscus. In most instances, the absence of hollow viscus injury is associated with a lower risk of infection than the risk of antibiotics themselves, so that these should be discontinued in the immediate postoperative period if no contamination is present in the abdomen. Blunt trauma, with the exception of compound pelvic fracture, does not require antibiotics postoperatively.

The patient with chest wall injuries should be mobilized early. Painful ventilation can be managed with careful titration of small doses of narcotic and with supplementation of intercostal rib block as necessary.

Abdominal wall injuries rarely constitute a postoperative problem, the patient should be mobilized promptly and can usually be discharged within a day or two if the injury is limited to this area. Devitalizing injuries, such as avulsion injuries, or wounds, such as those associated with tangential shotgun damage, may of course, need extensive time to heal and may require skin grafting.

The primary postoperative or post-injury problems come with management of the pelvic fracture. The unstable fractures and the compound fractures require intensive care unit monitoring, not only because of the possibility of continued blood loss but also because of complications, including the respiratory distress syndrome.[4] Prophylaxis of this last involves careful titration of vascular volume, so as to maintain a good urine output in excess of 0.5 cc/kg/hr, and the introduction of mechanical ventilation if progressive deterioration in pulmonary function is evident. The criteria for mechanical ventilation are shown in Table 4-3. In stable pelvic fractures, the patient can be mobilized as rapidly as other injuries permit and he will usually require several days of bedrest for the acute discomfort. Compound and unstable fractures require two to four weeks of bedrest, with or without traction, until there is evidence of stabilization of the injury on stress testing. A colostomy should not be closed until healing of the perineal laceration is complete or nearly complete, the pelvic injury is stable, and the patient has returned to normal activity. This process usually requires six weeks to three months.

COMPLICATIONS

The complications associated with rib fractures can be respiratory complications or bleeding. These can be manifest acutely with pneumothorax. If not present initially, pneumothorax can complicate the patient's course at any time, particularly when mechanical ventilation is instituted for anesthesia or for postoperative management. This should be considered whenever there is sudden unexplained deterioration of the patient. For this reason, chest tubes are used liberally when chest wall injury is present.

Table 4-4   COMPLICATIONS

	No. of Patients
Pulmonary (Total 53)	
Respiratory distress syndrome	22
Pneumonia	20
Pulmonary emboli	8
Severe atelectasis	3
Urinary tract infection	18
Sepsis	5
Congestive heart failure	4
Hemo-pneumo thorax	3
Delirium tremens	4
Wound infections	3
Complications directly related to pelvic fracture	
Pelvic abscess	1
Perirectal abscess	1
Flaccid bladder	2
Sciatic nerve palsy	1
Meningitis	1
Spontaneous abortion	2
All other complications	15

Hemothorax, which results in significant obliteration of the sulcus in the upright chest x-ray or partial opacification of the chest in the supine position, should be treated also by the placement of a chest tube for evacuation and monitoring of intrapleural bleeding.

Atelectasis should be prevented or treated by encouraging the patient to deep breathe and cough. Should major pulmonary collapse occur, this should be treated with tracheobronchial aspiration or bronchoscopy as necessary to remove mucous plugs. The ability of the patient to deep breathe and cough may be facilitated by appropriate application of intercostal nerve block and/or titration with small doses of narcotic.

Pelvic fractures are complicated by respiratory failure, infection, and thromboembolic problems (Table 4-4). The fat embolism syndrome or the respiratory distress syndrome (RDS) of shock and trauma follows major fractures, including those of the pelvis.[26] Demonstration of fat in urine and sputum after trauma does not, in itself, correlate with the development of RDS; this requires a combination of, and is directly proportional to, the degree of shock and soft tissue injury. Failure to promptly treat one or both of these problems results in a marked increase in the incidence and virulence of this syndrome. In patients with major injuries who require surgery, the endotracheal tube is best left in place 24 hours as pulmonary function is monitored. At the end of this time, if there is no evidence of deterioration of pulmonary function and the chest film remains clear, extubation can be carried out. Conversely, in the presence of progressive pulmonary infiltrates, or the persistent requirement of 40 percent oxygen or more to maintain normal blood gases in the first 24 hours postinjury, mechanical ventilation should be continued. The addition of positive end expiratory pressure (PEEP) prevents the progressive closure of lung units, increases Functional Residual Capacity and has resulted in a marked decrease in mortality from the progressive pulmonary failure which characterizes the post-traumatic respiratory distress syndrome.

Infection can complicate any penetrating wound. Generally, clean wounds have a low incidence of infection and can be closed; dirty wounds should be left open and allowed to drain. Infection rarely complicates closed pelvic fractures whereas the compound pelvic fracture is associated with a 50 to 70 percent incidence of virulent pelvic infection. This is because it is a contaminated wound in proximity to an extensive hematoma which dissects internally and externally around the fracture sites. If the infection is associated with spiking fevers and systemic toxicity, surgical intervention may be required, with exploration of the perineum and pelvic wound under general anesthesia. This is to establish drainage of all loculations and pockets and to localize and drain intrapelvic collections.

Thromboembolic complications are not complications associated with abdominal wall injury, but they are associated with major soft tissue injuries and major thoracic injuries and, unfortunately, often complicate pelvic fractures.[26]

In the previously healthy patient, pulmonary embolism rarely occurs before the fifth to seventh postoperative day. A sudden change in vital signs without explanation; particularly cardiac arrhythmias, the onset of respiratory distress, agitation, or apprehension should be considered to be due to pulmonary embolism until proven otherwise. A fall in arterial blood gases is a frequently associated manifestation of major pulmonary embolism but embolism can occur in the absence of arterial blood gas changes and in these instances, would be manifested by cardiac arrhythmias, apparent right-sided failure, and evidence of acute cor pulmonale. Treatment, unless a contraindication exists, consists of a large bolus of anticoagulant-20,000 units of heparin in the average adult, followed by 2,000 to 4,000 units of heparin per hour. Tests of clotting such as the activated clotting time (A.C.T.) or the activated partial thromboplastin time (A.P.T.T.), should be taken several times a day to make sure that there is anticoagulant effect. We have found that arbitrarily high doses of heparin are more effective than simple titration to a given level of A.C.T. or A.P.T.T. This consists of a bolus injection of 300 u/kg followed by 50 u/kg/hr by continuous intravenous infusion. The patient usually improves dramatically on this regimen and after 24 to 48 hours, the doses of heparin can be cut to conventional levels such as 20 to 30u/kg per hour by continuous pump infusion or controlled by the A.C.T. or the A.P.T.T. To avoid severe bleeding complications, the hematocrit should be monitored at least twice daily, along with platelets, and the patient treated in an intensive care unit setting.

REFERENCES

1. Allen RE, Eastman BA, Halter BL, Conolly WR: Retroperitoneal hemorrhage secondary to blunt trauma. Am J Surg 118:558, 1969.
2. Batalden DJ, Wickstrom PH, Ruiz G, et al: Value of the G Suit in patients with severe pelvic fracture. Arch Surg 109:326, 1974.
3. Bryan WJ, Tulles H: Pediatric pelvic fractures: Review of 52 patients. J Trauma 19:799, 1979.
4. Conolly WB, Hedberg EA: Observations on fractures of the pelvis. J Trauma 9:104, 1969
5. Cullen TS, Bordel M: Lesions of the rectus abdominis muscle: Simulating acute intra-abdomial conditions. Bull Johns Hopkins Hosp 61:295, 1937.
6. Bunn AW, Russo CL: Central acetabular fractures. J Trauma 13:695, 1973.
7. Fleming WH, Bowen JC: Control of hemorrhage in pelvic crush injuries. J Trauma 13:567, 1973.
8. Flint LM, Brown A, Richardson JD, Polk HC: Definitive control of bleeding from severe pelvic fractures. Ann Surg 189:709, 1979.
9. Hauser CW, Perry JR Jr: Control of massive hemorrhage from pelvic fractures by hypogastric artery ligation. Surg Gynecol Obstet 121:313, 1965.
10. Hawkins L, Pomeranta M, Eiseman B: Laparotomy at the time of pelvic fracture. J Trauma 10:619, 1970.
11. Hubbard SG, Bivins BA, Sachatello CR, Griffen WO: Diagnostic errors with peritoneal lavage in patients with pelvic fractures. Arch Surg 114:844, 1979.
12. Kalisman M, et al: Treatment of extensive avulsions of skin and subcutaneous tissues. J Dermat Surg Oncol 4:322, 1978.
13. Lucas GL: Missle wounds of the bony pelvis. J Trauma 10:624, 1970.
14. Margolies MN, Ring EJ, Waltman AC, Kerr WS, Baum S: Arteriography in the management of hemorrhage from pelvic fractures. NEJM 287:317, 1972.
15. Maull KI, Sachatello CR: Current management of pelvic fractures: a combined surgical angiographic approach to hemorrhage. South Med Journal 69:1285, 1976.
16. Paster SB, Van Houton F, Adams DF: Percutaneous balloon catheterization: A technique for the control of arterial hemorrhage caused by pelvic trauma. JAMA 230:573, 1974.
17. Petersen FR, Sheldon GF: Morbidity of a negative finding at laparotomy in abdominal trauma. Surg Gynecol Obstet 148:23, 1979.
18. Ravitch MM: Hypogastric artery ligation in acute pelvic trauma. Surg 56:601, 1964.
19. Ring FJ, Athanasculis C, Waltman AC, et al: Arteriographic management of hemorrhage following pelvic fracture. Radiology 109:65, 1973.
20. Rothenberger DA, Fischer RP, Strate RG, Velasco R, Perry JF: The mortality associated with pelvic fractures. Surg 84:356, 1978.
21. Rothenberger DA, Fischer RP, Perry JF: Major vascular injuries secondary to pelvic fractures. Am J Surg 136:660, 1978.
22. Seavers R, Lynch J, Ballard R, et al: Hypogastric artery ligation for uncontrollable hemorrhage in acute pelvic trauma. Surg 55:516, 1964.
23. Sheldon GF, Winestock DP: Hemorrhage from open pelvic fracture controlled intra-operatively with balloon catheter. J Trauma 18:68, 1978.
24. Sherman RT, Parrish RA: Management of shotgun injuries. J Trauma, 3:76, 1963.
25. Smith K, Ben-Menachem Y, Duke JH, Hill GL: The superior gluteal artery: an artery at risk in blunt pelvic trauma. J Trauma 16:273, 1976.
26. Trunkey DD, Chapman MW, Lim RC, Dunphy JE: Management of pelvic fractures in blunt trauma injury. J Trauma 14:912, 1974.

Chapter Five

GASTRIC, ESOPHAGEAL, DIAPHRAGMATIC AND OMENTAL INJURY

RICHARD A. CRASS

Although Celsus, in the first century, advocated excising devitalized omentum which might herniate through a stab wound, not much progress was made in the management of penetrating wounds of the upper abdomen until the eighteenth century. [5] There is a report by Schenk of a spear wound to the abdomen in a Bohemian hunting accident in the late sixteenth cenury that resulted in a gastric fistula with survival of the victim.[15] Two centuries later, a shotgun wound to Alexis St. Martin produced a similar outcome and was to provide Beaumont with a means of making his pioneering observations on gastric physiology. Nolleson in 1767 reported a saber wound to a Palatine soldier named Rumpf that pierced the stomach and was sutured, after which procedure the patient survived.[14] Although some enthusiasm existed for laparotomy for penetrating abdominal injuries during the nineteenth century, the frequently fatal outcome resulted in generally conservative management of penetrating abdominal injuries up to the First World War. Prompt exploration, improved technique, and superior postoperative care reduced the mortality rate from isolated gastric injuries from 29 percent during World War I to essentially zero percent during World War II.[12]

The sheltered location of the intra-abdominal esophagus and diaphragm and the pliability of the stomach and omentum make penetrating injury to these organs more common than blunt injury. The major problem with injuries to this group of structures is recognition preoperatively (and in the case of diaphragm and esophagus, intra-operatively), while once identified, treatment is usually straightforward.

Gastric injuries are much more commonly due to penetrating than to blunt trauma. A full or distended stomach can, however, be ruptured by blunt trauma. Cardiopulmonary resuscitation, if performed incorrectly, can result not only in gastric distention but in gastric perforation. Gastric necrosis can result from corrosive ingestion, and laparotomy should be undertaken without delay in any patient who develops peritonitis after accidental or intentional ingestion of a corrosive. [1,3,4,6,8,16,18]

The combination of good blood supply, relative sterility of the empty organ, and ease of recognition of injury results in a good prognosis in isolated gastric injuries. This, of course, is not the case if any injury is overlooked.

Diaphragmatic injury should be searched for in all penetrating injuries involving the lower chest or upper abdomen. Rupture of the diaphragm can also result from blunt thoracoabdominal trauma.[13] If overlooked, the injury can result in a hernia with a significant potential for early and late strangulation of viscera.[9,11]

The omentum is most commonly injured by penetrating trauma, but it can be injured with blunt trauma, especially if fixed to a previous laparotomy wound. Bleeding from epiploic vessels is the only consequence of omental injuries.

The incidence of injury to the stomach from penetrating trauma is approximately 19 percent of all intra-abdominal organ injuries, whereas the incidence of injury from blunt trauma is less than 1 percent.[2,10]

The incidence of injury to the abdominal esophagus from blunt or penetrating trauma is miniscule because of the minimum amount of esophagus in the abdominal cavity and because of its protected position. However, when it does occur it is almost always due to penetrating injury, although compression of a full stomach can result in a disruption akin to emetogenic injury (Boerhaave Syndrome).[17]

Diaphragmatic injuries are common following penetrating trauma averaging about 6 percent of all intra-abdominal organ injuries.[2] The incidence is perhaps related to how assiduously the injury is looked for. Blunt injuries, while relatively rare (1 percent of all blunt abdominal injuries), are complications of violent injury and are seen most commonly following high-speed motor vehicle accidents[7,10].

ANATOMY

The abdominal esophagus emerges from the esophageal hiatus, where it is supported by the phrenoesophageal ligament, to course for 2 to 4 cm within the abdominal cavity before joining the stomach. The posterior surface of the intraabdominal esophagus overlies the aorta. Only the anterior surface is covered by the peritoneum. Accompanying the esophagus through the hiatus are the anterior and posterior vagus nerves.

The stomach occupies the left upper quadrant of the abdomen and topographically consists of the cardia, adjacent to the esophageal junction, the fundus, that portion craniad to the esophagastric junction, the pyloric antrum, extending from the angular incisure to the pylorus, and the body. The stomach is suspended from the gastrohepatic ligament above, the gastrocolic ligament below, and the splenic ligament to the left. Aside from these attachments, the stomach is totally invested in peritoneum with the anterior surface facing the general peritoneal cavity and the posterior surface facing the lesser sac. The generous blood supply of the stomach includes the left and right gastric arteries to the lesser curvature and the left and right gastroepiploic and short gastric arteries to the greater curvature. (Figure 5-1) The left gastric artery is a branch of the celiac axis, the right gastric artery arises from the common hepatic artery, the right gastroepiploic from the gastroduodenal artery, and the left gastroepiploic and short gastric arteries from the splenic artery. The venous drainage is through the coronary vein to the portal vein for the lesser

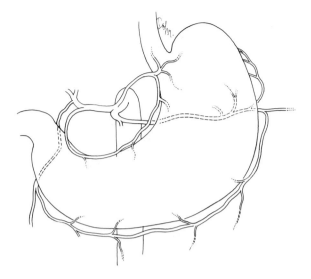

Figure 5–1 Blood supply of the stomach.

curvature and right and left gastroepiploic and short gastric veins for the greater curvature, the last two emptying into the splenic vein (Figure 5-1).

The omentum is a double layer of peritoneum and adipose tissue that takes origin from the greater curvature of the stomach and drapes over and has avascular attachments to the transverse colon. It forms an anterior apron over the contents of the peritoneal cavity and projects as far as the pelvis. The blood supply is from branches of the right and left gastroepiploic arteries.

The diaphragm is a musculotendinous dome-shaped structure which is attached posteriorly to the first, second and third lumbar vertebrae, anteriorly to the lower sternum, and lateral to the costal margins (Figure 5-2). It contains three foramina. The aortic hiatus is located posterior at the level ot T12 and contains the aorta, thoracic duct, and azygous veins. Anterior and slightly to the left is the esophageal hiatus, at the T10 level. To the right of the esophageal hiatus, at the T9 level, is the vena cava foramen. Except for the bare area of the liver, the inferior surface of the diaphragm is covered by peritoneum. The course of the phrenic nerve should be borne in mind during diaphragmatic incisions (i.e., circumferential detachment is more likely to avoid injury than radial incision). The phrenic nerves course through the thorax along the middle of the pericardium on both sides. Soon after reflecting onto the diaphragm, the major phrenic trunk divides into an anterior and a posterior branch.

ASSESSMENT

Intra-abdominal esophageal or gastric injuries rarely present problems in diagnosis. The patient will usually have peritoneal signs due to the release of gastric contents. A plain abdominal film will usually demonstrate free air (Figure 5-3). If there is doubt about the possibility of esophageal injury, especially with penetrating chest injuries, a water-soluble contrast swallow is helpful.

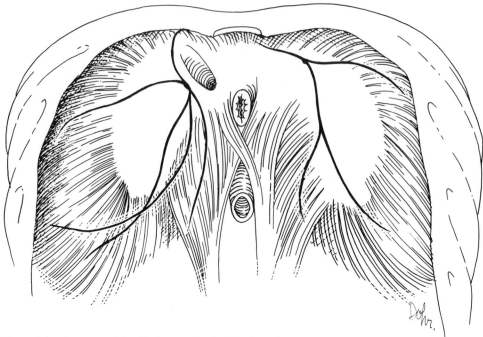

Figure 5–2   Anatomy of the diaphragm showing location of the phrenic nerves.

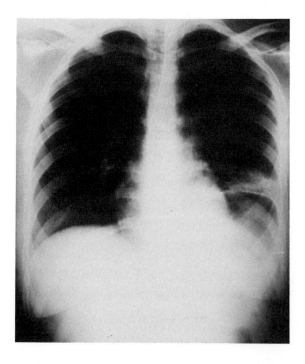

Figure 5–3 Chest x-ray shows the air under the diaphragm.

We generally perform endoscopy upon patients who have ingested corrosives to assess the extent of disease. These patients should then be observed closely for the development of peritonitis or mediastinitis.

Diaphragmatic injuries may be easily appreciated if abdominal viscera are seen on a chest film, or if the nasogastric tube is seen coiled in the left chest (Figure 5-4). Injury is evident if abdominal viscera are palpated or gastrointestinal contents are noted during chest tube placement.

There is nothing specific to implicate an omental injury prior to exploration unless there is obvious evisceration. Signs of intraperitoneal bleeding, as manifested by hypotension or peritoneal irritation may be present if a major epiploic vessel is injured.

Following placement of a chest tube for hemothorax a repeat chest x-ray should be obtained since herniated viscera may be obscured by blood on the initial film. Hemothorax and/or pneumothorax is usually present with diaphragmatic rupture.

Most diaphragmatic injuries, however, are not so easily appreciated—especially if due to penetrating trauma. Adjacent structures are usually sucked into the laceration and may provide a temporary seal. One should be aware of the fact that during expiration, the domes of the diaphragm reach the 5th intercostal space so that a high index of suspicion of diaphragmatic violation is appropriate in penetrating injuries of the lower chest. With the pressure gradient across the diaphragm, the tendency is for small diaphragmatic lacerations to enlarge with time as more and more viscera insinuate into the defect. Therefore, all diaphragmatic injuries, no matter how small, should be searched for at the time of laparotomy and repaired. In massive right diaphragmatic laceration with herniation of the liver, the chest film may look completely normal except for an apparently elevated right diaphragm.

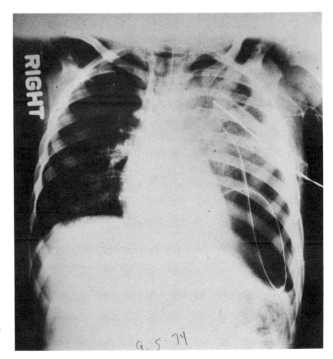

Figure 5–4 The presence of the nasogastric tube in the left pleural space documents the presence of diaphragmatic laceration.

PRE-OPERATIVE PREPARATION

In any patient in whom there is a possibility of esophageal, gastric, or diaphragmatic injury, a nasogastric tube should be inserted to aspirate gastric contents, in order to prevent further contamination of the peritoneal cavity and to provide diagnostic information (e.g., blood in stomach, tube above the diaphragm). Intravenous fluids should be administered in quantities sufficient for resuscitation and broad spectrum antibiotics should be given prior to exploration.

When diaphragmatic injury is suspected or when esophageal injury contaminates the pleural space, a chest tube should be placed in the appropriate pleural cavity, either prior to induction of anesthesia or immediately following it. Blood should be typed and crossed, given the potential for associated injury.

EXPLORATION

An upper midline incision is preferred and should be extended as necessary to achieve adequate exposure. The anterior surface of the decompressed stomach is flattened out with the surgeon's hand as an assistant retracts on the greater curvature with Allis or Babcock clamps or by traction on the omentum to visualize the entire anterior stomach. The esophagus, cardia, and fundus are the most difficult areas to visualize, often requiring careful flattening with sponge sticks. Any serosal blood staining requires careful inspection of the area, often requiring taking down the short gastric arteries and/or the triangular ligament of the left lobe of the liver to expose the esophageal cardiac junction. The spleen should be carefully protected during left upper quadrant exploration.

Examination of the posterior surface of the stomach requires opening of the lesser sac. This can be done by incising the gastrocolic omentum below the gastroepiploic arcade or by detaching the avascular attachments of the omentum to the transverse colon. The gastroepiploic arcade should be preserved to minimize the risk of devascularization of the stomach. Filmy adhesions may be present between the posterior stomach and pancreas, and should be taken down sharply. Utilizing narrow retractors and/or sponge sticks, (Figure 5-5) the entire posterior surface of the stomach is visualized. If injury should be detected in the cardia or fundus of the stomach, the upper portion of the greater curvature should be mobilized. This can be accomplished by sequentially dividing the short gastric vessels and mobilizing the fundus medially and anteriorly or, alternatively, by mobilizing the spleen and tail of the pancreas along with the greater curvature upward and medially into the wound. The latter risks splenic injury and must be done carefully after dividing the splenocolic attachments.

The esophagus is exposed utilizing the approach for the anterior wall of the stomach. Evidence of hemorrhage or staining in the esophagocardiac area requires further mobilization, including inspection of the posterior wall of the stomach and the cardiac area through the lesser sac. When there is any uncertainty regarding esophageal injury, complete mobilization of the intra-abdominal esophagus is essential. This is accomplished using the approach utilized for vagotomy. The peritoneum over and lateral to the esophagus and above the fundus is opened sharply or bluntly and the esophagus encircled by blunt dissection with the index finger. The left lobe of the liver is retracted medially with division of the triangular ligament if

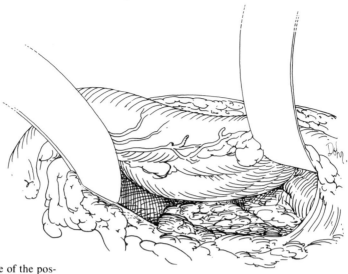

Figure 5–5 Exposure of the posterior wall of the stomach through the lesser sac.

necessary, and the encircling maneuver completed with two fingers, which are then used to draw a Penrose drain around the esophagus for downward traction. Exposure of an injury is facilitated by having the anesthesiologist pass a large-bore tube, such as a 36F Ewald tube or dilator, through the esophagus. The esophagus then is rotated about the tube in the distended esophagus to facilitate recognition of the extent of the injury for subsequent repair.

Diaphragmatic injury, especially if due to penetrating trauma, can only be ruled out by visualization of its entire peritonealized surface. Palpation alone is not sufficient and will result in injuries being overlooked. The diaphragm over the bare area of the liver is not routinely explored, except during access to a hepatic injury, since overlooked diaphragmatic injury in this area, unless massive, will not result in herniation of viscera.

Access to the pericardium can be obtained by incising the diaphragm in the midline. This allows cardiac injury from penetrating injury to be ruled out in selected patients. Such a patient would be one with a left lower chest penetrating injury who, during exploratory laparotomy, develops an unexplained rise in central venous pressure or deteriorates rapidly. Another patient in whom this might be applicable is one with multiple pentrating injuries requiring laparotomy with one of the wounds in the precordium.

The omentum usually presents no problem in identifying injury. It is readily inspected during exploration.

OPERATIVE TREATMENT

Esophageal injuries are best closed over a large-bore nasogastric tube (Ewald) or dilator to assure that the lumen is not compromised by closure. One layer of interrupted nonabsorbable 3-0 or 4-0 through-and-through suture is sufficient. A second layer adds no strength, owing to the absence of serosa, and may narrow the lumen. If a portion of esophageal wall is lost due to the injury or must be excised due to devitalization, the fundus of the stomach can be brought up as a Thal patch or the area encircled with the fundus as with a Nissen fundoplication.

As regards the stomach, any devitalized tissue should be excised. This is seldom necessary with stabwounds but may be necessary with rupture from blunt trauma or high velocity gunshot wounds.

A two-layer closure is optimal for gastric injuries to avoid postoperative mucosal hemorrhage. If the mucosa cannot be visualized owing to small wound, one should not hesitate to extend the wound. Running absorbable 3-0 or 4-0 suture through all layers is used for the inner layer with interrupted 3-0 or 4-0 Lembert nonabsorbable sutures for the outer layer. The presence of one gastric wound demands thorough search for a second. The occasional complex wound involving antrum, duodenum, and pancreas presents a formidable challenge. This is dealt with in Chapter 6. If a necrotic stomach is found following ingestion of corrosive material, total gastrectomy without anastomosis is prudent. A duodenostomy or jejunostomy will decompress the distal bowel and allow enteral alimentation up to the time of reconstruction. A transnasal sump tube can be left above the esophageal closure for proximal decompression, or the esophagus drained to the flank, using a right-angled chest tube inserted into the esophagus from below.

Diaphragmatic lacerations are best repaired with interrupted 2-0 nonabsorbable sutures or, alternatively, interrupted horizontal mattress sutures. This is facilitated by grasping the cut edges with Allis clamps. Access to posterior lacerations can be helped by the application of a series of Allis clamps to draw the wound forward. Big bites are necessary due to the low tensile strength of the muscle. An associated gastric injury makes intrapleural soilage with gastric contents a possibility that necessitates pleural lavage through the diaphragm wound with pleural drainage by one or two large-bore chest tubes.

When hemostasis is achieved in bleeding omentum, one should be certain that any devitalized omentum is excised. Small rents in the omentum should be closed to prevent intestinal herniation and obstruction.

A final step for exploration at which peritoneal contamination is found to be present is lavage with copious amounts of balanced salt solution, with or without topical antibiotics. Closure can be handled on an individual basis. We use interrupted closure of fascia with nonabsorbable monofilament sutures such as wire. Whether or not skin closure is performed is dictated by the level of contamination. Drains are not used routinely but are individualized, based on degree of contamination, status of the esophageal or gastric closure, and duration from injury to treatment.

POSTOPERATIVE MANAGEMENT

We generally leave a nasogastric tube in place for 3 to 4 days following repair of gastric injuries. If the patient is multiply injured, antacid prophylaxis against stress ulceration is maintained as well until the patient is eating. Diet is begun when the patient passes flatus and is hungry. Following esophageal repairs, a contrast study is obtained about one week postoperatively to rule out a leak prior to feeding. Antibiotics are not continued for more than 24 hours postoperatively unless associated injuries, such as colonic perforation, are found. If the skin has been left open, we frequently inspect it on the fourth postoperative day and, if not infected, perform a delayed primary closure with skin tapes. If a chest tube (or tubes) has been placed, it is pulled when output is minimal, no air leak is present, and the lung has not collapsed after 24 hours on water seal.

COMPLICATIONS

Serious postoperative complications are rare following penetrating omental or diaphragmatic injury, whereas pulmonary complications are frequent after blunt injuries which involve the diaphragm and, in most instances, there is associated chest wall and commonly pulmonary injury. Careful monitoring of pulmonary function is essential and progressive deterioration in arterial blood gasses may require the addition or maintenance of mechanical ventilation. If a diaphragmatic repair disrupts, a diaphragmatic hernia results and should be repaired when recognized. Delayed recognition of diaphragm injury will result in progressive herniation of abdominal contents into the pleural space and should be treated by immediate laparotomy.

The attendant contamination of an esophageal or gastric injury can result in overt leakage with generalized peritonitis, with intra-abdominal abscess, or with gastric or esophageal fistulae. If suspected, these diagnoses can be assessed with plain abdominal films, water soluble, upper gastrointestinal series, sonogram, and CT scans. When infection is evident and not responding to conservative management, or progresses, operative drainage is indicated. Although a posterior approach is preferred if the collection is in the right subphrenic or subhepatic space, left subphrenic or lesser sac abscesses require exposure from an anterior approach to avoid injuring the spleen, pancreas, or splenic flexure of the colon. This can optimally be done by reopening the midline incision and then establishing posterior or dependent drainage through the bed of the 12th rib or a generous subcostal incision.

When breakdown of a gastric or esophageal repair occurs, reclosure is seldom possible. The best approach is to establish adequate drainage—the resultant fistula will usually close spontaneously with adequate drainage, nasogastric suction, and intravenous nutrition.

Suture line bleeding is extremely unusual if proper closure of gastric wounds is accomplished but, on rare occasions, re-exploration for control of bleeding may be required. In such cases, preoperative endoscopy is useful to exclude other sources of the hemorrhage such as stress ulceration or hemobilia.

REFERENCES

1. Allen RE, et al.: Corrosive injuries of the stomach. Arch Surg 100:409, 1970.
2. Anderson CR, Ballinger WF: Abdominal injuries. In The Management of Trauma. Zuidema GF, Rutherford RB, Ballinger WF (eds.). Philadelphia, WB Saunders, p. 431, 1979.
3. Asch MJ, Coran AG, Johnston PW: Gastric perforation secondary to blunt trauma in children. J Trauma 15:187189, 1975.
4. Bussey HJ, McGehee RN, Tyson KRT: Isolated gastric rupture due to blunt trauma. J Trauma 15:190-191, 1975.
5. Celsus: De Medicina, with an English Translation by WC Spencer, 3 vols., Cambridge, Harvard University Press, VII, 16, 1938.
6. Citron RP, et al: Chemical trauma of the esophagus and stomach. Surg Clin N Am 48:1303, 1958.

7. DiVincenti FC, et al.: Blunt abdominal trauma. J Trauma 8:1004, 1968.
8. Garfinkle ES, Matolo NM: Gastric necrosis from blunt abdominal trauma. J Trauma 16:406-407, 1975.
9. Gourin A, Garzon AA: Diagnostic problems in traumatic diaphragmatic hernia. J Trauma 14:20-31, 1974.
10. Griswold RA, Collier HS: Blunt abdominal trauma. Int Abstr Surg 112:309, 1961.
11. Hill LD: Injuries of the diaphragm following blunt trauma. Surg Clin N Am 52:611-624, 1972.
12. Howard JM, et al.: Studies of adrenal function in combat and wounded soldiers: A study of the Korean Theatre. Ann Surg 141:314-320, 1955.
13. McCune RP, Roda CP, Eckert C: Rupture of the diaphragm caused by blunt trauma. J Trauma 16:531-537, 1976.
14. Nolleson Le Fils: Surg une plaie d'estomac guerie la suture de pelletier. J Med Chir Pharm 27:595, 1767.
15. Schenk J: Observationum medicarun, rosarorum, novarum, admirabilium, et monstrosatum. Frankfurt; p. 38., 1609.
16. Vassy LE, et al.: Traumatic gastric perforation in children from blunt trauma. J Trauma 16:184-186, 1975.
17. Worman LW, et al.: Rupture of the esophagus from external blunt trauma. Arch Surg 85:333, 1962.
18. Yajko RD, Seydel F, Trimble C: Rupture of the stomach from blunt abdominal trauma. J Trauma 16:177-183, 1975.

Chapter Six

TRAUMA TO THE PANCREAS AND DUODENUM

CHARLES FREY

INTRODUCTION

The pancreas and duodenum, both retroperitoneal organs in intimate proximity to one another, present unique problems in diagnosis and treatment. These organs, because of their relatively protected location, are infrequently injured, and constitute no more than 3 to 12 percent of all abdominal injuries.[15,19,64,88] However, if the possibility of trauma to these structures is not considered and appropriate studies are not obtained, either pre-operatively or at operation, significant injuries, associated with high morbidity and mortality, may be missed during routine laparotomy.[3,18,46]

While the major pancreatic duct and duodenum and common duct may be injured separately, not infrequently the major pancreatic duct and duodenum are both injured (20 percent) or some other combination of injury, including all three structures, may occur.[37] These combined injuries, even when recognized promptly, or indeed any injury to either pancreas or duodenum missed on initial evaluation or at celiotomy present complex challenges to the trauma surgeon's judgement and technical ability, and to intensive care support facilities. The incidence of secondary life-threatening complications with pancreatic and duodenal injury is far higher than with any other comparable abdominal injuries. Delays in diagnosis are common and this increases the complexity of the treatment and greatly increases the chance of serious secondary complications.[2,14,16,46]

Mortality associated with pancreatic or duodenal trauma based on recent reports, is in the range of 16 to 20 percent. Over half these deaths result from massive hemorrhage and shock due to associated injuries to major vascular structures and death occurs intraoperatively or within 48 hours of injury. Duodenal and pancreatic injury has almost nothing to do with the fatal outcome in these early deaths.[16,37,70,73] Sepsis, the second most common cause of death after hemorrhage, is most often seen in patients with hemorrhagic shock in the preoperative and operative period and in those with colon injury or those in whom the gastrointestinal tract has been opened.[33,37,74,89]

As regards the historical aspect of these injuries, an intoxicated woman struck in the chest and abdomen by a stagecoach wheel and brought to St. Thomas' Hospital was reported by Travers in the 1827 Lancet.[82] She was the first recorded victim of blunt injury to the pancreas. At autopsy, hours after the injury, a transverse tear of the pancreas as well as an hepatic laceration were found. The cause of death was intra-abdominal hemorrhage from an associated hepatic injury.

The first recorded description of a penetrating injury and surgical resection of a portion of the pancreas is credited by Otis (who edited the *Medical and Surgical History of the War of Rebellion* (Civil War) in 1876) to Kleberg of Odessa.[58] Kleberg described, in 1868, a 60-year-old soldier who fell among thieves and was stabbed in the abdomen. The protruding exteriorized pancreas was later ligated and excised. The patient had an uncomplicated course after discharge.

Similarly, the only survivor among five patients reported with pancreatic injury during the Civil War had a portion of protruding pancreas excised and ligated. The other four patients reported by Otis had survived long periods of delay (the shortest of which was one and a half days) between the time of injury and definitive hospitalization, only to die from late complications of injury, peritonitis, and hemorrhage, which in three of the four cases resulted from associated injuries to liver, stomach, or splenic vessels.[58]

While the significance of an intact pancreatic duct was not fully appreciated by Otis, he described two patients who had at autopsy a ball (bullet) lodged in the pancreas the main duct of which, in both cases, was intact but no evidence of pancreatic inflammation or necrosis, and who, in fact, died of associated injuries; Case 506, "The pancreas was perforated at about its middle but except in the immediate track of the ball, gave evidence of no departure from its healthy standard;" and Case 418, The pancreas was rather large, seven inches long; weight five ounces (weighed with the ball embedded). There was nothing abnormal in its appearance except the presence of the foreign body . . . On examining the specimen microscopically, no deviation from the normal structure is found in sections made from tissue taken from the left end or tail of the viscera and from the middle part or body. The coat of the great arteries with which the ball was in apposition were uninjured."[58] Otis then went on to quote several surgical treatises and textbooks of surgery which outline the problems and importance of diagnosing pancreatic injury, the consequences of not doing so, and what constitutes a significant pancreatic injury. [58] These concepts only recently have been reaffirmed and generally recognized as valid more than 150 to 200 years after the original publication. Bell, H: A System of Surgery, volume V, published in 1787 says, "As the pancreas lies deeply covered with the other viscera, wounds of it can seldom be discovered: but as a division of the duct of this gland will prevent the secretion which it affords from being carried to the bowels, this may, by interrupting or impeding digestion, do much injury to the constitution; and as the liquor will be effused into the cavity of the abdomen, it may thus be productive of collections, the removal of which may ultimately require the assistance of surgery."

Gooch (Chirurgical Works, 1792, volume I, p 99), declares that "wounds of the pancreas are to be concluded mortal if its duct or blood vessels are injured, whence the succus pancreaticus or blood may be discharged into the cavity of the abdomen and there putrefying, cause inevitable death."

Little progress was made in either the recognition or management of pancreatic injuries during World War I. Only five cases with one survivor were described by the British, a record similar to that observed in the Civil War.

Poole's World War II report on the Second Auxillary Surgical Group in 1944 and 1945 recorded 62 pancreatic injuries associated with a 56 percent mortality.[63]

The importance of associated injuries as factors contributing to mortality received appropriate emphasis, as only one of the 62 patients was noted to have an isolated pancreatic injury. Thirteen of the 35 deaths were associated with major vascular injury and a correlation was noted between the number of viscera injured and mortality. The mortality rose progressively from 33 percent with one associated injury, to 50 percent with two viscera, to 60 percent with three viscera, to 100 percent with four viscera injured in addition to the pancreas.

During the Korean conflict, the mortality of nine pancreatic injuries was reduced to 22 percent, according to Sako, reporting the experiences of the surgical research team in Korea of the Army Medical Service Graduate School, United States Army.[64] There was no evidence of any enhanced awareness of the appropriate operative management of the surgical injuries included in the report. The decreasing mortality of pancreatic injury, as well as of other injury, was attributed accurately to improvements in supportive care, including resuscitation, fluid replacement, antibiotics, and improved management of associated injuries.

A major step in improved diagnosis of pancreatic injury following blunt trauma to the pancreas was the observation by Elman in 1929 that the serum amylase became elevated in some pancreatic injuries if the duct was injured or obstructed. [20] This observation was later confirmed by McCorkle and Goldman in 1942 and reaffirmed the following year in a report by Naffziger and McCorkle.[48,55]

Walton, in 1923, recommended pancreatic resection of the portion of the pancreas distal to the fracture and oversewing the proximal end of the pancreas as the safest form of management of injuries to the body and tail of the pancreas in which the pancreatic duct was severed.[85] The report by Kerry and Glas in the Archives of Surgery in 1962 emphasized the significance of injury to the major ductal system of the pancreas through clinical and laboratory investigations and has become a landmark in establishing appropriate operative management of patients with complex pancreatic injuries and associated injuries to duodenum and common bile ducts.[40]

A major problem related to pancreatic injuries is the high incidence of associated injuries (Table 6-1). Mortality relates to the nature of the pancreatic injury, the number and type of associated injuries, and the wounding agent (Table 6-2). The immediate cause of death is uncontrollable hemorrhage from the pancreas and associated injury in 56 percent of patients, as a result of the secondary complications of sepsis and abscess formation in 30 percent, organ failure in 10 percent, and miscellaneous causes, such as central nervous system injury and secondary hemorrhage in the remaining 4 percent (Table 6-3).

Duodenal Injuries

Although blunt trauma to the abdomen resulting in duodenal perforation was associated with a mortality of over 86 percent in the period preceding World War I, the mortality had been reduced to 50 percent by the time of World War II, which closely paralleled the experience with penetrating injuries of the duodenum reported in military casualties, 56 percent. [52, 62,66] By the time of the Korean conflict, the mortality of duodenal injuries from blunt trauma had been reduced to 20 percent although the mortality of penetrating injuries remained at 43 percent, despite advances in resuscitation, fluid replacement, and antibiotic therapy.[15,64]

Table 6–1 PANCREAS ASSOCIATED INJURIES

Author		Number of Patients	Major Vascular	Liver	Stomach	Spleen	Duodenum	Common Duct	Kidney	Colon
Jones	Penetrating	226	129	125	117	45	51	5	49	55
	Blunt	74	6	24	0	21	5	2	4	1
Werschky	Penetrating	117	59	63	61	29	31	3	27	24
	Blunt	23								
Wilson	Penetrating	45	11	19	17					7
	Blunt	39		10		9	11			
Steele	Penetrating	55		34	26	24				
	Blunt	30								
Stone	Penetrating	56	19	30	35	16	13	1	17	8
	Blunt	6								
Thompson	Penetrating	39	10	20	16	7	9		10	13
	Blunt	48	2	8	2	7	6		1	1
Heitsch	Penetrating	77								
	Blunt	23								
White	Penetrating	36	16	15	18		8			11
	Blunt	27		7	0	5	6			0
Karl	Penetrating	14	8	10	6	4	2	1		7
	Blunt	11	2	2	1	5	2	1		1
Bach	Penetrating	10	6	7	8	7	7	4	4	2
	Blunt	34								
Babb	Penetrating	55	18	23	29	18	15		21	11
	Blunt	21		6		4	5			
TOTAL		1066	286	405	336	216	171	20	135	141

Table 6–2 PANCREATIC INJURY WOUNDING AGENT AND MORTALITY

Author	Penetrating	(% Died)	Stab	(% Died)	Gunshot	(% Died)	Shotgun	(% Died)	Blunt	(% Died)
Jones			46	(7%)	156	(19%)	24	(58%)	74	(18%)
Werschky			39	(10%)	71	(24%)	7	(29%)	23	(18%)
Wilson			24	(8%)	20	(45%)	1	(100%)	39	(38%)
Steele	55	(27%)							30	(27%)
Stone			12	(8%)	41	(20%)	3	(100%)	6	(17%)
Thompson			12	(16.6%)	27	(29%)			48	(10.4%)
Heitsch	77	(20%)	8		51				23	(9%)
White	36	(13.8%)							27	(3.7%)
Karl	14	(14%)							11	(18%)
Bach	10	(20%)			7		3		34	(20%)
Babb	55	(5%)	23		28		4		21	
TOTAL	247		164		401		42		336	

Table 6–3 PANCREATIC INJURY CAUSE OF DEATH

Author	Hemorrhage and Other Associated Injuries	Pancreatic Injury Intra-Abdominal Abscess and Sepsis	Organ Failure	Miscellaneous
Jones	34	13	7	4
Werschky	19	3	3	–
Wilson	15	15	–	–
Steele	10	7	5	1
Stone	8	5	–	–
Thompson	2	6	5	2
Heitsch	15	13	3	1
White	6			
Karl	3	1		
Bach	1	8		
Babb	16			
TOTAL	129 (56%)	71 (30%)	23 (10%)	8 (4%)

In 1964, Cocke and Meyer identified the retroperitoneal rupture of the duodenum as a special problem which, if not suspected and operated on, or if not recognized at operation (as occurred in 15 percent of patients) was, as a result of the delay, associated with extensive retroperitoneal inflammation and an operative mortality of 71 percent.[14]

As is true of the pancreas, the location of the duodenum in a relatively protected position results in a high incidence of associated injuries (Table 6-4). The wounding agent plays a major role in subsequent mortality, that from knives being negligible, shotgun wounds being highly lethal (Table 6-5). The cause of death is similar to that following pancreatic injury, consisting of hemorrhage in 43 percent, duodenal fistula in 37 percent, sepsis in 8 percent, organ failure in 8 percent and other causes in the remaining 4 percent (Table 6-6).

Combined Pancreatic and Duodenal Injuries

The basis of our understanding of these complex injuries involving duodenum, pancreas, and common bile duct was derived in large part from the 1962 report of Kerry and Glas.[40] These authors defined which lesions of the pancreas or duodenum resulting from blunt or penetrating trauma required resection of the duodenum or pancreas in order to ensure survival.

ANATOMY

The junction between the stomach and duodenum is marked by the pyloric vein, which courses inferiorly upward from the pancreas, transversely across the duodenum at the distal end of the pyloric muscle. The first portion of the duodenum is that portion between the pyloric muscle and the common duct superiorly and the gastroduodenal artery inferiorly. The second portion of the duodenum extends from the common duct and gastroduodenal artery to the ampulla of Vater. The third portion of the duodenum extends from the ampulla of Vater to the mesenteric vessels and the fourth portion of the duodenum extends from the mesenteric vessels to the point at which the duodenum emerges from the retroperitoneum at the ligament of Treitz. The duodenum shares a common blood supply with the pancreas, so that while it is possible to remove the duodenum from the pancreas, it is not possible to remove all the head of the pancreas with out irreversibly devascularizing the duodenum. This is why 5 percent of the pancreas along the rim of the inner aspect of the duodenal 'C' is preserved during a 95 percent resection of the pancreas for chronic pancreatitis, as penetrating within its substance are the anterior and posterior branches of the inferior and superior pancreaticoduodenal arcade.

The first portion, the distal third portion and all of the fourth portion of the duodenum lie over the vertebral column and are particularly vulnerable to injury by abdominal trauma that compresses them against the vertebral column. The mesocolon lies over and prevents direct inspection of the third and fourth portions of the duodenum, and the omentum and transverse colon overlie much of the second and, occasionally, the first portion of the duodenum. The duodenum is essentially entirely

Table 6-4 DUODENUM—ASSOCIATED INJURIES

Author		Number of Patients (%)	Major Vascular (%)	Lung (%)	Liver (%)	Stomach (%)	Spleen (%)	Pancreas (%)	C.D. (%)	Kidney (%)	Colon (%)	S.B. (%)
Stone	Penetrating	299 (74%)	Artery (31%) Vein (33%)	21%	63%	33%		34%	25%	21%	34%	50%
	Blunt	27 (26%)			63%		33%	26%		26%		
Snyder	Penetrating	190 (78%)	43%		43%	26%		28%	16%	23%	32%	26%
	Blunt	54 (22%)										
Flint	Penetrating	56 (75%)	17%		41%	32%		27%	15%	16%	39%	33%
	Blunt	19 (25%)										

Table 6-5 DUODENUM: WOUNDING AGENTS AND MORTAL INJURY*

Author	Penetrating	(% Died)	Stab	(% Died)	Gunshot	(% Died)	Shotgun	(% Died)	Blunt	(% Died)
Stone			31	(0%)	239	(11%)	24	(46%)	27	
Snyder			23	(0%)	143	(10%)	14	(29%)	44	
Flint	55	(20%)	4		51	(11%)			19	(11%)
TOTALS	55		58		433		38		90	

*Late deaths only—excludes 19 early deaths from major vascular injuries.

Table 6-6 DUODENUM DEATHS

Author	Hemorrhage	Duodenal Dehiscence or Fistula	Intra-Abdominal Sepsis	Organ Failure (Liver, Lung, Kidney)	Miscellaneous
Stone	19	5	3	2	4
Snyder	19	27	–	–	–
Flint	5	5	5	2	–
TOTAL (Percent)	43%	37%	8%	8%	4%

retroperitoneal, although the anterior half of the circumference of the first and second parts of duodenum can be visualized through the thin overlying translucent peritoneum in most patients. The third part of the duodenum can be visualized by mobilizing the cecum and distal ileum as described by Braach.

The pancreas is divided anatomically into a head, body, and tail. The junction between the head and the body, the neck, can be identified by the groove through which the superior mesenteric artery and vein run on their way to the small bowel mesentery. The neck of the gland and a portion of the proximal body directly overlie the vertebral column and mesenteric vessels. The *uncinate process* is the posterior part of the head of the pancreas and is derived from the ventral pancreas, bulging to the patient's left posteriorly under the mesenteric vessels superficial to the aorta.[29] The body of the pancreas extends laterally, dorsally, and superiorly from the neck and blends into a distal, more narrow portion of the pancreas or tail, which constitutes approximately the lateral one-third of the length of the gland.

The distal portion of the body and the tail of the gland overlie the left adrenal and superior pole of the kidney. The tail of the pancreas, containing the highest concentration of islets in the gland, overlies the superior pole of the kidney and ends at the hilum of the spleen.[90]

The pancreatic duct, which represents the fusion of the duct of Santorini supplying the body and tail with the duct of Wirsung, which supplies the head, runs longitudinally through the gland, entering the duodenum at the ampulla of Vater. Numerous lobular ducts come off at right angles to the main duct. Both the pancreatic duct and common duct enter the duodenum through a common channel in 85 percent of patients at the ampulla of Vater. In another 5 percent of patients, the two ducts enter the duodenum on the same papilla but through separate channels.[50] In 10 percent of patients, the bile duct and pancreatic duct enter the duodenum separately.[51] This is because the major pancreatic duct may be derived from the dorsal pancreas and enter the duodenum separately in a more proximal location closer to the pylorus.[32] In this 10 percent of cases, an accessory pancreatic duct, derived from the dorsal pancreas (the duct of Santorini) drains a major portion of the gland.[32,51] The duct enters the second portion of the duodenum, where it is vulnerable to injury. Injury to either of the pancreatic ducts anywhere in their course through the pancreas sets the stage for pancreatic ductal obstruction with all its attendant complications, such as pancreatitis, pancreatic fistula, pancreatic pseudocyst and pancreatic abscess.

Experience with Endoscopic Retrograde Cholangiopancreatography has confirmed the important observation first made by Cross that there are small accessory pancreatic ducts that enter the duodenum independent of the main duct in most patients.[17] These can become dilated and form small pseudocysts that are not decompressed by filleting open the main pancreatic duct, as is done in the Puestow ductal decompression operation.

The pancreas and duodenum are abundantly supplied with blood vessels (Fig. 6-1). The largest vessel in intimate relationship with the pancreas is the splenic artery, one of the main branches of the celiac axis which joins the superior aspect of the gland near, but lateral to, the junction of the head and body and runs in the groove within the superior substance of the gland to the tail, giving off two to ten branches at right angles to the long axis of the pancreas along the way in 75 percent of patients. Then it leaves the pancreas to enter the spleen. In 25 percent of patients, the splenic artery gives off virtually no branches to the pancreas, except a large

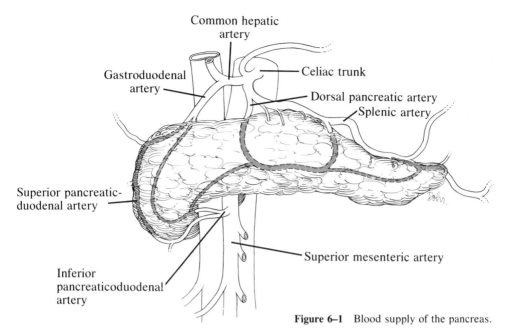

Figure 6–1 Blood supply of the pancreas.

branch, the dorsal pancreatic, which joins the transverse pancreatic artery which supplies the pancreas.[68] Short gastric branches are given off by the splenic artery to the greater curvature of the stomach as the splenic artery leaves the tail of the pancreas. Most proximal to these is the left gastroepiploic artery, which supplies the greater curvature of the stomach and the omentum, and in 75 percent of patients a major branch, the dorsal pancreatic, joins to the transverse pancreatic artery which runs parallel and inferior to the splenic to the tail of the gland. The splenic artery, but not the splenic vein, may be ligated without compromising the viability of the spleen or distal pancreas.[68]

The first branch of the hepatic artery is the gastroduodenal artery. This courses from its hepatic artery origin at the superior surface of the duodenum under the second portion of the duodenum to enter the pancreas just below and opposite the common duct above the duodenum. In the pancreas, this artery divides into the superior pancreaticoduodenal artery and the right gastroepiploic artery. This latter vessel leaves the pancreas adjacent to the duodenum and supplies the greater curvature of the stomach and the omentum. The pancreaticoduodenal artery curves through the head of the pancreas near the duodenum, giving off multiple branches to the pancreatic head, many of these anastomosing with the inferior pancreaticoduodenal artery. The latter, a branch of the superior mesenteric artery, arises off the superior mesenteric just as it emerges from the inferior surface of the pancreas. In 5 percent of patients, an anomalous common hepatic artery or, in 25 percent of patients, an anomalous right hepatic artery arises from the superior mesenteric artery. It is crucial for the surgeon to be aware that both the anamolous common or right hepatic artery may pass through the head portion of the uncinate process of the gland and be injured during resection of the uncinate process when the short, direct branches to the uncinate from the superior mesenteric artery and vein are being divided or ligated.[49,79]

The major vein draining the pancreas is the splenic vein, which runs longitudinally in a groove up the mid- to upper portion of the posterior surface of the gland from the spleen to its junction with the portal vein posterior to the pancreatic neck. The portal vein is constituted by the joining of the splenic and superior mesenteric vein. The latter vessel courses under the pancreas, following the same pathway in the opposite direction as the superior mesenteric artery. It joins the splenic vein near the superior border of the gland. The first portion of the portal vein and distal portion of the superior mesenteric vein receive veins draining the uncinate portion of the head of the pancreas. The superior mesenteric and portal veins pass under, and are in intimate contact with, the posterior surface of the neck of the gland. The portal vein emerges from the superior surface of the duodenum most often just posterior to and between the common bile duct on the right and the hepatic artery on the left. The inferior mesenteric vein joins the superior mesenteric or splenic vein as does the coronary vein, which may, in some cases, enter the portal vein. The pancreas is entirely covered by the retroperitoneum of the lesser sac and, anterior to this, another layer consisting of the stomach and gastrohepatic ligament. Much of the body may be visible through the gastrohepatic ligament superiorly and through the base of the mesocolon inferiorly in the vicinity of the ligament of Treitz.

The common bile duct enters the posterior substance of the head of the pancreas in 83 percent of patients after it passes under the duodenum.[29,69] After piercing the capsule of the gland posteriorly, it courses down within the pancreatic substance a centimeter or two from the curve of the duodenum, entering the duodenal lumen at the junction between the second and third portion of the duodenum approximately 20 to 25 centimeters from the pylorus.[68]

ASSESSMENT OF PANCREATIC OR DUODENAL INJURY

The pancreas and duodenum are injured either by blunt or penetrating trauma. The likelihood of penetrating injury occurs whenever a missile or penetrating object passes in the vicinity of the pancreas or duodenum. Since penetrating injury is usually obvious and is usually associated with clinical findings which demand exploration, the primary problem in diagnosis is the recognition of blunt injury to the pancreas or duodenum. This is particularly true when the injury is confined to either of these two organs, both of which lie in a relatively protected position and are usually injured only by a direct blow that compresses them against the vertebral column.

Classically, with injuries to the retroperitoneal pancreas or duodenum, abdominal discomfort may be out of proportion to the abdominal findings and the patient usually has abdominal tenderness and an absence of bowel sounds. The protected position of the pancreas and duodenum does not result in peritoneal irritation as severe as more common intra-abdominal injuries, as the extravasated blood, enteric contents, or enzymes are initially contained retroperitoneally. Unless the surgeon has a high index of suspicion, these injuries may not be recognized immediately. It is important for the surgeon to understand the mechanism of blunt injury to pancreas and duodenum and, therefore, to know why the presenting signs and symptoms may not reflect the seriousness of the injury.

The typical blunt trauma resulting in injury is a blow to the abdomen. Most commonly, in our experience, this has been due to impalement of a driver of a motor vehicle on the steering wheel of the car.[18,37,70] History of a severe blow to the upper abdomen should lead to the suspicion that pancreatic or duodenal injury may exist. In children, bicycle handlebar injuries or any fall against an object are the most common cause of pancreatic and duodenal injuries other than being a passenger in an automobile.[22,30,47,62,68] Tenderness in the anatomic location of either of these two organs should suggest the possibility of pancreatic or duodenal injury.

In blunt trauma, the duodenum or head, body, or tail of the pancreas are injured, depending on which direction the impinging force is directed at the vertebral column. If the force is sufficient, fracture of the pancreas or duodenum may result, between the steering wheel compressing the abdominal wall and the unyielding spinal column. The spinal column is like the hub of a wheel around which the pancreas is wrapped. If the patient has his left side between the steering wheel and his vertebral column, the tail of the pancrease will be injured; if his right side is forward, then the head of the pancreas and duodenum are at risk; if he is struck in the midepigastric region, the neck of the pancreas may be divided over the mesenteric vessels. The major pancreatic duct is a more rigid, brittle structure than are the vasculature, the capsule, and pancreatic parenchyma. Often the duct is fractured in the absence of appreciable hemorrhage or capsular disruption, a fact which must be appreciated if significant injury to the pancreas is not to be overlooked at operation (Figure 6-2). If the major duct is fractured, the injury is significant owing to the leakage of enzymes and ductal obstruction which result, among the sequelae of which are pancreatic fistula, pseudocysts, and pancreatitis. If the major duct is intact, pancreatic injury is not significant. Extravasation of pancreatic secretion from the tributary ducts or obstruction of the tributary ducts cause self-limited fistula or pancreatitis.

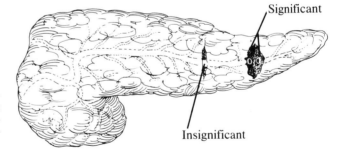

Significant

Insignificant

Figure 6–2 Demonstration of significant (disruption of pancreatic duct) versus proximal insignificant injury (in which duct is intact).

The duodenum may be ruptured if compression of the abdominal wall by the impinging force traps the distal end of the duodenum against the vertebral column at the time the pylorus is shut, creating a closed loop while the duodenum is full of fluid.[14,18] This type of closed loop injury leads to extravasation of digestive enzymes in the retroperitoneum and is most often associated with severe symptoms and so is usually suspected and diagnosed. However, in instances when the duodenum is crushed against the vertebral column, the nonviable crushed wall may remain intact for a period of hours, or even days, until it is digested by a combination of gastric juice and pancreatic enzymes. In such instances, while the necrotic wall is still intact, initial abdominal findings may be minimal.

A less common problem is intramural hematoma of the duodenal lumen. The vomiting of bile or gastric juice following epigastric trauma should lead to the suspicion of the possibility of duodenal obstruction.[36] This is particularly likely if there is very little associated abdominal distention. If there is a question of intramural duodenal hematoma, a gastrointestinal series, with soluble radio-opaque material demonstrating the characteristic inverted fir-tree sign due to swelling of the plicae of the duodenal mucosa, will lead to the diagnosis.[36]

Pancreas injury resulting from blunt trauma should be suspected by the presence of tenderness over the anatomical distribution of the pancreas. Pancreatic injury is often associated with accompanying ileus and very frequently the serum pancreatic enzymes (amylase and lipase) are elevated This does not provide any clues as to the magnitude of pancreatic injury and is not specific for the pancreas, since any upper gastrointestinal enteric perforation may release pancreatic enzymes in the free peritoneal cavity and their absorption by the abdominal lymphatics will result in elevation of the serum enzymes. Mild trauma that is of no clinical significance may, on occasion, be associated with amylase elevations.[53]

Patients with isolated duodenal or pancreatic compression injuries are often hemodynamically stable and sometimes may initially have no abnormal abdominal findings.[3,70] Diagnostic peritoneal lavage may well be normal (returns of which should also be checked for elevated amylase level) because of the retroperitoneal position of the pancreas and posterior aspect of the duodenum or because of an initially intact, but necrotic, duodenal wall. In such patients, where there is no immediate indication for operation, the serum amylase or urine amylase is a very useful test with which to follow the patient.[2,3,88] If the serum or urine amylase is noted to progressively increase, on the basis of serial determinations every three to four hours, or remain elevated, then the duodenum and pancreas should be examined at operation in the absence of other indications for operation. If an initially elevated serum amylase declines and there is no other indication for operation, none should be undertaken. A single amylase determination should not be used as a basis for deciding whether the patient does or does not need an operation.[53] In many patients with total disruption of the pancreatic ductal system, the serum amylase will not become elevated until 24 to 48 hours after injury.[3] White has noted serum amylase levels tend to rise more with ductal injuries of the head and body then with injuries of the tail.[88] This is understandable. The serum amylase is a measure of ductal obstruction. The more proximal the fracture of the duct to the duodenum, the more gland there is secreting behind the obstruction or ductal disruption. The amylase behind an obstructed duct diffuses into the interstices of the gland and may be picked up and returned to venous stream by the pancreatic venous capillaries and lymphatics, or if the duct draining the distal pancreatic segment is pouring its contents in the abdominal cavity, the amylase will be picked up by the abdominal lymphatics and returned to the blood venous circulation, raising serum levels of amylase. Knowing these facts, it should be no surprise why the amylase may remain normal if the tail of the gland is shot away. First, there is no proximal obstruction, so that pancreatic juice in the uninjured body and head continue to flow into the duodenum, not retrograde into the area of injury. Second, with the tail shot away, there are no viable acinar cells left to produce a pancreatic secretion containing amylase, even if the duct of the distal segment was fractured and obstructed.

In patients who are hemodynamically stable and in whom there is no other indication of injury or need for celiotomy, other than a progressive increase in amylase, E.R.C.P., if available, can be employed to ascertain whether the pancreatic ductal rupture suspected has occurred and its location, that is, the head, body, or tail.[27,76]

There are no specific diagnostic tests for pancreatic injury. CT scanners and peritoneal lavage are being used with increasing frequency to evaluate abdominal trauma and retroperitoneal edema in the vicinity of the pancreas and may lead to suspicion of pancreatic injury. However, we do not believe that injury can necessarily be ruled out should the scan or peritoneal lavage be interpreted as normal, particularly with early assessment of the injured patient.

In the final analysis, the diagnosis of pancreatic or duodenal injuries rests with a high index of suspicion leading to laparotomy. Whether the injury is due to blunt or penetrating trauma, there is no substitute for exploration of the abdomen.

PRE-OPERATIVE PREPARATION

As with any patient about to undergo laparotomy, good reliable access to the vascular system should be obtained for fluid and blood infusion, preferably by at least one good cutdown in an upper extremity.

A nasogastric tube should be placed pre-operatively if pancreatic or duodenal injury is suspected, to decompress the stomach to prevent a leakage of gastric juice from the ruptured duodenum. In blunt trauma, pre-operative antibiotics are not indicated. In penetrating trauma, broad spectrum antibiotics are usually administered prior to surgery, in anticipation of a possible hollow viscus injury and intraperitoneal or retroperitoneal contamination. Blood should have been sent for typing and cross-match. Routine CBC, white count, and urinalysis are necessary and helpful in the evaluation of associated injuries. Routine chest x-ray should be obtained in all penetrating trauma and is often helpful in blunt trauma. Intravenous pyelograms should be obtained if penetrating trauma passes anywhere near the vicinity of a kidney or kidney hilum, as is usually the case when pancreatic injuries are suspected or are present. Hematuria suggests renal damage and is an indication for pre-operative intravenous pyelograms, if for no other reason than to verify the presence of two functional kidneys. The patient, as is true in all trauma cases, should be prepped from clavicles to pubis and from bedline to bedline to permit posterior drainage should this be necessary.

OPERATIVE EXPLORATION AND EVALUATION OF
THE PANCREAS AND DUODENUM

The routine laparotomy incision for most trauma is a midline abdominal incision. When there is tenderness in the upper abdomen, and the most likely source is in this region, the initial incision should be generous and carry at least from the xiphoid to umbilicus. It should then be extended well below the umbilicus once the presence of injury or reasonable probability of injury has been verified.

The patient should be eviscerated promptly to permit a thorough abdominal exploration with inspection of the retroperitoneum. All blood and clots should be rapidly evacuated from the peritoneal cavity. Any injury other than catastrophic bleeding should be temporarily isolated with packs to avoid missing more major sources of hemorrhage. Following verification that no injury to intra-abdominal

structures exists or following assessment and treatment of the injuries that do, particularly injuries to major vascular structures, which are the principal cause of mortality (Tables 6-1 and 6-2) attention should be directed toward the retroperitoneum
and the duodenum and pancreas. Since injuries of these structures rarely produce
catastrophic hemorrhage in themselves, they do not have high priority in the initial
exploration.[67,72] The site of injury in duodenum and pancreas from collected reviews
of pancreatic and duodenal injuries are shown in Figure 6-3.

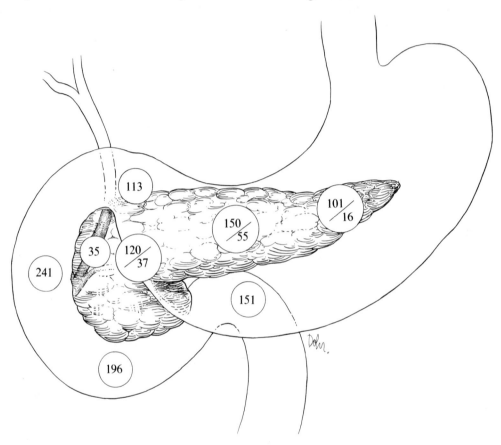

Figure 6–3 The number of injuries from collected reviews is shown in the circles. The mortality for
injuries to the head, body and tail is shown below the slash in the larger circles. The relative frequency
of injuries should be considered separately for pancreas and duodenum; the former (large circles) is much
more frequent than the latter (small circles).

The initial exploration of the free peritoneal cavity with the bowel eviscerated
permits inspection of the inferior aspect of the base of the mesocolon from the
ligament of Treitz outward to the left. Injury to the pancreatic ductal system is
suspected whenever a retroperitoneal hemorrhage can be seen thorough the base of
the mesocolon or gastrohepatic mesentery. Sometimes it is possible to visualize a
ductal injury in penetrating trauma or appreciate that the duct must be fractured if
the pancreas itself is more than half transected. A severely macerated gland or one
which has a central perforation should be assumed to have a ductal injury until this
is ruled out by pancreatogram or operative exploration.[27] In most patients, the pancreatic substance can be inspected along its inferior surface and injury to the body

and tail relatively well ruled out. Attention can next be directed toward the gastro-hepatic ligament, as in thin patients, the upper portion of the body and tail can often be visualized through the gastrohepatic ligament; once again, hemorrhage seen through the gastrohepatic ligament suggests the possibility of pancreatic injury.

Next, attention should be directed toward the duodenum, mobilizing the colon downward and, if necessary, sweeping the mesocolon down with sponges. The hepatic flexure of the colon should be mobilized when there is any reason to suspect injury to the duodenum or the head of the pancreas. By severing the lateral attachments of the hepatic flexure of the colon, the entire mesocolon can be mobilized downward to permit inspection of the anterior or lateral surface of the first, second, and third portion of the duodenum. Evidence of hemorrhage in the duodenum or posterior to the duodenum requires mobilization of the duodenum by severing its lateral attachments (Kocher Maneuver). These attachments should be cut from the foramen of Winslow around to the fourth portion of the duodenum. This permits the entire duodenum to be mobilized upward and the posterior surface inspected and palpated. It also permits evaluation of the head of the pancreas. If there should be even a small hematoma in the head of the pancreas, bi-manual palpation should be carried out to determine whether there is loss of substance or pulpification of the head. This finding is associated with the possibility of injury to major pancreatic ducts. The fourth portion of the duodenum can be inspected from the area of the liagment of Treitz. The absence of hemorrhage around the ligament of Treitz makes injury to the fourth portion of the duodenum unlikely. Should there be a suggestion of injury, the entire right colon and small bowel mesentery can be mobilized and swung upwards to permit exposure of the entire sweep of the duodenum.[11] When there is any reason to suspect the possibility of injury to the body and tail of the pancreas or when there is evidence of trauma to the head of the pancreas, the lesser sac should be opened and the entire pancreas exposed. This is best done by separating the omentum from the colon in the avascular plane of attachment or by ligating two to three arcades outside the gastric epiploic vessels in a relatively avascular area of the gastroepiploic omentum and coming down on the pancreas through the lesser sac. Once the lesser sac is entered in the right plane, the entire body and tail of the pancreas are open to view.

If there should be evidence of hemorrhage in the retroperitoneum, the entire transverse colon should be separated from the omentum to permit direct inspection of the entire anterior surface of the pancreas. Ecchymosis in the area of the neck, body, or tail of the pancreas requires an exploration. Bimanual palpation is another method for evaluating a pancreatic injury. This can best be done by sweeping the mesocolon downward, separating it from the inferior surface of the pancreas or by opening the mesocolon at its junction with the retroperitoneum inferiorly. The latter maneuver, unless carefully done, risks injuring the colonic arcade that provides collateral blood flow from the middle colic artery to the left colic artery. Once the colon and the mesentery have been separated from the body and tail of the pancreas, the body and tail of the pancreas can be rotated superiorly along its length without having to mobilize the spleen. The posterior aspect of the gland can be visualized and bi-manual palpation of the body of the tail of the pancreas performed. A loss of integrity of pancreatic substance provides indirect evidence of ductal injury. An alternative exploration for those experienced with pancreatic injury is accomplished by duodenotomy and retrograde pancreatogram through the ampulla of Vater using a Fogarty irrigating catheter. The pancreatic duct can also be intubated by incising the tail of the pancreas and using the Fogarty irrigating catheter to perform a pancreatogram.

EVALUATION OF THE PANCREATIC AND
DUODENAL INJURY

Absence of any hemorrhage over the pancreas and duodenum makes injury very unlikely. The only exception is the possibility of injury to the posterior aspect of the duodenum, although this is entirely unlikely if palpation of the duodenum does not reveal induration, crepitus, or bile staining nor, on inspection, the slightest trace of ecchymosis. Small, ecchyotic lesions, however, demand definitive evaluation, since injuries to the pancreas and duodenum are easily underestimated.[3,13]

Duodenal intramural hematomas and duodenal lacerations are relatively easily recognized: the former, by the presence of severe ecchymosis and induration of the duodenum, the latter, of course, by evidence of serosal damage and leakage of duodenal contents on mobilization of the duodenum.[36,73] The consequences of the injury may be difficult to evaluate in the duodenum if the time between injury and operation is short. If four or five hours have passed and there has been no evidence of duodenal obstruction, intramural hematomas of the duodenum can be left intact.[36] If, preoperatively, there has been evidence of obstruction, manifest by biliary drainage from the nasogastric tube or by x-ray studies, the serosa should be opened through the main area of the induration and the submucosal hematoma evacuated.[36]

The pancreas is the most difficult of all abdominal organs to evaluate. The pancreas can, in the dog, be pounded with a hammer, squeezed and macerated, its substance and capsule lacerated, yet no serious injury results as long as the main pancreatic duct remains intact, as Kerry and Glas demonstrated.[40] The same situation seems to apply to humans. Conversely, a seemingly relatively minor injury may result in disruption or obstruction of a brittle main pancreatic duct, resulting in a leakage of pancreatic juice causing acute pancreatitis and if untreated, pancreatic pseudocysts, fistulas, ascites, abscesses, sepsis, and chronic pancreatitis.[3,6,22,25,30,33,37,39,71,72,88]

For all practical purposes, if the major pancreatic ductal system is intact, the pancreatic injury, be it capsular tear, hematoma, or laceration of its substance, is not significant. Any leakage of pancreatic fluid from a tributory duct will resolve spontaneously, usually in less than four to six weeks, if drainage is instituted. Hematomas of the pancreas and capsular injuries of the pancreas, if encountered at operation, ought to be drained even if the pancreatic ductal system is intact, in order to avoid collections that predispose to abscess formation. If the major pancreatic ductal system is disrupted, it is essential the injury be recognized and appropriately treated, to prevent mortality and serious morbidity.

RATIONALE FOR CHOICE OF OPERATION

We feel the rationale for the choice of operation in duodenal and pancreatic trauma, which may occur either independently or together or in association with common duct injury, should be reconstitution of enteric and ductal integrity based on the anatomy of injury and preservation of function. However, our first priority should be to save a life and, in a hemodynamically unstable patient with severe associated injuries to major vascular structures, definitive therapy of the pancreatic or duodenal injury may have to be delayed in order to shorten operating time.

Some useful concepts in the management of pancreatic trauma which can be applied to the individual patient are discussed in the following paragraphs.

1. At operation, the diagnosis and management of pancreatic and duodenal injuries should be deferred in the patient with multiple injuries until hemorrhage from associated injuries, such as to major vessels or liver and spleen, is controlled. This recommendation is based on the knowledge that the single most frequent cause of death in pancreatic and duodenal injury is hemorrhage and shock from associated injuries. (See Tables 6-3, and 6-6). Most of the deaths from these injuries occur within 48 hours of injury. [1,6,12,13,16,19,28,31,34,37,42,45,56,70,72,73, 75,87,92]

2. Definitive management of pancreatic injuries in the absence of injury to the common duct or duodenum requires recognition of pancreatic ductal injury and, generally, either resection of the distal segment if less than 50 to 60 percent of the gland, or drainage of the distal segment if it exceeds 60 to 70 percent of the gland by means of a Roux-en-Y limb of jejunum. The pancreaticojejunosotomy should be an end-to-side duct to an jejunal mucosa anastomosis.[10] While most patients do not become diabetic unless 80 percent of the gland is resected, an occasional patient may do so with what is judged to be less than an 80 percent resection.[25] Aside from the fact that we have no way of knowing whether these patients were prediabetic, it seems prudent, particularly in the young, to leave some margin of protection for the surgeon's estimate of what constitutes an 80 percent resection in a particular gland. When a gland lacks an uncinate process there is a marked decrease in volume of the head of the pancreas. The surgeon may not recognize this normal variation and assume a resection of the neck of the gland is removing 60 to 65 percent of the gland when it is more likely, in the congenital absence of the uncinate, 70 to 80 percent of the gland being removed.

While definitive therapy of the pancreatic injury is an important goal in pancreatic injury, the first priority is to save the patient's life and in the event the patient's condition is precarious from associated injuries and operative time needs to be minimized, the pancreatic ductal disruption can be managed by sump drainage.[37,38,72,74] Creation of a controlled fistula will prevent loculated collections which otherwise could culminate in pseudocyst or abscess formation.

3. Most duodenal injuries (85 percent) can be managed by debridement and simple closure.[70,73] However, those few patients with 75 percent circumferential crush injuries, large lacerations with loss of tissue, or devascularization of a large segment of duodenum require an operative solution tailored to the anatomy of the injury.[70] No one operation for duodenal repair is suitable for all duodenal injuries. Therefore, the trauma surgeon, to do best by the patient, must be familiar with those operative procedures most appropriate for injuries of different size and shape in a variety of duodenal locations, as well as taking into account the patient's general condition from associated injuries or preexisting illness.[16,18,54,70,73]

4. In an injury of the common duct and duodenum in association with a pancreatic ductal disruption, there is potential for much mischief from the devastation created by uncontrolled loss of a combination of gastric, duodenal, pancreatic, and biliary secretions, which may lead to fluid and electrolyte disorders, dehydration,

digestion of skin, intraabdominal collections, abscesses, and sepsis. Therefore, it is essential intestinal and ductal integrity be established by pancreaticoduodenectomy or diversionary drainage, separating the secretions if the patient is judged by the operating surgeon to be unable to tolerate pancreaticoduodenectomy.[1,3,9,12,24,26,28,31,37,45,50,56,59,65,75,87,89,93]

PANCREATIC INJURY AND ITS OPERATIVE MANAGEMENT

Types of Trauma

Suburban hospitals receiving auto accident victims tend to report a higher incidence of blunt than penetrating injuries of the pancreas.[3] In trauma centers located in the metropolitan areas, most injuries result from penetrating trauma.[34,74,87]

One factor that contributes to the mortality of patients with pancreatic trauma are the nature of the wounding agent, with shotgun injuries being the most lethal and stab wounds the least (Table 6-2).[37] Likewise, the condition of the patient on arrival in the emergency department and in the operating room is important; if in shock from associated injuries to major vessels of liver or spleen, the patient's mortality is six times higher than for the patient who is normotensive during preoperative and operative management.[37,74,89] The massive tissue destruction associated with shotgun injuries (58 percent mortality) and the presence of shock are not usually a reflection of the severity of the pancreatic injury, but of the injuries to major vessels or liver and spleen.[28,37,87,89] Sepsis, the second most common cause of death after hemorrhage, is most often seen in patients who are in hemorrhagic shock pre and postoperatively, and in those with associated bowel injuries.[33,37,74,89] Factors related to the pancreas that adversely affect survival are the location of the wound in the head of the gland with injury to the major duct and overlooked injuries of the major duct. [3,70,80] We prefer posterior drainage of the pancreas below the 12th rib. When the major pancreatic duct is intact, leakage from tributary ducts will be short-lived and drainage may be expected to subside in four to six weeks. If a major ductal injury is recognized but the patient's condition is unstable, prohibiting definitive treatment, and the injury is drained, then it is advisable to employ a sump drainage. With injury to the major duct, these controlled fistulae are often persistent and further operative management may be required after the patient is fully recovered from any associated injuries.

Injuries Limited to the Pancreas

The junction of the neck and body of the pancreas is the most common site of injury (see Figure 6-3). The portion of pancreas distal to the neck and body constitutes about 60 to 65 percent of the mass of the pancreas and can, therefore, be resected with little immediate or late morbidity from pancreatic exocrine or endocrine insufficiency (Fig. 6-4). [25] Distal pancreatic resection is the treatment of choice for any

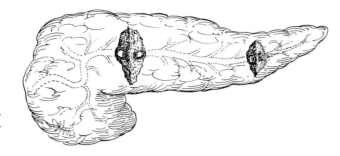

Figure 6-4 Lesions readily amenable to treatment by distal pancreatic resection.

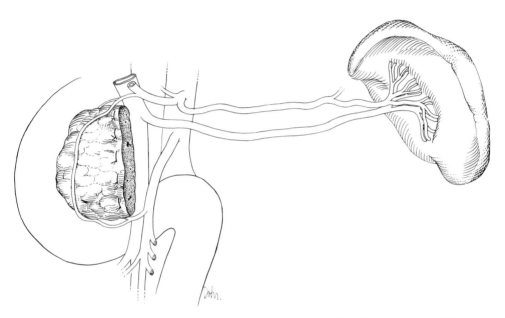

Figure 6-5 An example of extensive distal pancreatic resection (80%) with preservation of the spleen and its blood supply. The preservation of the splenic vein is crucial and the dissection is difficult and indicated only in good risk patients with isolated pancreatic injury.

injury involving the neck, body, or tail of the pancreas from either penetrating or blunt trauma (Figure 6-5).

The pancreas is usually resected with the spleen in continuity. Short gastrics are divided and the attachments between the splenic flexure and the colon and the spleen are severed. The spleen and tail of the pancreas are mobilized and rotated left to right, the splenic artery is divided as it joins the body of the pancreas, and the pancreas is transected at the point of the laceration. Interrupted, interlocking mattress sutures of 2-0 silk on an atraumatic needle is the preferred method of closing the severed distal end of the pancreas. The main pancreatic duct should be identified and separately ligated. In isolated injuries of the pancreas, it is possible to preserve the spleen by ligating and dividing the branches of the splenic vein and artery to the tail of the pancreas.

Eighty to 95 percent resection of the distal portion of the pancreas can be carried out in injuries involving the major pancreatic duct in the head of the gland. However, because of the high incidence of pancreatic endocrine and exocrine insufficiency,

80 to 95 percent resection should only be carried out when the patient is unstable and preferrably already a diabetic and a short operation is essential for survival. For the proximal pancreatic ductal fractures, there is a better option than 80 to 95 percent distal resection, that is, oversewing the proximal severed end of pancreas with interlocking mattress sutures of 2-0 silk and then anastomosing the distal end of the pancreas end-to-side into a Roux-en-Y limb of jejunum in a duct to jejunal mucosa anastomosis (Figure 6-6). We do not recommend placement of a Roux-en-Y jejunal limb blindly over fresh lacerations and stellate fractures in lieu of a duct to jejunal

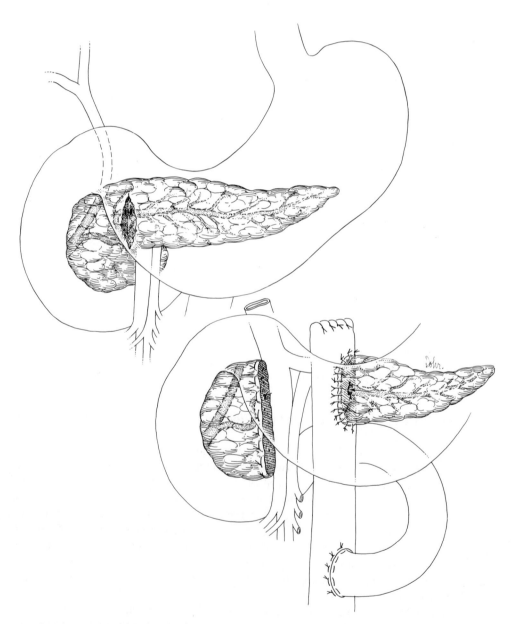

Figure 6–6   In many instances of injury to the head of the pancreas, preservation of the tail of the pancreas may be indicated to prevent diabetes.

mucosal anastomosis nor do we recommend trying to drain the proximal portion of the pancreas into the Roux-en-y limb as well as the distal segment in a T-type anastomosis. Draining the proximal segment of the pancreas with a Roux-en-Y limb is unnecessary and may compromise the anastomosis of the distal segment of pancreas with a Roux-en-Y limb. There is the additional risk of gastrointestinal contamination from two rather than one suture line. If the duodenum and common bile duct are intact, pancreaticoduodenectomy is not indicated for a major pancreatic ductal injury in the head of the gland. In the very occasional patient, in whom there has been minimal trauma to the adjacent pancreatic tissue, a primary repair of the fractured duct may be considered.[24,47]

DUODENAL INJURIES

Mortality

In major trauma centers, half the deaths, 8 percent of cases in which the duodenum is injured, occur early from massive hemorrhage and shock due to associated extra-duodenal injuries (see Table 6-6). Most of these patients die in the operating room or within 72 hours of injury. The duodenal injury in these instances has little to do with the fatal outcome.[16,70,73]

Factors that contribute to a fatal outcome in the other 8 percent of patients include delays in operative treatment owing to failure to diagnose the injury or to recognize it at operation. The operative mortality in these patients, most of whom have had blunt trauma, is 40 to 50 percent if the delay in operative therapy is 24 hours or longer.[16,46,70] The location of the duodenal wound and the size of the wound are believed to influence the mortality.[70,74] The larger the duodenal wound, the more complex the operation is to reconstitute intestinal continuity. The wounding agent is also important, in that the agent affects the size of the wound, shotgun wounds being most lethal and stab wounds the least (Table 6-5).

Associated Injuries

Penetrating wounds most frequently affect liver, small and large bowel, pancreas, and stomach. The great vessels are always involved in the early deaths. Blunt trauma more often effects the solid organs, that is, the liver, spleen, pancreas, and kidney.[18] Mortality of duodenal wounds increases as the number of associated injuries increases.

ISOLATED DUODENAL INJURIES IN THE ABSENCE OF INJURY TO THE PANCREAS OR COMMON BILE DUCT

The site and presence of duodenal injury may be identified at operation by tracing the missile track or noting the site of active bleeding or hematoma, or by bile staining or crepitation of surrounding tissues. A higher percentage of blunt injuries than penetrating trauma, 46 percent versus 7 percent, can be said to be extensive, extensive being defined as involving more than 75 percent of the circumference of the duodenal wall according to Snyder, and colleagues (Figure 6-7).[70] Fortunately, in most patients with penetrating duodenal injury, the wounds are not extensive and local debridement and duodenal closure in two layers is safe and sufficient therapy.[70,73] The closure of the duodenum should be performed without tension. This

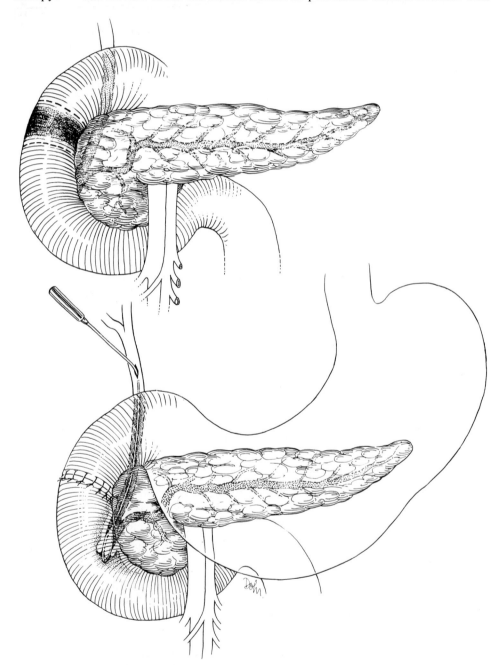

Figure 6–7 Lacerations of the duodenum may be treated by primary suture or by resection and reanastamosis if there is segmental circumferential injury.

may be accomplished by closing the duodenum either in a transverse or vertical direction according to Krauss and Gordon.[41] The mortality associated with duodenotomy is high but attributed to the condition that prompted duodenotomy.[35]

In larger defects, application of a serosal patch may be helpful. There is controversy over whether tube duodenostomy or gastrostomy is beneficial in these injuries.[46,70,73]

The more extensive duodenal wounds require segmental resection or Roux-en-Y duodenojejunostomy (Figure 6-8). Segmental resection and end-to-end anastomosis with standard two-layer closure is indicated in circumferential crush injuries. This can be accomplished in the first, second, third, or fourth portion of duodenum. In order to avoid injury to the common duct and ampulla, the distal bile duct can be intubated with a Bakes dilator passed into the duodenum and maintained there during the resection and anastomosis. If a large segment of duodenum has been devitalized and segmental resection performed, it may not be possible to mobilize sufficient duodenum to perform an end-to-end duodenostomy. This problem, particularly if the duodenal injury is distal to the ampulla, lends itself to Roux-en-Y duodenojejunostomy (Figure 6-9). The jejunum is divided 20 cm distal to the ligament of Treitz. The distal limb of the jejunum is advanced and anastomosed end-to-end to the proximal duodenum. Proximal jejunum is anastomosed end-to-side 30 cm from the site of duodenojejunostomy. The distal duodenum can be oversewn.

Duodenojejunostomy side-to-end has limited applicability except for injuries of the third part of the duodenum along its antimesenteric border (see Fig. 6-9). Occasionally useful is the duodenal patch by Roux-en-Y duodenojejunostomy. Patients having more than one duodenal perforation or extensive loss of duodenal tissue may be candidates for the diverticulization procedure as originally described by Berne and simplified by Graham, Maddox, Vaughan, and Jordon (Figure 6-10).[7,28] The diverticulization procedure is only applicable if closure of the duodenum is still possible. As described by Berne, the procedure included antrectomy, gastrojejunostomy, end tube duodenostomy, T-tube biliary drainage, and oversewing the duodenal lacerations.[7] Mortality associated with its use is reported to be 16 percent.[8] Diverticulization avoids stimulation of the pancreas by preventing hydrochloric acid entering the duodenum. If the duodenal repair fails, diversion of gastric secretion from the duodenum converts a potentially lethal duodenal leak into a more benign fistula.

We do not ordinarily recommend gastrostomy or conventional tube jejunostomy for simple duodenal wounds, as the chance of peritoneal contamination is increased which would outweigh any benefits derived from their use.

MAJOR PANCREATIC DUCTAL DISRUPTIONS IN PANCREAS HEAD WITH ASSOCIATED DUDOENAL LACERATION

Except under unusual circumstances, neither 80 to 95 percent distal pancreatectomy nor pancreaticoduodenectomy is indicated.

Segmental resection and end-to-end repair of the duodenum is often possible in the duodenum even in the second portion close to the ampulla of Vater. A Fogarty irrigation catheter may be employed to intubate the ampulla of Vater through the

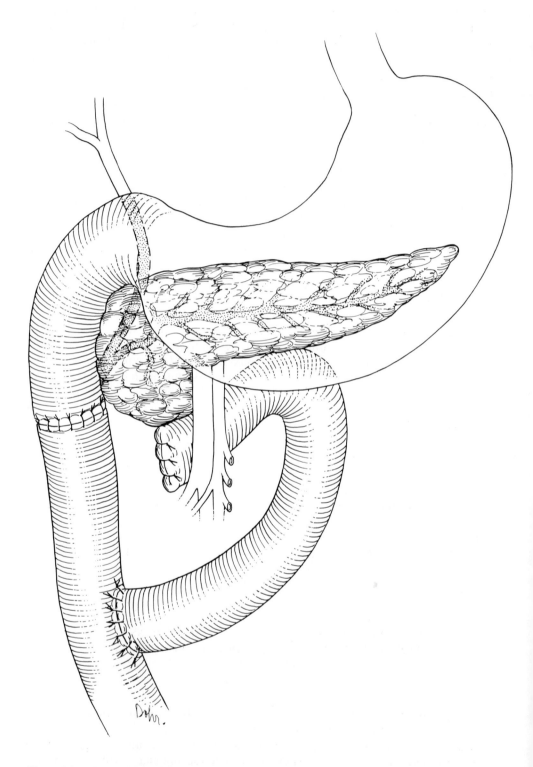

Figure 6–8   Distal duodenal injuries may be treated by resection and duodenal jejunal anastomosis.

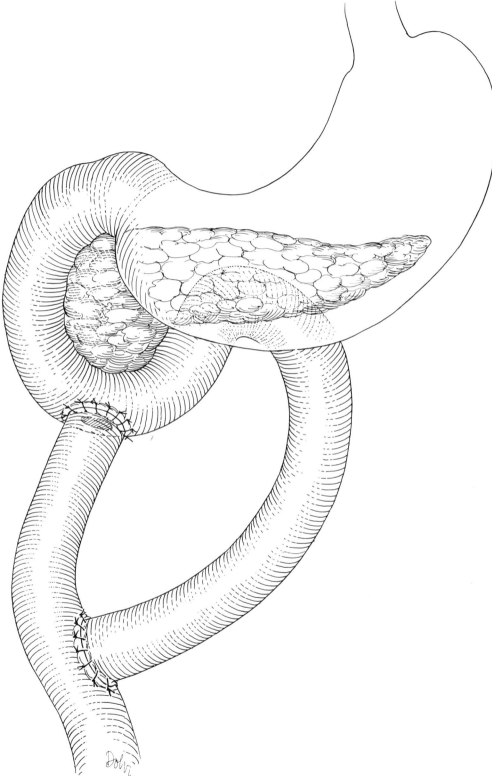

Figure 6–9 In rare instances, localized duodenal injuries may be treated by jejunal patch or Roux-en-Y duodenal anastomosis as shown here.

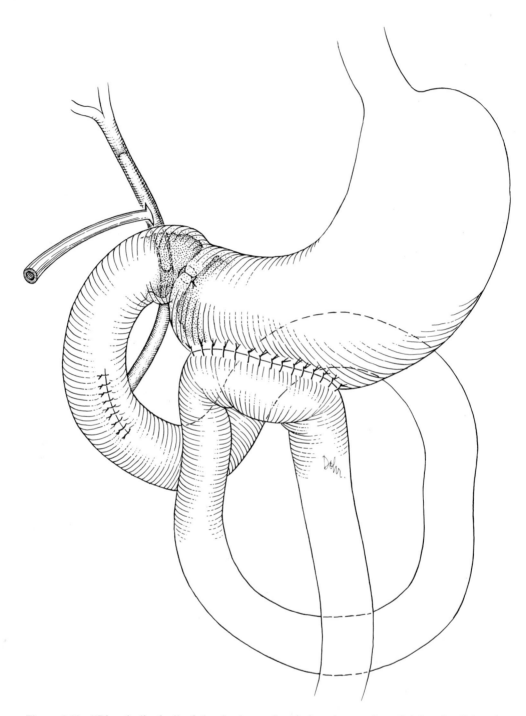

Figure 6–10 "Diverticulization" of the duodenum in this instance consists of defunctionalizing the duodenal injury by sewing the pylorus shut from inside utilizing a distal gastrotomy, then following this with a gastrojejunostomy.

duodenal wound to obtain an on-the-table pancreaticogram or to ascertain the integrity of the pancreatic duct. If the duct is found to be injured in the head of the gland, a Roux-en-Y jejunal limb may be used to drain the distal segment of pancreas. The proximal end of the pancreas is oversewn (Figure 6-11).

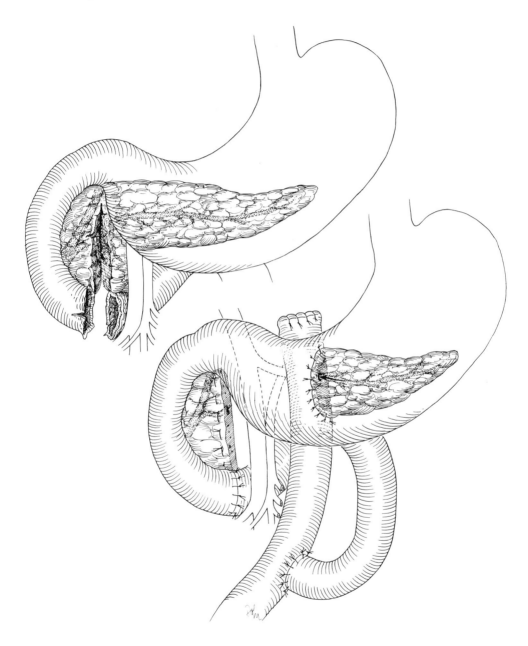

Figure 6–11   Combined duodenal pancreatic ductal injury is treated by resection of the body of the gland, repairing the duodenum and draining the distal pancreas into a Roux-en-Y jejunal limb.

When the duodenum is extensively lacerated, but repair is still possible but tenuous and the pancreatic duct is transected in the head of the pancreas, the surgeon is faced with a dilemma. There is no really ideal operation that deals with both a major duodenal injury and major pancreatic duct injury. The surgeon must weigh the risk of a less extensive procedure, such as duodenal exclusion or diverticulization, which does not adequately deal with the major pancreatic duct fracture as Jones has noted, against that of a procedure, pancreaticoduodenectomy, which does deal with the problem but has the disadvantage of requiring a biliary anastomosis when none is required by the injury.[37]

Duodenal diverticulization as described by Berne is effective in the management of duodenal laceration, as it diverts gastric and biliary secretions from the duodenum.[7] Likewise, temporary pyloric exclusion, described by Graham and colleagues, which includes sewing the pylorus shut with absorbable suture is an effective method for dealing with major duodenal injury.[28] However, neither of these operations provide for management of an associated major ductal injury of the pancreas except by Penrose or sump drainage. Therefore, we must remain skeptical that pyloric exclusion or diverticulization of the duodenum is a procedure with a major role in the management of both a major duodenal injury and major pancreatic duct fracture, because neither operation addresses the problem of major pancreatic ductal disruption.

Injuries of the pancreas in which the major pancreatic duct remains intact are not associated with serious sequelae, and should not be considered significant injuries. Patients whose duodenal wound was treated definitively but in whom the injury to the major pancreatic duct was treated by suction, may require re-operation if the fistula from the distal pancreas has not closed in three to four months.

COMBINED DUODENAL AND BILIARY TRACT
INJURIES

These serious injuries fortunately occur in only about 5 percent of all duodenal injuries.[70] In patients with injury to the duodenum and common duct, it may be possible to perform duodenal closure and an end-to-side choledochojejunostomy to a Roux-en-Y limb of jejunum after injury to the major pancreatic duct has been ruled out by retrograde pancreaticogram (Figure 6-12). Rarely, avulsion of the ampulla in association with duodenal injury may occur. This injury has also been treated by closure of the duodenum, and placement of the ampulla of Vater end-to-side to a Roux-en-Y jejunal limb, however, more than likely, combined duodenal and biliary tract injuries will require pancreaticoduodenectomy if the duodenal injury is major.[21,43] Pancreaticoduodenectomy is justified in patients with this injury, which has a serious prognosis. Pancreaticoduodenectomy for trauma has a 30 percent mortality associated with its use, but with other forms of treatment, the mortality is closer to 100 percent. [37,40,45,79,89,92] The common duct is usually of normal caliber and therefore not as easy to anastomose successfully through an isolated loop of bowel as is the obstructed duct associated with pancreatic tumor or chronic pancreatitis. Nonetheless, a pancreaticoduodenectomy can and should be carried out when indicated. While the antrum of the stomach is resected in pancreaticoduodenectomy for cancer, it is not necessary in trauma and, as Traverso and Longmire have shown, the antrum can be preserved.[83]

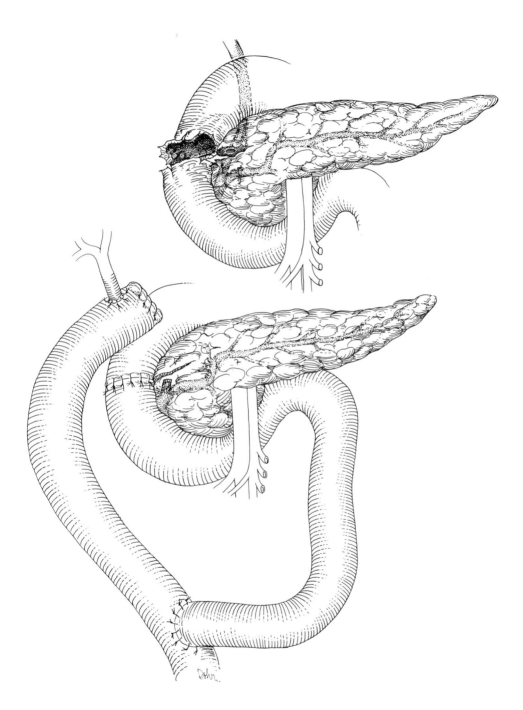

Figure 6–12 The combined duodenal biliary lesion is treated by duodenal repair and choledochojejunostomy using a Roux-en-Y limb.

The maximal length of common duct should be preserved by carrying the dissection of the common duct under the duodenum before dividing it. The pancreatic head should be mobilized carefully from the portal vein and the gastroduodenal artery ligated as it passes under the duodenum. The uncinate process can then be mobilized from the mesenteric vessels after the mesocolon is retracted downward and separated from the body of the pancreas and it is divided at the site of the fracture. During the dissection of the uncinate, careful attention must be paid to the possibility of a right hepatic, accessory hepatic, or totally replaced hepatic artery arising from the superior mesenteric artery and transversing the uncinate portion of the head of the pancreas.[49,50,79] The splenic vein is preserved at its junction with the superior mesenteric vein. In freeing up the distal segment of pancreas from the splenic vein, numerous small veins entering the pancreas directly from the splenic vein need to be divided and ligated. After removal of the head and uncinate, the distal end of the pancreas is anastomosed end-to-side to the Roux-en-Y jejunal limb in a duct-to-jejunal mucosal anastomosis performed with 4-0 or 5-0 braided polyester sutures. An end-to-side anastomosis between the common duct and the jejunal limb can then be performed 10 to 15 cm distal to the pancreatic anastomosis using a precise two-layered anastomosis. Twenty to 30 centimeters further distal, an end-to-side gastrojejunostomy or pylorojejunostomy can be carried out (Fig. 6-13).

COMBINED DUODENAL, COMMON BILE DUCT, AND MAJOR PANCREATIC DUCTAL INJURIES

Combined duodenal, common bile duct, and major pancreatic ductal injuries of the head of the pancreas (Figure 6-13) are fatal if treated by drainage alone and are best managed by a pancreaticoduodenectomy as recommended by Kerry and Glas and others (Figure 6-14).[1,3,5,6,112,23,24,26,31,34,37,40,45,56,65,75,80,89,92]

In the most severe combined pancreatic, duodenal, and biliary tract injuries also involving severe associated injuries to the liver and major vascular structures, it may be necessary to resort to a series of exteriorization procedures as recommended by Owens and Wolfman until the patient is stable enough to restore ductal and enteric continuity of the GI tract. [59,91]

POSTOPERATIVE CARE

In patients with pancreatic injuries, the gastrointestinal tract is kept at rest until the ileus has subsided. For major pancreatic injuries, we maintain the patients on nasogastric suction to avoid acid stimulation of the duodenum and bicarbonate secretion by the pancreas. For duodenal injuries we keep the gastrointestinal tract decompressed by nasogastric tube for an equivalent period of time. The patient is maintained on intravenous fluids. Should there be any overt evidence of complications, as manifest by severe ileus or infection, intravenous hyperalimentation is initiated four or five days postoperatively. If a duodenal diverticulization or pancreaticoduodenectomy has been performed, hyperalimentation may be initiated as soon postoperatively as the patient is hemodynamically stable.

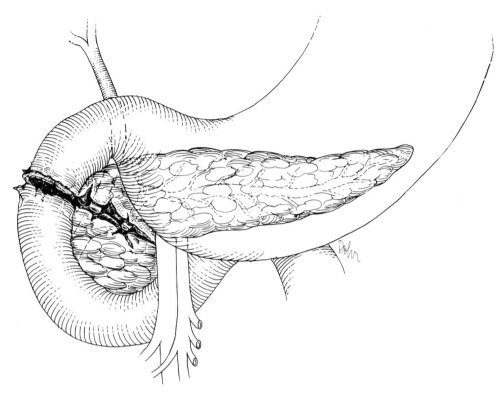

Figure 6–13 Demonstrates a combined duodenal, biliary and pancreatic ductal injury which is best treated as shown in Figure 6–14.

If, after five to seven days, the patient's condition is benign, nasogastric suction is discontinued. If this is not followed by symptoms and the patient's ileus has subsided, the patient may be started slowly on oral nutrition. Initially, clear liquids are given followed by a regular diet if the former is tolerated. Drains may be left in place until the patient is back on full activity and tolerating a regular diet without overt complications. This can involve the use of drains for ten days to two weeks or even longer if drainage persists. In such cases, drains are often removed on a return visit after hospital discharge. Ordinarily, if drainage has ceased by the fourth or fifth day or none has developed, the drains can be removed.

The possibility of infection should be anticipated. However, we do not use prophylactic antibiotics in clean injuries, that is, injuries limited to the pancreas alone. If penetrating trauma was the cause of injury or duodenal injury suspected pre-operatively, then antibiotics should be initiated pre-operatively. When duodenal injuries are encountered at operation, antibiotics should be started in the operating room when the injury is discovered.

COMPLICATIONS

The complications of pancreatic and duodenal injury are duodenal fistula, duodenal obstruction, pancreatic fistula, pancreatitis, pancreatic abscess and intraper-

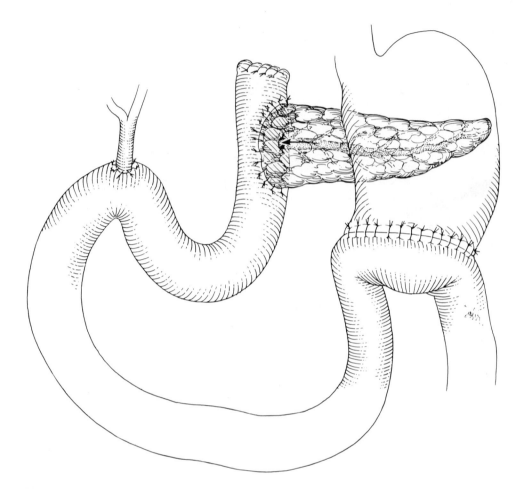

Figure 6–14 Showing a pancreatic duodenal resection followed by reanastomosis of pancreatic duct, common duct and gastrojejunostomy.

itoneal abscess and infection, pancreatic pseudocyst, and chronic pancreatitis. Complications most frequently associated with pancreatic injury are: pancreatic fistulas, the incidence of which is reported to be 3.6 to 35 percent; pancreatic abscesses, 2.3 to 20 percent; acute pancreatitis, 4.3 to 26 percent; and pseudocysts, 1.1 to 9.1 percent. Pancreatic fistulas and pseudocysts are most common after blunt trauma.[87] Abscesses and sepsis are most frequently associated with shock on admission to the hospital from hemorrhage due to associated injuries to major vessels as well as liver and spleen and the presence of colon injuries or contamination created by placement of jejunostomy or gastrostomy tubes.[30,33,37,39,72,73,74,80,87,88,89]

Complications most often noted in association with duodenal injuries are: duodenal fistulas, 3.6 to 7 percent; duodenal obstruction, 1.1 to 1.7 percent; intra-abdominal abscess, 10.9 to 18.4 percent; recurrent pancreatitis, 2.5 to 14.9 percent; common bile duct fistula, 1.3 percent.[70,73] The incidence of duodenal fistulas was lowest when jejunostomy and gastrostomy were employed by Stone, 3.6 percent.[73] However, he also had the highest rate of intra-abdominal abscess, 18.4 percent which may have resulted from contamination as a result of opening the GI tract to perform duodenal decompression.[73] Snyder, on the other hand, reported the adjunctive use of duodenal decompression, when used selectively, was associated with an incidence of duodenal fistula of 9 percent, two and a half times higher than Stone's and higher at his own institutions than in patients in whom no duodenal decompression was employed (5.6 percent).[70,73] The incidence of intra-abdominal abscess in Snyder's experience was 10.9 percent.[70]

In patients with combined pancreaticoduodenal injury (in the abscence of common duct injury), the combination alone does not increase mortality, however, associated injuries are more common than in either pancreatic or duodenal injuries alone and are more likely to involve the aorta and inferior vena cava.[28,70]

When the common duct is also injured in a pancreaticoduodenal injury or in association with duodenal injury without major pancreatic ductal injury, the complication and mortality rate are higher (Stone, 43 percent; Snyder and Graham, 26 percent) than in pancreatic or duodenal injuries alone or combined.[28,70,73] The incidence of duodenal, biliary, or pancreatic fistulas has been reported as high as 38 percent and the mortality rate between 15 and 40 percent.[73]

These complications occur with greater frequency following pancreatic and duodenal injuries combined with common duct injuries than with any other intra-abdominal injuries, and the lethality is secondary only to that following leakage of a colon anastomosis. In these massive combined injuries, there is no substitute for a definitive operation, that is, pancreaticoduodenectomy other than complete separation and diversion of bile, pancreatic, and gastric contents as described by Owens and Wolfman.[59] Simple drainage of these combined injuries is not adequate therapy.[40]

If the pancreas and duodenum are well drained posteriorly, the consequence of duodenal or pancreatic fistula are usually relatively benign. However, if the proximity of the drains to the area of leakage are remote, then there may not be immediate egress of pancreatic or duodenal secretions, resulting in severe complications such as retroperitoneal sepsis. Therefore, if the patient develops evidence of sepsis postoperatively, this is an indication for immediate reoperation and institution of posterior drainage.

Pancreatitis is a complication that results from obstruction of the pancreatic duct and should not occur if the injury to the duct was noted and appropriate operative treatment initiated at the time of initial injury. It is unlikely that edema and hemorrhage in an area adjacent to the duct results in sufficient obstruction to the duct to cause more than a self-limited pancreatitis.

However, in some patients, although an injury to the major pancreatic duct is identified at operation, the surgeon may feel the patient's condition is too unstable, owing to associated injuries, to withstand more than drainage.

Treatment in pancreatitis is initially supportive, maintaining the patient on nothing by mouth, nasogastric suction, and intravenous support, waiting out the complications. Intravenous hyperalimentation should be started once the patient has gone more than four or five days post-injury with no immediate prospect of taking food by mouth. Pancreatic ductal discontinuity is the cause of pancreatic fistulas after trauma, the most common complication of pancreatic injury, and wholly avoidable if detected and treated at operation.[3,4] If the patient's condition at time of operation does not permit definitive repair, sump drainage should be instituted to create a controlled fistula. Re-operation will usually be required at a later date to drain any fistula from a major pancreatic duct into a Roux-en-Y limb or resect the distal portion of gland responsible for the fistula secretion. Pancreatic ascites occurs when the ductal discontinuity leads to the pancreatic secretion from the distal segment of pancreas entering freely into the abdominal cavity.[31,61] The whole abdomen, in effect, becomes a pseudocyst.

Pancreatic ductal disruption may also lead to the complications of pancreatic pseudocyst or pancreatic abscess or pancreatitis.[23,33,70,73,83,88] Generally, a well-drained pancreas is not susceptible to these complications, even if the ductal injury is overlooked or couldn't be dealt with because of the patient's condition at the time of initial injury and operation. A pancreatic pseudocyst following trauma is usually associated with blunt injury and results from the accumulation of undrained enzymes secreted from the distal portion of the severed gland.[2,87] A persistent ileus in the absence of overt infection suggests the possibility of a local accumulation of pancreatic enzymes, which has become walled off in the form of a pseudocyst. Scintillation scans and CT scans may permit localization of the pseudocyst or abscesses and provide an indication for reoperation. Frequently, the primary manifestation of inflammation around the pancreas is pleural. A collection of fluid in the left pleural space following pancreatic injury is a manifestation of the collection of enzymes dissecting beneath the posterior portion of the diaphragm into the chest. Failure of the patient to respond to a conservative therapy is an indication for re-operation and drainage of the subphrenic space or internal drainage of the pancreatic pseudocyst. Occasionally, patients with traumatic pancreatitis, particularly children, will manifest osteolytic lesions that resolve spontaneously over time.[57]

Secondary intraperitoneal infection with abscess formation is not unusual following pancreatic injury.[37,73] An indication for re-operation in this instance is uncontrolled sepsis.

Persistent gastrointestinal obstruction, mechanical or functional, due to altered motility may develop secondary to pancreatitis or inflammation around a duodenal injury.[70] Generally this type of obstruction can be treated conservatively and will resolve spontaneously in four or five days to a week or two at most. The status of the GI tract can be assessed by x-ray contrast studies of the gastrointestinal tract. A few patients with pancreatic injury who have not been initially treated appropriately will go on to develop chronic pancreatitis associated with severe pain.[25] These patients must be treated as are other patients with chronic pancreatitis.[25]

In addition to specific complications related to the pancreas and duodenal injury, other complications such as respiratory failure, renal failure and, particularly, diffuse sepsis are complications of this major injury. These are treated as described in the previous section.

REFERENCES

1. Anderson CB, et al.: Combined pancreaticoduodenal trauma. Am J Surg 125:530-533, 1973.
2. Babb J, Harmon H: Diagnosis and management of pancreatic trauma. Am Surgeon 390-394, 1976.
3. Bach RD, Frey CF: Diagnosis and treatment of pancreatic trauma. Am J Surg 121:20-29, 1971.
4. Baker RJ, et al.: External pancreatic fistula following abdominal injury. Arch Surg 95:556-566, 1967.
5. Baker RJ, et al.: The surgical significance of trauma to the pancreas. Arch Surg 86:1038-1044, 1963.
6. Balasegarem M: Surgical management of pancreatic trauma. Am J Surg 131:536-540, 1976.
7. Berne CJ, Donovan AJ, Hagen WE: Combined duodenal pancreatic trauma: The role of end to side gastrojejunostomy. Arch Surg 96:712-722, 1968.
8. Berne CJ, et al.: Duodenal "diverticulization" for duodenal and pancreatic injury. Am J Surg 127:503-507, 1974.
9. Brawley RK, Cameron JL, Zuidema, GD: Severe upper abdominal injury treated by pancreatic duodenostomy. Surg Gynecol Obstet 126:516-522, 1968.
10. Cattel RB: A technique for pancreaticoduodenal resection. Surg Clin N Am 28:761-775, 1948.
11. Catell RB, Braasch JW: Technique for exposure of the third and fourth portion of the duodenum. Surg Gynecol Obstet 111:378, 1960.
12. Chambers RT, Norton L, Hinchey EJ: Massive right upper quadrant intra-abdominal injury requiring pancreaticoduodenectomy and partial hepatectomy. J Trauma 15:741-719, 1975.
13. Cleveland HC, Waddell, WR: Retroperitoneal rupture of the duodenum due to nonpenetrating trauma. Surg Clin N Am 43:413-431, 1963.
14. Cocke WM Jr, Meyer KK: Retroperitoneal duodenal rupture proposed mechanism: Reviews of literature and report of case. Am J Surg 108:834-839, 1964.

15. Cohn I, Hawthorne AR, Frofere AS: Retroperitoneal rupture of the duodenum. Am J Surg 84:293, 1952.
16. Corley RD, Norcross WJ, Shoemaker WS: Traumatic injuries to the duodenum: A report of 98 patients. Ann Surg 181:92-98, 1975.
17. Cross KR: Accessory pancreatic ducts: Special reference to the intrapancreatic portion of the C.D. Arch Path 61:323, 1956.
18. DeMars JJ, Bubrick MP, Hitchcock, CR: Duodenal perforation in blunt abdominal trauma. Surg 86: 632-638, 1979.
19. Doublier L, Garren A: LesPlaies duodeno-pancreatoques par projectiles. Lyon Chir 65:842-854, 1969.
20. Elman R, Arnesan N, Graham EA: Value of blood amylase estimations in the diagnosis of pancreatic disease. Arch Surg 19:943, 1929.
21. Fish SC, Johnson GL: Rupture of duodenum following blunt trauma: Report of a case with avulsion of papilla of Vater. Ann Surg 162:917-932, 1965.
22. Fraser CG: Handlebar injury of the pancreas. J Ped Surg 4:216-219, 1969.
23. Freeark RJ, et al.: Unusual aspects of pancreaticoduodenal trauma. J Trauma 6:482, 1966.
24. Freeark RJ, et al.: Traumatic disruption of the head of the pancreas. Arch Surg 91:5-13, 1965.
25. Frey CF, Child CG, Fry W: Pancreatectomy for chronic pancreatic. Ann Surg 184:403-414, 1976.
26. Gibbs BF, Crow JL, Rupnik ET: Pancreaticoduodenectomy for blunt pancreaticoduoenal injury. J Trauma 10:702-705, 1970.
27. Gougeon TW, et al.: Pancreatic trauma: A new diagnostic approach. Am J Surg 132:400, 1976.
28. Graham JM, et al.: Combined pancreaticoduodenal injuries. J Trauma 19:340-345, 1979.
29. Gray SW, Skandalakis JE: Embroyology for Surgeons, WB Saunders, Philadelphia, 1972.
30. Grosfeld JL, Cooney DR: Pancreatic and gastrointestinal trauma in children. Ped Clin N Am 22:365-377, 1975.
31. Halgrimson CG, et al.: Pancreaticoduodenectomy for traumatic lesions. Am J Surg 118:877-882, 1969.
32. Heiss FW, Shea JA: Association of pancreatitis and varient ductal anatomy, dominant drainage of the duct of Santorini. Am J Gastro 70:158-162, 1978.
33. Heitsch RC, et al.: Delineation of critical factors in the treatment of pancreatic trauma. Surgery 80:523-529 1976.
34. Heyse-Moore GH: Blunt pancreatic and pancreaticoduodenal trauma. Br J Surg 63:226-228, 1976.
35. Hutchinson WB: Duodenotomy. Am J Surg 122:777-780, 1971.
36. Janson KL, Stockinger F: Duodenal hematoma. Am J Surg 129:304-308, 1975.
37. Jones RC: Management of pancreatic trauma. Ann Surg 187:555-564, 1978.
38. Jordon GL, Overton R, Werschky LR: Traumatic transaction of the pancreas. South Med J 62:90-93, 1969.
39. Karl HW, Chandler JG: Mortality and morbidity of pancreaticoduodenectomy. Am J Surg 134:549-554, 1977.
40. Kerry RL, Glas WW: Traumatic injuries of the pancreas and duodenum. Arch Surg 85:813-816, 1962.
41. Kraus M, Gordon RE: Alternate techniques of duodenotomy. Surg Gynecol Obstet 139:417-419, 1974.
42. LaLaoude J, Segal P, Evaard C: Les traumatiques du pancreas a propes de 11 observations. Ann Chir 27:278-284 1973.
43. Lee D, Zacher J, Vogel TT: Primary repair in transection of duodenum with avulsion of the common duct. Arch Surg 111:592-593, 1976.
44. Letton, AH, Wilson VP: Traumatic severance of pancreas treated by Roux-en-Y anastomosis. Surg Gynecol Obstet 109:473-478, 1959.
45. Lowe RJ, Saletta JD, Moss GS: Pancreaticoduodenectomy for penetrating pancreatic trauma. J Trauma 17:732-747, 1977.
46. Lucas CE, Ledgerwood AM: Factors influencing outcome after blunt duodenal injury. J Trauma 15:839-846, 1975.
47. Martin LW, Henderson BM, Welsh N: Disruption of the head of the pancreas caused by blunt trauma in children: A report of two cases treated with primary repair of the pancreatic duct. Surgery 63:697-700, 1968.
48. McCorkle H, Goldman L: The clinical significance of the serum amylase test in the diagnosis of acute pancreatitis. Surg Gynecol Obstet 74:439-445, 1942.
49. Michels NA: The hepatic, cystic and retroduodenal arteries and their relation to the biliary ducts. Ann Surg 133:503, 1951.
50. Michels NA: Blood supply and anatomy of the upper abdominal organs. JB Lippincott, Philadelphia and Montreal, 1955.
51. Millbourn E: On excretory ducts of pancreas in man, with special reference to their relation to each other, to common bile duct and to duodenum. Radiological and anatomical study. Acta Anat 9:1-34, 1950.
52. Miller RT: Retroperitoneal rupture of the duodenum by blunt trauma. Ann Surg 64:550, 1916.
53. Moretz JA III, et al.: Significance of serum amylase in evaluating pancreatic trauma. Am J Surg 13:739-741, 1975.
54. Morton JR, Jordon GL Jr: Traumatic duodenal injuries, review of 131 cases. J Trauma 8:127-139, 1968.
55. Nafziger HC, McCorkle HJ: The recognition and management of acute trauma of the pancreas, with

particular reference to the use of the serum amylase test. Ann Surg 118:594-602, 1943.
56. Nance FC, DeLoach DH: Pancreticoduodenectomy following abdominal trauma. J Trauma 11:577-585, 1971.
57. Neuer FS, Roberts FF, McCostle V: Osteolytic lesions following traumatic pancreatitis. Am J Dis Ch 131: 738-740, 1977.
58. Otis GA (ed.): The Medical and Surgical History of the War of the Rebellion, Part II, Vol II. Chapter VI: Penetrating wounds of the abdomen; surgical history. Government Printing Office, Washington D C, 1876, pp. 158-161.
59. Owens MP, Wolfman EF: Pancreatic trauma: Management and presentation of a new technique. Surgery 73: 881-886, 1973.
60. Pantazelos HH, Kerhulos AA, Byrne JJ: Total pancreaticoduodenectomy for trauma. Ann Surg 170: 1016-1020, 1969.
61. Parrish RA, Humphries AL, Moretz WH: Massive pancreatic ascites. Arch Surg 96:887, 1968.
62. Pollock AV: Pancreatic trauma and idiopathic retroperitoneal fibrosis: Long term follow up study of 4 patients. Br J Surg 61:42, 1974.
63. Poole LH: Wounds of the pancreas (62 casualties). Surgical History of World War II, Chapter XXII, Office of the Surgeon General Government Printing Office. Washington DC.
64. Sako Y, et al.: A survey of evacuation, resuscitation, and mortality in a forward surgical hospital. Surgery 37:602-611, 1955.
65. Salyer K, McClelland RN: Pancreaticoduodenectomy for trauma. Arch Surg 93:636-639, 1967.
66. Schumaker ED: Zur duodenum chirurgie. Beitr Z Klin Chir 71:482, 1910.
67. Sheldon GF, Cohn LH, Blaisdell FW: Surgical treatment of pancreatic trauma. J Trauma 10:795-800, 1970.
68. Skandalakis JE, et al.: Anatomical complications of pancreatic surgery. Cont Surg 15:21-50, 1979.
69. Smanio T: Varying relations of the common bile duct with the posterior face of the pancreas in Negroes and White persons. J Int Coll Su 22:150, 1954.
70. Snyder WH, et al.: The surgical management of duodenal trauma. Arch Sur 115:422, 1980.
71. Stauffer VG, Grob M: Traumatiische: Pankreaspseudo zystem im kindesalter. Helv Paediat Acta 26:625-635, 1971.
72. Steele M, Sheldon GF, Blaisdell FW: Pancreatic injuries. Arch Surg 106:544-549, 1973.
73. Stone HH, Fabian TC: Management of duodenal wounds. J Trauma 19:334-339, 1979.
74. Stone HH, Stowers KB, Shippey SH: Injuries to the pancreas. Arch Surg 85:525-530, 1962.
75. Sturm JT, et al.: Patterns of injury requiring pancreaticoduodenectomy. Surg Gynecol Obstet 137:629-632, 1973.
76. Taxier M, et al.: ERCP in the evaluation of trauma to the pancreas. Surg Gynecol Obstet 150:65-68, 1980.
77. Thal AP, Wilson RF: A pattern of severe blunt trauma to the region of the pancreas. Surg Gynecol Obstet 119:773-778, 1964.
78. Thomassen B, et al.: Blunt pancreatic trauma. Act Chir Sc 139:48-54, 1973.
79. Thompson IM: On the arteries and ducts in the hepatic pedacle: A study in statistical human anatomy. U CA Publ Anat 1:55, 1953.
80. Thompson RJ, Jr, Hinshow DB: Pancreatic trauma: Review of 87 cases. Ann Surg 163:153-160, 1966.
81. Thomson RG, McFarland JB: Traumatic rupture of the pancreas with complications. Br J Surg 56:117-120, 1969.
82. Tavers B: Rupture of the pancreas. Lancet 12:384, 1827.
83. Traverso W, Longmire W: Preservation of the pylorus during pancreaticoduodenectomy. Surg Gynecol Obstet 146: 959, 1978.
84. Walters RL, Gasperd DJ, Germann TD: Traumatic pancreatitis. Am J Surg 111:364-368, 1966.
85. Walton AJ: A Textbook of the Surgical Dyspepsias. Edward, Arnold Co, London, 1923.
86. Weitzman JJ, Rothschild PD: The surgical management of traumatic rupture of the pancreas due to blunt trauma. Surg Clin N Am 48:1347-1352, 1968.
87. Werschky LR, Jordon GL: Surgical management of traumatic injuries to the pancreas. Am J Surg 116: 768-772, 1968.
88. White PH, Benfield JR: Amylase in the management of pancreatic trauma. Arch Surg 105:158-163,1972.
89. Wilson RF, et al.: Pancreatic trauma. J Trauma 7:643-651, 1967.
90. Wittinger J, Frey CF: Islet concentration in the head, body, tail and uncinate process of the pancreas. Ann Surg 179:412-414, 1974.
91. Wurtz A, Henriet P, Ribet M: Fistuliarterio veinuse renocave traumatique et plaie duodenopancrea-tique. Chirurgie 99:489-493, 1973.
92. Yellin NE, Rosoff I: Pancreaticoduodenectomy for combined pancreaticoduodenal injuries. Arch Surg 110:1177-1182, 1975.
93. Yeo CK, McNorman J: Retroperitoneal rupture of the duodenum with complicating gas gangrene. Arch Surg 106:856-857, 1973.
94. Flint LM, et al.: Duodenal injury: Analysis of common misconceptions in diagnosis and treatment. Ann Surg 697-702, 1980.

Chapter Seven

INJURIES TO THE LIVER AND EXTRA HEPATIC DUCTS

ROBERT C. LIM, JR.

INTRODUCTION

The liver is the largest organ in the abdomen. It weighs approximately 1500 g and plays an essential role in carbohydrate, protein, and fat metabolism for sustaining life. Because of its size and vulnerability, it is probably the most frequently injured abdominal organ following penetrating and blunt trauma. Many minor injuries are undoubtedly not diagnosed, so that, statistically, the frequency of injury appears second to that involving the spleen.

In "Notes on the Arrest of Hepatic Hemorrhage Due to Trauma," J.H.Pringle (1908) discussed 8 patients whom he had treated and noted that when his 'assistant held the portal vein and the hepatic artery between a finger and thumb it completely arrested all bleeding."[1] He went on to state that this method was earlier described by Ponfick in animals and had disastrous results. However, when he performed his own experiments on rabbits to test out this method of vascular arrest and the use of large mass sutures to control bleeding from the amputated stump of the liver, all the animals survived. Subsequently, he applied these two techniques successfully on his patients. Other methods of compressing the liver edge, with strips of whale bone, as described by Cecherelli and Bianchi, or strips of magnesium, as described by Payr and Martina, were noted by Pringle; however, he did not believe these approaches had any permanent place in the surgery of the liver. He felt the method of mass suture, which was earlier described by Kusnetzoff and Pensky, would easily compress the margin of the liver. He described passing the suture a distance from the liver edge, tying it tightly to cut through the liver tissue so as to occlude the vessels. With release of the portal vessels little bleeding would be encountered. Pringle also described the use of packing for control of liver lacerations, which was the method of treating liver bleeding until the 1940s.

It was not until World War II that a group with extensive experience in caring for a large number of liver injuries logically analyzed their results and came forth with certain principles in surgical management, i.e., early operative treatment, avoiding gauze packing in the wound, and adequate drainage of the injury.[2]

In the 1960s, with advances in surgical technique and anesthesia, hepatic resection was introduced into the management of severe liver trauma. Principles laid down by Quattlebaum (1959) were followed.[3] McClellan and colleagues described 259 patients, of whom 9.6 percent were treated by resection.[4] This method of management became popular and numerous reports of liver resection appeared in the literature during that decade.[5,6,7,8]

With early operative intervention, patients survived injuries which previously were fatal and injuries to the hepatic veins and inferior vena cava became the major challenge to the surgeon. Methods for vascular control were necessary to prevent exsanguinating hemorrhage during repair. Schrock and associates studied cadavers, recommended the use of a shunt through the atrium to permit caval isolation, and tried it on one patient.[9] Other reports on this same theme subsequently appeared.[10] At the present time, vascular isolation use is selective and is most applicable for caval hepatic vein injuries (See chapter 13).

During the same time, attention was focused on extra hepatic biliary injuries.[11,12] Although such injuries were rare, complications were frequent, so management was directed toward repair techniques and minimizing complications resulting from the repair techniques. Biliary fistula observed after liver trauma was thought to be due to intrabiliary pressure allowing persistent leakage through the damaged ductiles. Merendino and colleagues (1963) advocated routine T-tube drainage to decompress the biliary system.[13] Lucas and Walt, in experimental and clinical studies, showed that the complication rate was higher in those with T-tube drainage.[14] However, the experience in the Vietnam conflict showed no difference between using biliary drainage and not using it.[15]

In 1967, Mays published a series of articles describing the efficacy of hepatic artery ligation in the management of exanguinating wounds of the liver.[16] He later refined his method to selective lobar artery ligation as the optimal location for hepatic artery control. Others have found this method a major adjunct in the management of massive bleeding from the liver.[17,18]

Since then, emphasis has been placed on postoperative management following liver trauma. Lim and associates described the use of fresh blood in these massively transfused patients.[18] Treatment of the consumptive coagulopathy which developed in these patients consisted of the use of fresh blood, fresh frozen plasma, or platelet concentrates or some combination of these agents. Meticulous monitoring of the patient's hemodynamic status to ensure adequate blood flow was essential, especially for patients after liver resection. Glucagon was introduced to increase total liver blood flow, primarily following major hepatic resection.[20,21] Early use of intravenous hyperalimentation has also become an important adjunct in the trauma surgeon's armamentarium.[22] Miller and colleagues have shown that immunocompetence is seriously compromised in these trauma victims.[23] Their studies in animals show that it can be reversed by the early institution of intravenous hyperalimentation.

In spite of these advances, injuries to the liver often still result in mortality. Although overall mortality was 60 to 65 percent in the pre-1940 era, it has stabilized at about 15 percent today. The mortality average from blunt trauma is 25 percent and from penetrating injury it is 5 percent. The mortality in penetrating wounds depends largely on the type of weapon used. In stab wounds from knives or in low-velocity gunshot wounds the primary problem relates to obtaining hemostasis, and complications are low. Often, these injuries are singular and recovery is uneventful. However, in high-velocity gunshot wounds or shotgun wounds, extensive parenchymal damage usually results, which necessitates extensive debridement or formal hepatic lobectomy. The mortality rate from these latter injuries is high, at about 50 percent, and the incidence of associated injuries is in the range of 75 to 80%. Associated injuries involving the gastrointestinal tract are particularly lethal because they often result in death from sepsis or multiple organ failure.

Hepatic trauma from blunt injury is more serious than from penetrating injuries. Thirty-one percent in Morton and colleagues' report on blunt trauma died, whereas in their series on penetrating injuries, the mortality rate was only 3 percent from stab wounds and 15 percent from gunshot wounds. [24] In spite of the large size of the liver, it lies under and is protected by the right lower rib cage. However, if the force of injury is great, the liver is often crushed under the ribs. In a study by Trollope, on primates, it was noted that the force necessary to create a liver injury appears to be less when transmitted directly onto the liver than directly against the abdominal wall over the liver.[25]

With blunt trauma to the liver, the liver may fracture in several patterns. It will often have multiple linear lacerations with a gross picture of a "bear-claw" injury (Figure 7-1). If the trauma is more severe, there may be devastating pulverization of the parenchyma, with the manifestation of a stellate fracture of the capsule. Complicated to manage, and fortunately less commonly encountered, are the large, transverse tears across both the right and left lobes of the liver. Technical difficulties in controlling hemorrhage from this type of injury are formidable; and, if associated injuries of the hepatic veins or inferior vena cava exist, the salvage rate will be small.

In addition to direct impact on the liver, with a sudden deceleration of the type associated with motor vehicle collisions or falls from heights, sheer force plays a

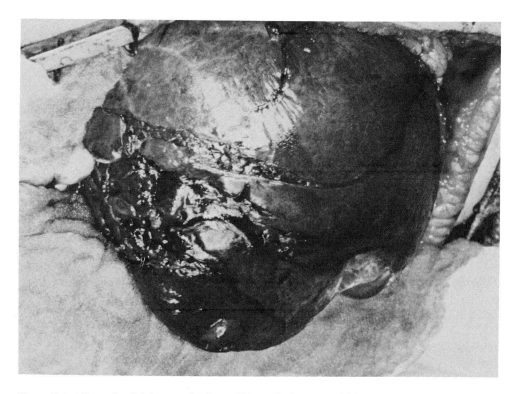

Figure 7–1 "Bear-claw" injury to the liver. This explosive type of injury produces marked hepatic parenchymal disruption.

major role in the avulsion of the liver and hepatic veins from their attachments to the diaphragm and the inferior vena cava.

Death from hepatic injury is usually due to uncontrollable hemorrhage. With improvements in transportation and resuscitation, there has been an increasing number of patients arriving at the hospital alive. It is reported that approximately only 50 percent of patients with major injuries now survive to arrive at the hospital. Frey and associates reported that, if patients had a systolic blood pressure of less than 80 mm Hg, the mortality rate was 80 percent.[26] No deaths occurred in patients who on arrival to the emergency room were not in shock.

The majority of patients with liver injury have an uncomplicated course. In penetrating injuries, the mortality ranges between 3 percent and 15 percent. In blunt trauma, expecially from motor vehicle accidents, the outcome is more serious, with an overall mortality rate of 20 to 40 percent. In the 10 percent of liver injuries where major resection is necessary for the management of the injury, the mortality rate is 50 to 60 percent. Studies on long-term survivors after liver trauma showed no sequelae from the damaged liver with or without major resection. Clinical tests noted no compromise of hepatic function and it is apparent that liver regeneration will occur if the patient survives the initial post-injury period.[22]

SURGICAL ANATOMY

As stated earlier, the liver is the largest glandular organ in the body, with an average weight of 1500 g. The shape of the liver is pyramidal or wedge-shaped, with the apex or the thin edge to the left. It has three major surfaces; the superior and inferior surfaces meet anteriorly in a sharp, well defined margin, whereas the remaining posterior surface is rounded (Figure 7-2).

The liver is held in its upper abdominal position by reflections of the parietal peritoneum which coalesce as ligaments. The coronary ligament occupies the superior surface of the right lobe of the liver, securing it to the diaphragm superiorly and posteriorly. This surrounds the bare area of the liver in which the inferior vena cava and hepatic veins are located. At the extreme left, the two leaves of the coronary ligament join laterally to form the triangular ligament. This provides the attachment of the left lobe to the diaphragm. The falciform ligament and the ligamentum teres form an anterior attachment to the abdominal wall and extend upward to join the coronary ligament and downward into the groove between the medial and lateral segments of the left lobe of the liver. The obliterated umbilical vein (ligamentum teres) enters the liver along the inferior margin of the falciform ligament.

The liver is divided into right and left surgical lobes by a plane or fissure that is not apparent on the external surface. This extends roughly from the middle of the gallbladder fossa inferiorly to the inferior vena cava superiorly forming an angle of about 35 degrees with the vertical plane and 25 degrees with the sagittal plane (Figure 7-3). This plane is devoid of anatomy except for the middle hepatic veins. The hepatic veins, as is true of the lungs, drain the external portions of segments and fissures. The right lobe is divided into anterior and posterior segments by a plane which runs from a posterior superior position inferiorly and anteriorly to the porta hepatis. One can readily demonstrate in corrosion casts that the fissure is complete and is rarely crossed by branches of either hepatic artery, portal vein, or ramifications of the bile

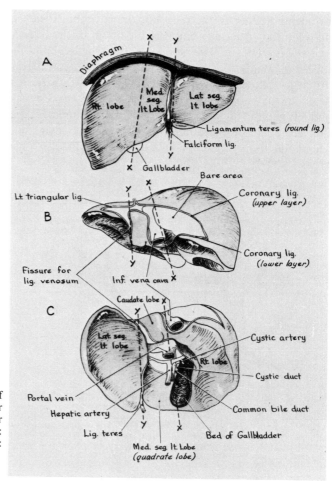

Figure 7–2 Surface anatomy of the liver. *A,* anterior, *B,* superior and *C,* interior surfaces of the liver (from Madding and Kennedy: *Trauma to the Liver.* Philadelphia: W.B. Saunders Co., 1971).

Figure 7–3 Segmental anatomy of the liver. The right segmental fissure separates the anterior and posterior segments of the right lobe. The intralobar fissure the right and left lobes and the left intrasegmental fissure the lateral from the medial segment of the left lobe.

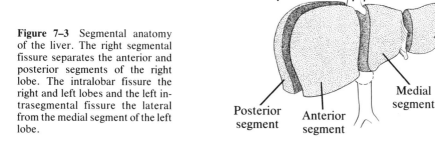

duct. The left lobe is divided into two segments, a medial segment and lateral segment, by a vertical plane continuous with the falciform ligament to the ligamentum venosum. The inferior surface of the liver is composed of the undersurface of the left lobe laterally and the quadrate lobe which makes up most of the medial segment of the left lobe lying between the vena cava and the falciform ligament. The caudate lobe, because of its bilateral blood supply and drainage, is really a separate lobe belonging to neither the right nor the left lobe. It lies superior to the quadrate lobe between the structures entering the hilum of the liver and the diaphragm.

BILE DUCTS. The blood supply to the liver and the bile drainage from the liver follow a common anatomical pathway (the portal triad) (Figure 7-4). The biliary drainage follows a segmental and lobar pattern with no evidence of a functional anastomosis between the right and left lobes except across the junction of the right and left hepatic ducts of the porta hepatis. Similarly, there is no connection between the bile ducts of the anterior and posterior segment of the right lobe across the segmental fissure, except in a small percentage of cases where small ducts may cross.

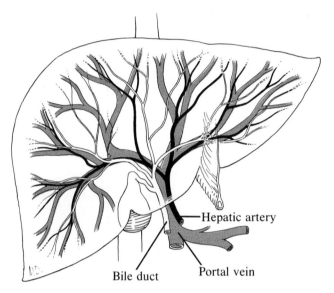

Hepatic artery

Bile duct Portal vein

Figure 7–4 Demonstrates the anatomy of the portal triad-bile ducts, hepatic arteries and portal vein which accompany one another and supply the segmental anatomy of the liver.

The right hepatic duct, which averages 9 mm in length, is formed by the union of the anterior and posterior segmental ducts near the porta hepatis. However, in nearly 30 percent of cases, either the posterior or anterior segment duct crosses the lobar fissure to drain directly in to the left hepatic duct. When this anomaly is present, a left lobectomy would obstruct drainage from either the anterior or posterior segment of the right lobe, resulting in the possibility of atrophy of the entire segment. The lateral segment of the left lobe is drained by two segmental ducts, a more extensive inferior duct and a smaller superior duct which unite at the line of the segmental fissure. The left lobe medial segmental drainage is more variable, however, in the majority of cases, all four of the area ducts join to form a single medial segment duct. The lateral segment duct runs medially and inferiorly and joins the medial segment duct to form the left hepatic duct. In half of the cases, this occurs in the segmental fissure but, in a large number of cases, this is to the right and, in a few cases, to the left of the fissure. Drainage of the caudate lobe is variable and drainage into both the right and left hepatic ducts occurs. The common hepatic duct is formed in the transverse fissure of the liver by the union of the left and right hepatic ducts and varies in length from 1 to 5 cm, being an average of 2.5 cm. The common bile duct averages 2 to 7 cm in length and is remarkably consistent in course and arrangement. It is a continuation of the common hepatic duct from the point of junction of that duct with the cystic duct and descends in the free margin of the lesser omentum and passes behind the first part of the duodenum, to enter in the back of the head of the pancreas downward and slightly to the right, to end in the posterior-medial portion of the second part of the duodenum. The duct in the lesser omentum is lateral to the hepatic artery and anterior to the portal vein. While the duct is in the head of the pancreas, the inferior vena cava is posterior and the pancreatico-duodenial artery is medial to it.

The gallbladder is the reservoir in which bile from the hepatic duct is stored and concentrated. It is a small, piriform sac, holding about 30 to 60 cc of bile. It rests in a fossa in the visceral surface of the liver at the plane between the right and left lobes of the liver. Occasionally, it is partially embedded in the liver parenchyma or it may be freely attached by a short peritoneal mesentery. It is obliquely oriented, with its long axis directed posteriorly and superiorly to the right of the porta hepatis (Figure 7-2). The gallbladder is divided into a body, fundus, and neck. The fundus is most anterior and is the wide end protruding beyond the edge of the liver. The body is in contact with the liver and the neck, the narrowed end, is continuous with the cystic duct.

The cystic vein enters into the right branch of the portal vein before entering into the liver parenchyma. The branches of the hepatic artery are in front of the veins. The cystic artery usually comes off the common hepatic artery superior to the cystic duct to enter into the gallbladder. Occasionally, it may arise from the right hepatic artery. Anatomical variations in the arrangement of the original relations of the arteries to the duct can prove troublesome to the surgeon, who must be constantly aware of the anatomic variations in this area.

ARTERIAL SUPPLY. The arterial blood supply to the liver is usually derived from the coeliac axis. The common hepatic artery courses through the lesser omentum at its superior border above the first portion of the duodenum and then gives rise to the right gastric artery and, at the junction of the first and second portions of the duodenum, the gastroduodenal artery. The vessel then proceeds on toward the porta hepatis as the proper hepatic artery left of the common bile duct and anterior to the portal vein. The hepatic artery ascends and bifurcates to the right and left branch. The bifurcation may occur at different levels. This variability is important to recognize when operating in this area (Figure 7-5).

The right hepatic artery, after originating from the proper hepatic artery, courses to the right behind the common hepatic duct. However, in approximately 10 percent of the cases, it may pass in front of the common hepatic duct. In 1 to 2 percent of the cases, there is no true right main hepatic artery present. Two vessels, anterior and posterior segmental arteries of the right lobe, take separate origin from the hepatic artery. The anterior segmental branch is usually inferior to the posterior segmental artery. It courses downward along the gallbladder fossa and is in close proximity to the cystic duct, which makes it vulnerable to injury during cholecystectomy. The posterior segmental artery courses alongside of the segmental hepatic duct along its inferior border. Its course is inferior and posterior.

The cystic artery, in the majority of cases, is an extrahepatic branch of the right hepatic artery as it courses along side of the common hepatic duct. It proceeds forward along the neck of the gallbladder in a superior position and divides into the superficial cystic artery. It then penetrates into and attaches itself to the wall of the gallbladder. In approximately 85 to 90 percent of the cases studied on gross dissection, there is a single cystic artery. However, there may be double cystic arteries

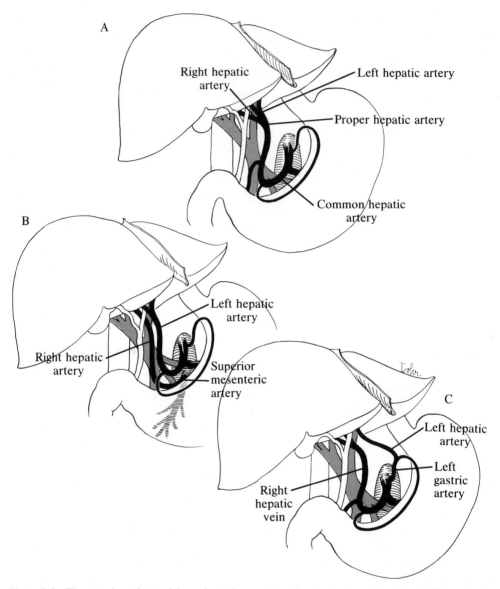

Figure 7–5 The extra hepatic arterial supply. *A* demonstrates the standard anatomy, *B* and *C* the variants each of which are present approximately 20% of the time. In *B* the right hepatic artery takes origin from the superior mesenteric artery. In *C*, the left hepatic artery originates from the left gastric artery.

in approximately 10 to 15 percent of the cases, which take separate origins from the hepatic artery.

The left hepatic artery, after taking origin from the proper hepatic artery in the porta hepatis, courses upward and obliquely to the left and divides into two terminal branches, the medial and lateral segmental arteries. In half of the cases, the left hepatic artery may divide early, to the right of the left segmental fissure.

The medial segmental artery normally arises from the undersurface of the left hepatic artery and descends into the portion of the liver described as the quadrate lobe. There it divides within the liver parenchyma into superior and inferior branches.

The medial segmental artery has also been termed the medial hepatic artery or the quadrate lobe artery.

The lateral segmental artery originating in the region of porta hepatis is usually located inferior to the corresponding hepatic duct. It extends obliquely towards the upper, outer aspect of the lateral segment accompanying the bile duct. It divides into superior and inferior branches in the region of the segmental fissure. The inferior lateral branch descends to the lateral segment, curving towards the left, again corresponding to the bile duct in that region.

The blood supply to the caudate lobe is variable and originates both from the right and left hepatic arterial branches. The usual pattern is that there is a single branch arising from the right hepatic artery or segmental branch in that region. In approximately 35 percent of the cases, the entire blood supply of the right caudate lobe comes from the right hepatic artery and, in 12 percent entirely from the left hepatic artery.

Atypical arterial vessels may replace the usual anatomical arrangement. As mentioned earlier, the right hepatic artery may take its origin from the superior mesenteric artery; this occurs in approximately 20 percent of cases. The vessel in this case usually courses anteriorly, to the right of the portal vein in the hepataduodenal ligament. This variance is important to be aware of in operating in this region, especially in cases of portal hypertension. In approximately 20 percent of cases, the origin of the left hepatic artery may be the left gastric artery. This similar variation must be kept in mind in taking down the gastrohepatic ligament.

PORTAL VEIN. The portal vein returns blood to the liver from the mesentery bed draining the gastrointestinal system (Figure 7-6). It is formed by the junction of the superior mesentery vein and the splenic vein anterior to the vena cava and posterior to the head of the pancreas. It emerges from behind the duodenum, and traverses through the gastrohepatic omentum lying posterior to the common duct and the hepatic artery. In the porta hepatis, the portal vein enters the hilum of the liver and divides into the right and left trunk. The left trunk is longer than the right, and is made up of the transverse portion, which lies in the hilum, and an umbilical portion, in the region of the falciform ligament. The umbilical portion gives off a branch to the superior area of the lateral segment and another branch posteriorly that drains into the posterior medial segment.

The right trunk of the portal vein courses laterally from its portal origin and divides into an anterior and posterior segment to supply blood to those areas. There are very few anastomoses between branches of the portal vein.

THE HEPATIC VEINS. The venous drainage of the liver is arranged in a very simple fashion and empties into the inferior vena cava. A major portion of the venous drainage is returned by three major veins: the right, middle, and left hepatic veins (Figure 7-7). The right hepatic vein, largest of the three, drains the posterior and anterior aspect of the right lobe of the liver. The middle and left hepatic veins enter the inferior vena cava frequently as a single trunk, but may be separated just at the juncture of its confluence to the cava. The middle hepatic vein drains the superior aspect of the anterior segment of the right lobe. The venous drainage of the caudate lobe is less consistent and may drain through several veins directly into the vena cava. The left hepatic vein drains a portion of the superior aspect of the medial segment and lateral segment of the left lobe. These veins are frequently injured when dividing the left triangular ligament because of their close proximity to it. There are anastomoses between the hepatic venous system and direct communication between the portal system and the hepatic venous system.

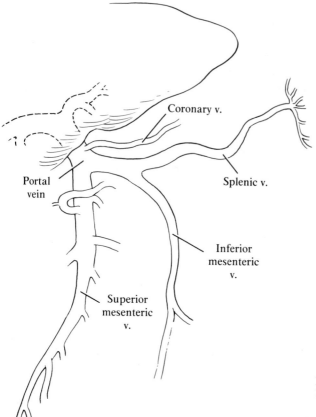

Figure 7–6   Anatomy of the extra hepatic portal vein.

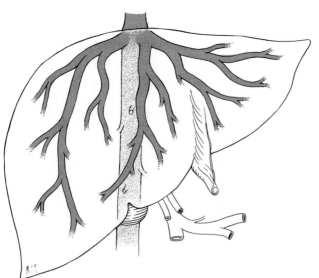

Figure 7–7   Anatomy of the hepatic veins. Knowledge of the location of the middle hepatic vein is critical. It courses between the right and left lobes entering the vena cava separately or, more commonly, the left hepatic vein a variable distance from its insertion into the cava.

DIAGNOSIS

In simple injuries, where the trauma is confined to the abdomen, the diagnosis of liver injury should be made on clinical grounds. In evaluating penetrating trauma in the vicinity of the right upper quadrant, the possibility of liver injury should always be considered.

In blunt trauma, diagnosis may not be as clear. Blunt trauma may produce liver injury by a number of means. A blow to the chest, sufficient to produce fractures of the lower six ribs on the right, may injure the liver by bursting compression or by a sharp fractured rib end. Falls from heights, particularly when the subject lands feet first, can be associated with avulsion injuries of hepatic veins from the vena cava. Enlarged congested liver is particularly vulnerable to lesser degrees of blunt trauma.

On examination, the patient with liver trauma may have a paucity of findings, even when 1 to 2 liters of blood may be lost into the peritoneal cavity. Usually, examination will disclose tenderness over the lower six ribs or in the right upper quadrant, which suggests the probability of underlying liver injury. Referred shoulder pain may or may not be present. The common manifestation of liver injury is bleeding into the peritoneal cavity or into the right chest when there is associated diaphragm laceration. Persistent thoracic bleeding or hemothorax associated with abdominal tenderness should always lead to suspicion that liver injury has occurred. Blunt trauma sufficient to injure both diaphragm and liver is usually obvious and is not a diagnostic problem. Small amounts of blood in the free peritoneal cavity may result in a rise in white count. In most instances, intraperitoneal bleeding will be associated with a fall in hematocrit. When such a fall occurs without obvious source one should be alert to the possibility of intraperitoneal bleeding. This is especially pertinent when there has been evidence of trauma in the vicinity of the right upper quadrant. Therefore, injuries to the lower right chest or right upper abdomen resulting in a fall in hematocrit should lead to the diagnosis of liver injury and a laparotomy should be performed promptly.

When there are multiple injuries, and in particular, when there is bleeding from other sites such as fractures of the femur or scalp lacerations, the reliability of the hematocrit to verify abdominal bleeding is lost. When there is altered consciousness so that the reliability of abdominal examination is questionable, another dimension of clinical assessment is lost. In these instances, peritoneal lavage is an excellent diagnostic procedure and is often very helpful (See Chapter 3). A positive lavage commits the surgeons to perform prompt laparotomy. X-ray examination of the chest and abdomen (flat and upright or decubitus) are of value in evaluating the trauma patient and should be done on all patients who are stable. The presence of hemothorax, reaction above the diaphragm, or evidence of fluid in the abdomen are all compatible with intraperitoneal liver injury. Liver function studies are of no value in the initial assessment. Special diagnostic procedures, such as peritoneal lavage, scintillation scans, CT scans, and arteriography, are not usually necessary for the diagnosis of liver injury—all are associated with false positives and false negatives and should not replace clinical acumen. When the multiple trauma patient has been conservatively managed for 12 to 14 hours and has been relatively stable, but suspicion of injury to the liver exists and peritoneal lavage is contraindicated, then CT body scan or scintillation scans may contribute to diagnosis.

In certain complex injuries, arteriographic assessment of the liver may be of great value. When there is doubt about the internal integrity of the liver or evidence of vascular injury, as noted by a bruit at operation in an area where the anatomy is unclear, arteriograms may be of value (Figure 7-8). This is best carried out in the x-ray department with selective catheterization of hepatic vessels. If, in the post-operative period, the patient manifests hematobilia or persistent bleeding from liver drains, arteriography is often very helpful in defining the specific bleeding site for resection or ligation of the bleeding vessel. As noted earlier under the section on anatomy, as the circulation of the liver is variable, the source of the right hepatic artery may be the superior mesenteric artery or the left hepatic artery may have its origin from the left gastric artery. Selective injection of the superior mesenteric vessels may be of value to assess the portal venous system for signs of injury as manifested by obstruction or intrahepatic parenchymal bleeding.

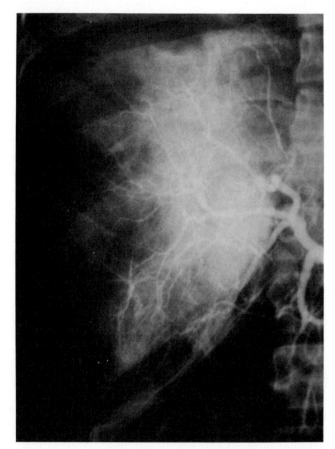

Figure 7–8 Arteriogram demonstrates the lack of vascularity of the right lobe of the liver. The findings at operation were similar to that shown in Figure 1.

PRE-OPERATIVE PREPARATION

If the patient's condition is stable, associated injuries should be assessed, and blood should be sent for type and cross-match while x-ray examination is being performed. All patients assumed to have major abdominal injury should have access to the vascular system provided by the placement of at least one cut-down. Our preference is a cut-down performed on the anticubital fossa and the passage of a 5 F infant feeding tube proximally into a central venous position. This permits monitoring of central venous pressure and the rapid infusion of fluids. If the patient presents in severe shock and major blood loss is evident, a second cut-down should be placed in the saphenous vein in the ankle. This vein usually will accept the entire cross-sectional diameter of an intravenous tube and permits rapid resuscitation of any patient in shock with reversible injuries. Though there is a possibility that the vena cava may be injured (the incidence is less than 5 percent), saphenous cut-down provides the most rapid access to the vascular system in severely injured patients and will function even if caval occlusion is required.

If injuries are extensive, the patient's condition unstable, and major liver injury is presumed, an arterial catheter may be of value to permit serial monitoring of blood gases and direct measurement of arterial pressure. It can be done percutaneously, utilizing the radial artery, or a cut-down can be performed on the same vessel. However, this procedure is best reserved for placement in the operating room while the patient is being prepared for surgery.

The unstable patient should be resuscitated with Ringer's lactate; 2000 cc can be administered in 5 to 10 minutes in the average adult. If the patient stabilizes, definitive evaluation can be carried out. If the patient fails to respond to therapy, the patient *must* be taken immediately to the operating room while resuscitation is continued. If the patient's response to fluid resuscitation is brief, major bleeding should be assumed and prompt surgery is indicated.

If penetrating trauma is present, pre-operative broad spectrum antibiotics should be administered to cover aerobic and anerobic enteric organisms. The association with gastrointestinal injury is usually the rule. Blunt trauma rarely produces hollow viscus perforation and a clean injury, such as liver injury, does not usually require pre- or postoperative antibiotics.

Provided there are no unnecessary delays in getting the patient to surgery, blood should be reserved for administration in the operating room. In urgent cases, type specific un-crossmatched blood can be started as control of hemorrhage is obtained. O-negative low-titer blood can also be utilized as an alternative.

In patients with multiple thoracic injuries in association with liver injury, the airway assumes top priority. Endotracheal intubation may be appropriate in the emergency department. This permits stabilization of thoracic injuries and may allow time to complete the assessment of the patient. Once positive pressure ventilation has been introduced, the possibility of producing a tension pneumothorax in patients with pulmonary contusion must be watched for. Placement of a chest tube in the right pleural space is often indicated, especially when there is evidence of pneumothorax or hemothorax. Since there is a high incidence of associated rib fracture in liver injury, placement of a right chest tube in the operating room would give some assurance to the anesthesiologist that the problem is not related to the thoracic cavity if the patient's condition becomes unstable.

SURGICAL APPROACH

Our routine laparotomy incision is a midline abdominal incision. For exposure of a complex liver injury, the abdominal incision should extend from the xiphoid, two-thirds to three-fourths of the way inferior to the pubis. For complex injuries, particularly those involving the vena cava or hepatic veins, it may be necessary to extend the midline abdominal incision superiorly as a sternal splitting incision. In these circumstances, we usually divide the sternum from the xiphoid to sternal notch. This can be rapidly done with a Leibsche knife or an electric sternal saw (should this be readily available). Upon entering the peritoneal cavity, rapid exploration should be carried out, unless hemorrhage in the vicinity of the liver is massive. The intestines should be eviscerated and all quadrants of the abdomen inspected. If the hemorrhage in the abdomen is massive, the four corners of the abdomen should be packed to isolate and localize the source of hemorrhage. All too often, the surgeon falls into the trap of assuming that an obvious injury such as the liver laceration is the only source of hemorrhage. Our studies show an incidence of 65 to 70 percent associated injuries and a significant number of them were other vascular injuries. If these other injuries are not identified, they may continue to bleed massively while attention is inappropriately directed to the liver injury.

The liver should be inspected in its entirety. The examining hand is rapidly passed over the dome of the liver. The undersurface is inspected directly and the left lobe viewed in its entirety. If there is a laceration that is bleeding, attempts should be made initially to stop the hemorrhage by compressive packing with lap pads while complete assessment of the remainder of the liver is carried out. Under certain circumstances, where hepatic artery ligation may be indicated to control bleeding, the liver should not be freed up by dividing the ligamentous attachments to the diaphragm. Interruption of this potential source of collateral flow may increase the morbidity of hepatic artery ligation.

If bleeding is not readily controlled by the application of packs and direct pressure, the portal triad should be occluded with a vascular clamp (Pringle maneuver) (Figure 7-9). If hemorrhage is controlled, the bleeding can be assumed to be from either the hepatic artery or portal vein. If bleeding is not alleviated, hepatic veins or collateral vessels are the most likely source of the bleeding. When bleeding is controlled by the application of the vascular clamp, the depths of the laceration can be inspected and definitive bleeding points secured by the direct application of sutures or hemostatic clips. If necessary, the laceration may be extended along anatomical lines or to the free edge to permit inspection of the depth of the laceration. Simple penetrating injuries, from which bleeding in the depths of the liver is difficult to identify, may best be controlled by hepatic artery ligation; under these circumstances, as mentioned previously, the liver attachments in the diaphragm should not be mobilized and divided.

In posterior injuries that are not readily exposed, the liver should be mobilized by dividing its ligamentous attachments to the diaphragm. With the attachments severed, traction can be exerted on the right lobe of the liver to rotate the liver upwards to the left. This permits access to, and inspection of, the entire right lobe. Almost all injuries to the liver except those related to the upper surface of the liver in the vicinity of the hepatic veins and vena cava, can be controlled from the abdominal approach.

OPERATIVE MANAGEMENT

Treatment of liver injury may involve any one of a number of possibilities. These include doing nothing to the liver directly, suture of bleeding points, placement of large mattress sutures, hepatic artery ligation, or resection of segments or lobes of liver.

Simple liver lacerations that are not bleeding at the time of operation should be left alone. If, on inspection of the laceration to determine the extent of injury, bleeding resumes, the area can be compressed temporarily with packs. Usually the hemorrhage will resolve. Reassurance is provided by the extent of the hemorrhage found at surgery. If it is under 200 cc it would be rare that a major hepatic vessel is lacerated. If there is no bile present, subsequent biliary leakage and peritonitis is unusual. The abdomen can be closed without drainage.

When blood loss is in excess of 500 cc or if there is evidence of biliary leak, even though spontaneous hemostasis has occurred, posterior drainage of the laceration should be done. Careful investigation of the laceration to secure the bleeding points with silver clips or sutures is also necessary. Sutures should be placed so as to secure the bleeding point but not to endanger or compromise other anatomical structures. As previously mentioned, suture of the bleeding vessels may be facilitated by the temporary application of a vascular clamp to the portal triad. Extension of the laceration may be necessary to facilitate exposure for suturing the bleeding vessel.

Large through-and-through mattress sutures are rarely indicated to treat bleeding from liver lacerations. The approximation of liver tissue over a bleeding artery risks serious or even fatal complications. Continued intraparenchymal hemorrhage can persist, with intrahepatic hematoma formation and the possibility of subsequent abscess or dissection of the bleeding into the biliary tract, resulting in hematobilia. Low-pressure bleeding from portal or hepatic veins rarely require this maneuver and high pressure, bleeding from the hepatic artery is rarely controlled by this manner unless the suture occludes the bleeding vessel. Should the mattress sutures be effective in controlling bleeding deep in the substance of the liver, there is also the danger that associated bile ducts and portal veins may also be encompassed. This will compromise parenchymal viability and obstruct biliary drainage.

On the occasions when the bleeding comes deep from the substance of the liver and the application of a portal triad clamp does not control the bleeding (see Figure 7-9), bleeding is presumed to be coming from injured hepatic veins. Documentation of the bleeding from the hepatic veins is possible (with the portal triad clamped) by instructing the anesthetist to temporarily discontinue positive pressure ventilation and restore spontaneous ventilation, thus creating a negative intrathoracic pressure upon inspiration. During this phase, pressure in the vena cava drops and hepatic venous bleeding will slow dramatically or stop. The choice is then to attempt to control the hepatic venous bleeding directly or to approximate liver tissue. Generally, the latter will be simpler and this is the only indication for blind approximation of liver tissue. This form of treatment is contraindicated if hepatic artery bleeding is also present, for the reasons previously given. One pitfall in this management is the anatomical variation of the hepatic arteries, which may not lend itself to be occluded at the portal triad. With application of the vascular clamp, bleeding will continue and may lead the surgeon to falsely direct his or her thinking to the hepatic veins.

Hepatic artery ligation may be of value in a limited number of injuries. The through-and-through wound of the liver is exemplified by stab wounds or low velocity wounds, which injure the hepatic artery with little damage to the liver substance. If the bleeding is brisk and is controlled by the Pringle maneuver, dissection and control of the hepatic artery will confirm that this is the source of the hemorrhage. The appropriate lobar artery should not be ligated until it is established that this is the source of hemorrhage. The right hepatic artery may be the source of the medial segmental artery to the left lobe or the vessel assumed to be the left lobar artery may in fact be the right lobar artery, with the left lobar artery coming into the liver through the falciform ligament (see the section on anatomic variations). In these circumstances of major hepatic arterial bleeding with minimal disruption of liver substance, hepatic artery ligation has constituted a major advance. Mortality and morbidity manifest by jaundice, and liver dysfunction has occurred primarily in those cases in which it is necessary to ligate the proper hepatic artery or in those cases in which the attachments of the liver were mobilized prior to making the decision to treat the bleeding with ligation. The surgeon dealing with the liver trauma should be fully familiar with the anatomical variables, since this is the key to successful operative treatment.

On rare occasion, somewhere between 0.5 and 1.0 percent of cases, there may be major disruption of hepatic veins at the undersurface of the liver, with massive hemorrhage from the vicinity of the vena cava. Attempts to expose this area directly are usually associated with exsanguinating hemorrhage. Usually, the bleeding can be controlled by pack and pressure, thus allowing time for restoration of circulating blood volume. The isolation of the liver is appropriate and this should be done before treatment attempts result in further exsanguination and prolonged shock. Managing these complex injuries requires vascular isolation of the liver by the use of an intracaval shunt combined with a portal triad occlusion. Approximately two-thirds of the venous return to the heart is through the suprarenal vena cava; therefore, in the hypovolemic trauma patient, temporary application of a clamp above the renal veins to isolate the intrahepatic vena cava usually results in profound hypotension and cardiac arrest. The occasional patient who has blood volume adequately restored may tolerate temporary occlusion and this has occasionally been successful in treating these complex injuries. For details of vascular isolation of the vena cava, see Chapter 13.

With the vascular isolation of the liver completed, the liver can be mobilized and retracted to visualize the depths of the laceration and provide access to the hepatic veins. If the injury to the undersurface is extensive and confined to the right lobe, a bloodless right hepatectomy can rapidly be carried out, permitting exposure of the vena cava for direct repair. Statistically, the right hepatic veins are most apt to be injured, so when there is doubt about the source of hemorrhage, it is the right lobe which should be sacrificed.

If the injured hepatic vein is on the left side, right lobectomy would not be necessary. Therefore, the liver should be split between the left and right lobes and the vena cava and confluence of hepatic veins exposed. The decision is then made on the need for lobectomy, depending upon the adequacy of the blood supply.

HEPATIC RESECTION

Resection of the liver is required in a relatively small percentage of cases; however, the surgeon who has occasion to deal with liver trauma should be throughly familiar with the anatomy of the liver (See section on anatomy). Generally, there has been a relatively high mortality with liver resection is to uncontrolled bleeding

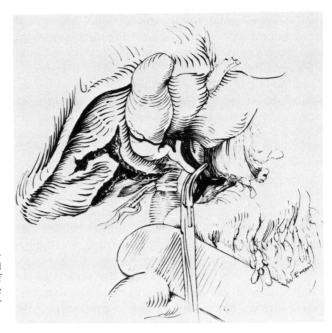

Figure 7-9 Application of a vascular clamp to the portal triad (Pringle maneuver). Cessation of bleeding strongly suggests the source of the hemorrhage is either hepatic artery or portal vein.

from raw surfaces with immediate demise, or to late complications from infection. The absolute indications for liver resection are dead or devitalized segments, inaccessible bleeding, or major intraparenchymal injury to large bile ducts. These constitute less than 10 percent of all liver injuries.

Generally the nature of the injury dictates the type of anatomical resection. Under emergency circumstances, it is theoretically possible to resect 85 percent of the liver, that is, all but the left lateral lobe. Practically speaking, injuries which dictate this extensive resection are rarely compatible with life. In most instances, the maximum resection required to treat trauma would be right or left lobectomy, right or left lateral segmentectomy, or nonanatomical resectional debridement. Temporary application of a clamp to the portal triad during resection may save considerable blood loss, permitting immediate control of all bleeding except that from the hepatic veins. The technique of vascular isolation just described has rarely been necessary for liver resection.

Major liver resection can be carried out adequately from the abdominal approach if the liver is mobilized by dividing its ligamentous attachments to the diaphragm and retroperitoneum. To mobilize the right lobe, the coronary ligament is divided to the midline and any attachments laterally to the diaphragm severed, permitting the right lobe to be lifted upward into the field. Dissection is carried superiorly, to identify the hepatic veins. In dealing with injuries to the left lobe, the triangular ligament should be cut and the liver mobilized medially to the vena cava. Care must be taken not to injure the left hepatic vein prior to making a definitive decision to resect the entire left lobe. In most instances, very little collateral supply exists for hepatic venous drainage on the left side, whereas on the hepatic veins draining the right lobe are numerous and potential collateral pathways are present.

The technique which facilitates the resection is for the surgeon to operate from the patient's left side for right lobar resections. This permits the surgeon to compress liver substance with the left hand while the surgical assistant retracts the lateral portion of the lobe in the opposite direction (Figure 7-10). The reverse is appropriate with the surgeon standing on the right side for left lobar resections. Once the capsule is incised, the scalpel handle is the optimal instrument to separate the liver tissue along the line of division from the free edge progressing up to the superior surface. Dissection of this type separates and isolates bile ducts and vessel sequentially so they can be clipped or clamped and serially ligated. As the resection is being carried out, small vessels can be coagulated with electrocautery and hemostats or hemostatic clips used on the larger vessels. If large veins are encountered, they can be ligated or oversewn with fine running vascular sutures.

It is imperative that the surgeon not be so conservative that major amounts of devitalized tissue are left behind. Safeguards include a thorough knowledge of liver anatomy for recognition of possible embryologic variation. When major vascular or biliary structures are encountered, these structures should be dissected for adequate distances to ensure that only those structures supplying the lobe or segments being removed are divided. This is particularly true when carrying out left lateral lobectomy near the falciform ligament, where the vessels in the intersegmental plane supply both the medial and lateral segments of the left lobe. During right lobectomy, the medial segment of the left lobe can be inadvertently devascularized, since the middle hepatic artery occasionally arises from the right hepatic artery to supply the left medial lobe. The safe ischemia time of the liver is probably thirty minutes; but, if the resection is done with the portal triad clamped, the operation must be carried out with dispatch to prevent severe portal and mesenteric congestion. Specific types of resection which are carried out consist of the following methods.

NONANATOMIC SEGMENTS (RESECTIONAL DEBRIDEMENT). In the removal of nonanatomic devitalized segments, the plane of the liver laceration is extended in the optimal direction to avoid leaving behind devascularized segments of liver. Resection must be minimal, including only small amounts of viable and non-injured portions of the liver. This usually involves completion of the laceration so as to leave a minimal cross-section of raw surface. In the course of nonanatomic segmentectomy, large vascular structures may be encountered. These can be dissected for short distances to permit identification of the anatomy and preservation of the blood supply to adjacent segments. A thorough familiarity with liver anatomy facilitates a decision regarding the direction the resection should take from any given laceration.

LEFT LATERAL SEGMENTECTOMY. Lateral anatomic segmentectomy consists of the removal of the portion of the liver to the left of the falciform ligament. The left lobar vessels branch in the plane of this ligament to supply the medial and lateral left lobar segments. The line of resection should be carried just lateral to the falciform ligament. As the vascular structures are encountered, these should be preserved to avoid compromise of the circulation to the medial segment. If the left lobe is well mobilized prior to the initiating resection, the medial lobe can be compressed manually to provide excellent hemostasis during the resection, thus avoiding the need to apply portal triad clamps and produce ischemia to the remainder of the liver. It may be possible to mobilize the falciform ligament in a manner so that it can be reflected down over the raw surface of the liver to cover the bare area after the resection is completed.

LEFT LOBECTOMY. Although successful resection of the medial segment of the liver has been carried out with preservation of the lateral segment, this is not

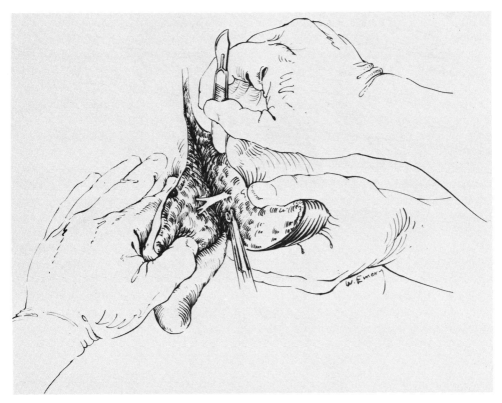

Figure 7–10 Technique of liver resection. The liver is compressed with one hand while the assistant compresses and retracts with the other. Hepatic parenchyma is divided bluntly until major structures are encountered.

feasible in trauma patients. Thus, when the medial segment of the left lobe of the liver is injured, it is not practical to attempt to preserve the lateral segment. A total left lobectomy is therefore indicated (Figure 7-11).

The anatomic division between the right and left lobe extends upward from the gallbladder fossa inferiorly to the vena cava superiorly. The one anatomic structure that must be identified during left lobectomy is the middle hepatic vein. This vein joins the left hepatic vein in most instances and drains the superior segment of the right lobe of the liver. If this vein can be preserved, the integrity of the superior segment can be assured. For this reason, the left lobectomy should be carried out just to the left of the anatomic division. When the large middle hepatic vein is encountered, it should be preserved, if technically feasible, by careful dissection to its juncture with the left hepatic vein. The left hepatic vein can then be identified and divided proximally to the middle hepatic vein. If the middle hepatic vein is injured, ligation is usually necessary. This is relatively well tolerated. The left hepatic artery can be relied upon to supply blood only to the left lobe, whereas the left portal vein may provide a branch to the anterior segment of the right lobe. Proximal ligation of the left portal vein should be deferred until adequate exposure is obtained by division of sufficient liver tissue to expose the hilum widely. Precautions should be taken as the hilum is approached through the line of the incision, because the right lobar hepatic artery and portal vein can be inadvertently included in ligatures or

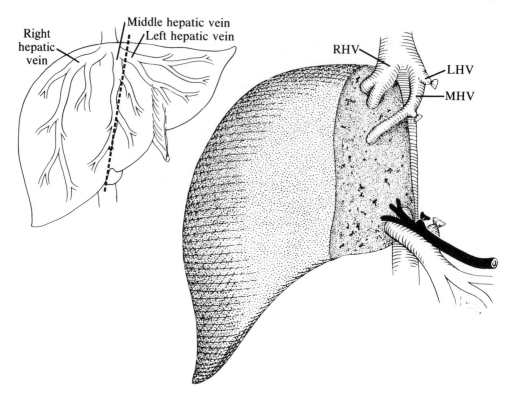

Figure 7–11 Left lobar resection. The line of resection passes to the left of the middle hepatic vein.

large sutures. This is more apt to occur in left, rather than right lobectomy, because the hilum is to the left of the anatomic division of the lobes. The small vessels and ducts are ligated with 4-0 silk or electrocoagulated, or clipped. The hepatic artery is ligated with 2-0 ligatures and the bile ducts and portal vein are usually oversewn with fine synthetic vascular sutures.

RIGHT LOBECTOMY. Precautions for right hepatic lobectomy are similar to those for left hepatic lobectomy. It must be remembered that the middle hepatic vein usually joins the left hepatic vein prior to entering the vena cava. One should not risk ligating the left hepatic vein, but divide the middle hepatic vein early in the dissection (Figure 7-12). If possible, the dissection is carried to the right of the deeper portion of the middle hepatic vein. Anatomic variations can occur, and it is essential that the surgeon be thoroughly familiar with these. Inadvertent compromise of any portion of the left lobe may produce hepatic insufficiency and liver necrosis. The right hepatic artery ordinarily supplies only the right lobe, although it may on occasion give rise to a branch to the left medial segment. The right lobar branch of the portal vein can be relied upon to supply only the right lobe, although its segmental branches can be variable. As in left lobectomy, the right hepatic artery and portal vein can be dissected and ligated in advance of the lobectomy. This is feasible if portal triad occlusion is not necessary for hemostasis. We prefer to perform the Pringle maneuver in most instances, to initiate right hepatic lobectomy promptly rather than prolonging dissection in the depths of the incision and liver substance. The location of the vena cava should always be kept in mind when dividing the liver.

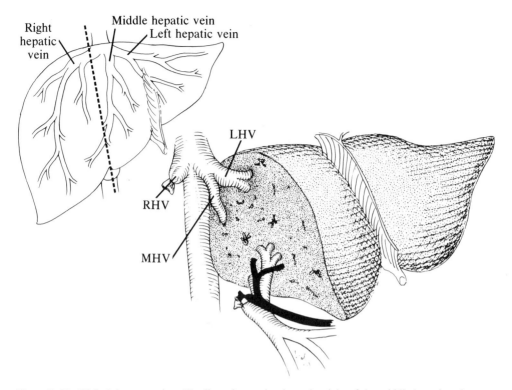

Figure 7–12 Right lobar resection. The line of resection is to the right of the middle hepatic vein.

This may be facilitated by freeing the posterior surface of the right lobe early in the dissection so the fissure for the vena cava can be palpated. If the right lobe is grasped firmly it can be rotated upward and to the left, exposing the posterior surface. As the cleavage plane is created through the liver substance, it should emerge posteriorly along the right lateral margin of the inferior vena cava.

If total isolation of the liver has not been carried out and the intrahepatic vena cava has not been bypassed with the shunt, the major right hepatic veins may be ligated posteriorly before division of the liver substance is initiated. This avoids considerable blood loss during lobectomy, and also helps prevent intravascular coagulation, which results from embolism of small particles of liver. Vessels and bile ducts are managed in similar fashion of that described for left lobectomy.

DRAINAGE

In all circumstances where drainage is indicated, we believe there is no acceptable alternative to wide posterior dependent drainage. This is best accomplished by a posteriolateral flank incision along the inferior border of the 12th rib. The muscles of the flank must be separated to admit three to four fingers. Five or six large, soft, Penrose drains (2 inches wide) should be placed in the vicinity of the injury and in the subhepatic space. We frequently drain injuries of the left lobe through the right subhepatic space, to avoid the risk of injuring the spleen or diaphragm. Although left lateral drainage is feasible, this, of necessity, must be lateral rather than posterior.

Injuries in Porta Hepatis

Injuries to the porta hepatis usually present with formidable hemorrhage. Because of the close proximity of the bile duct, hepatic artery, and portal vein, careful and direct contról is required. Adequate exposure to define the injured structures is paramount. Injuries to the hepatic artery should be approached with a goal of repair or reconstruction, especially when the portal vein is involved. If the portal vein is intact, the latitude in whether to repair or revascularize *versus* ligation is greater than when the portal vein is injured.

Hepatic artery repair should be attempted whenever possible. When the portal vein has been injured and hepatic artery ligation is necessary to control hemorrhage, postoperative precautions subsequently described must be strictly followed to avoid or minimize compromise of liver blood flow.

Injuries to the portal vein carry with them significant morbidity and mortality. Every attempt should be made to repair portal venous injuries. On occasion, it may be necessary to ligate the injured portal vein. When this is done in the presence of normal liver function, portal hypertension usually is minimal, and the long term consequence is small, since collateral pathways open and restore much of the liver flow.

Injuries to the Extrahepatic Biliary System

Penetrating injuries may involve the biliary system, including the right or left lobar duct, the hepatic duct, or the common bile duct and may, on very rare circumstances, be compromised by "stretch" injuries or blunt trauma. These injuries are identified by evidence of bile leakage from the lacerated ductal structures. When identified, they should be meticulously exposed and sutured. The development of hematobilia is unusual in injuries limited to the bile ducts, unless there is associated vascular injury in juxtapositon with the biliary injury. It is important to identify and control such bleeding associated with lacerated ducts and to drain the area properly. Later, if a biliary fistula should develop from the area of injury, a secondary procedure can be done at a later date, when the patient's condition is optimal. Usually these biliary fistulae will spontaneously close unless there is distal obstruction.

In cases where the porta hepatis is injured, and the main lobar hepatic ducts are involved or avulsed, liver resection may be necessary to gain exposure and identification of the duct. The lacerated duct or ducts must be carefully identified, the injured area debrided, and, if repair is possible, it should be done with fine nonabsorbable sutures with drainage of the duct by a soft T-tube. However, if extensive damage to the duct require resection of the damaged portion, immediate reconstruction with Roux-en-Y jejunal segment to the common hepatic duct or to the lobar segments is more likely to be successful than attempts at primary duct repair. If both right and left hepatic ducts should be injured, they may be anastomosed together into a common lumen for anastomosis into the Roux-en-Y segment.

In patients who are unstable, with multiple injuries, reconstruction of the biliary system should be delayed and temporary biliary drainage carried out by placing catheters into the injured ducts. These catheters should then be brought out of the abdominal cavity through separate stab wounds laterally and biliary output is monitored. Secondary reconstruction can be planned for in 2 to 3 months after complete recovery from other injuries. Meanwhile, biliary evaluation can be accomplished by catheter cholangiogram.

Injuries to the Gallbladder

Injuries to the gallbladder usually are best treated with cholecystectomy. However, in simple stab wounds or puncture wounds with minimal tissue damage, it may be repaired with one or two stitches. This assumes that the gallbladder is perfectly normal and the patient is stable, with minimal associated injuries or peritoneal contamination.

POSTOPERATIVE MANAGEMENT

The immediate operative problem relating to liver surgery is the development of a bleeding syndrome. This is most apt to result when vascular control has required temporary occlusion of the hepatic circulation or when the hepatic resection is completed. Diffuse oozing from all raw surfaces of the liver may represent a consumptive coagulopathy, and is the result from the combination of shock, extensive tissue trauma, and massive transfusions. Treatment of this syndrome requires maintenance of vascular volume utilizing fresh blood. When blood loss exceeds 5 units, as it usually does in cases requiring liver resection, an acquired platelet functional defect is likely. The anesthesiologist should be encouraged to request 6 to 10 units of platelet packs and these should be administered at the completion of hepatic resection or prior to peritoneal closure.

Upon accomplishment of hemostasis, the raw surface of the liver should be covered with tissue, as appropriate. The omentum is the optimal tissue and is readily available. It is swung upward, placed over the raw liver surface, and fixed with a few sutures to the liver capsule. In the absence of omentum, the falciform ligament, salvaged portions of liver capsule, or peritoneal grafts may be utilized.

In desperate situations, where massive, uncontrolled bleeding is present, it may be necessary to apply pressure with 3 or 4 warm laparotomy packs against the raw surface of the liver. They are left in place and the incision is closed without drainage. Re-operation is done in 12 to 24 hours to remove the packing. If bleeding is not well controlled, it may be necessary to replace the packs. In this situation, angiography is helpful to define the surgically correctable site while the patient's coagulation parameters are treated.

We do not drain the common duct with a T-tube as a matter of routine. Occasionally, in complex injuries when there has been biliary damage, or when it seems appropriate to monitor the status of bile ducts postoperatively, a small T-tube can be left in the common duct. However, it has been found that the complications associated with a T-tube placement outweigh its advantages.

As a matter of policy, whenever the status of the liver is unclear or questionable upon completion of operation, we have no hesitancy about re-operating on a planned basis, 24 hours later. This includes situations where there is any question of viability, in which hemostasis has been incomplete or external drainage has not been entirely satisfactory. We believe that, by so doing, subhepatic and subphrenic collections of blood may be identified, devitalized segments responsible for subsequent sepsis and mortality can be located, and unsuspected biliary leaks can be managed and drained appropriately when the patient is hemodynamically stable.

Immediate postoperative management includes careful monitoring of cardiovascular function, including urine output and peripheral perfusion. Maintenance of blood volume to insure good splanchnic and portal blood flow is important. The hematocrit should be obtained immediately after operation and every 4 hours if the patient is at all unstable. With major liver resections, blood glucose levels should be monitored and hypertonic glucose administered in quantities of one to two liters of 10 percent dextrose solution per 24 hours.

Platelet count and function, prothrombin time, and partial thromboplastin time should be monitored several times daily. Platelet transfusion and fresh frozen plasma should be administered to correct any deficiencies. Antibiotics are not used routinely unless there has been associated hollow viscus injury or severe shock. In these instances, broad spectrum coverage started in the operating room is continued post-operatively for 24 to 48 hours. Wound drainage should be cultured every two to three days and blood cultures should be obtained if fever spikes occur. Antacids and/or cimetadine should be administered prophylactically to prevent stress ulcer-ation and bleeding. Intravenous hyperalimentation is initiated within four to five days if the patient is not ready to resume diet by this time.

COMPLICATIONS

Bleeding, as described earlier, is the primary initial complication and uncon-trolled hemorrhage is the primary cause of early mortality. If good posterior drainage has been accomplished, bleeding can be monitored through a combination of serial hematocrits and observation of blood loss from the drains. Bleeding in excess of 500 cc/hour for more than several hours postoperatively demands re-operation, if only to insure that no major bleeding point has been left unsecured. Platelet function, prothrombin time, and partial thromboplastin time should be determined serially and appropriate hematologic corrective support, with platelet transfusion and fresh fro-zen plasma, should be provided.

Patients with major trauma can be expected to have respiratory difficulty, and are best treated by endotracheal intubation and positive pressure ventilation for a minimum of 24 to 36 hours. Should progressive deterioration of pulmonary function occur, positive end expiratory pressure may be necessary. The patient must be maintained on a ventilator until pulmonary function is restored.

Jaundice is a common postoperative complication, particularly when the patient has had severe shock and has received multiple transfusions or when major resection has been required. Liver function tests, including bilirubin, should be monitored every two days. In most instances, the jaundice is due to a combination of central lobular ischemia plus a high bilirubin load from the breakdown of the transfused red cells. If the circulation of the remaining liver is adequate, any liver failure which occurs will usually reach a peak at 7 to 10 days.

Biliary fistula is an occasional complication. Provided drainage has been ade-quate and no biliary obstruction exists, these fistulae are usually benign, and close spontaneously on conservative management.

Infections of the subphrenic and subhepatic space may result from an accu-mulation of bile and blood resulting from inadequate primary drainage. It may require secondary drainage procedures if sepsis develops. Sonography and CT body scans have been helpful in localizing these collections.

Infection rarely manifests itself before 4 to 5 days and is most apt to occur if posterior drainage has been inadequate. Subphrenic and subhepatic collections are usually manifest by the onset of fever 4 to 6 days postoperatively. An associated pleural effusion may be manifest on chest x-ray. Secretions should be cultured, and blood cultures taken at the time of temperature spikes. Specific antibiotic therapy will usually control the process but if the patient fails to respond after two to three days of therapy, exploration and drainage may be necessary. After 10 days, the patient who has not developed other secondary complications, such as pulmonary, hepatic, or renal failure, usually will have a relatively uneventful course.

REFERENCES

1. Pringle JH: Notes on the arrest of hepatic hemorrhage due to trauma. Ann Surg 48:541-549, 1908.
2. Madding GF, Kennedy PA: Trauma to the liver, Philadelphia, WB Saunders, 1971.
3. Quattlebaum JK, Quattlebaum JK, Jr: Technic of hepatic lobectomy. Ann Surg 149:648-656, 1959.
4. McClelland RM, Shires T, Poulos E: Hepatic resection for massive trauma. J Trauma 4:282-286, 1964.
5. Mays ET: Lobectomy, sublobar resection, and resectional debridement for severe liver injuries. J Trauma. 12:309-314, 1972.
6. Ackroyd F.W., Pollard J, McDermott WV Jr: Massive hepatic resection in the treatment of severe liver trauma. Am J Surg 117:442-447, 1969.
7. Donovan AJ, Michaelian MJ, Yellin AE: Anatomical hepatic lobectomy in trauma to the liver. Surgery 73:833-847, 1973.
8. Mayes ET: Hepatic lobectomy. Arch Surg 103:216-228, 1971.
9. Schrock T, Blaisdell FW, Mathewson C Jr: Management of blunt trauma to the liver and hepatic veins. Arch Surg 96:698-704, 1968.
10. Lim RC Jr, Lau G, Steele M: Prevention of complications after liver trauma. Am J Surg 132: 156-162, 1976.
11. Zollinger RM Jr, Keller RT, Hubay CA: Traumatic rupture of the right and left hepatic ducts. J Trauma 12:563-569, 1972.
12. Longmire WP Jr, McArthur MS: Occult injuries of the liver, bile duct, and pancreas after blunt abdominal trauma. Am J Surg 125:661-666, 1973.
13. Merendino KA, Dillard DH, Cammock EE: The concept of surgical biliary decompression in the management of liver trauma. Surg Gynecol Obstet 117:285-293, 1963.
14. Lucas CE, Walt AJ: Critical decisions in liver trauma. Arch Surg 101:277-282, 1970.
15. Carroll CP, Cass KA, Whelan TJ Jr: Wounds of the liver in Vietnam: A critical analysis of 254 cases. Ann Surg 177:385-392, 1973.
16. Mays ET: Observations and management after hepatic artery ligation. Surg Gynecol Obstet 124:801, 1967.
17. Aaron S, Fulton RL, Mays ET: Selective ligation of the hepatic artery for trauma of the liver. Surg, Gynec & Obstet 141:187-189, 1975.
18. Lewis FR, Lim RC Jr, Blaisdell FW: Hepatic artery ligation: Adjunct in the management of massive hemorrhage from the liver. J Trauma 14: 743-755, 1974.
19. Lim RC Jr, et al.: Platelet response and coagulation changes following massive blood replacement. J Trauma 13:577-582, 1973.
20. Kock NG, et al.: The effect of glucagon on hepatic blood flow. Arch Surg 100:147-149, 1970.
21. Darle N, Lim RC Jr, Blaisdell FW: Effect of glucagon on total liver blood flow in hemorrhagic shock. Acta Chir Scand 140:217-225, 1974.
22. Lim RC Jr, Guiliano AE, Trunkey DD: Postoperative treatment of patients after liver resection for trauma: A follow-up study. Arch Surg 112:429-435, 1977.
23. Miller CL, et al.: Evaluation of total parenteral nutrition by in vitro measurement of immune capacity. Surg Forum XXVIII, p. 81, 1977.
24. Morton JR, Roys GD, Bricker DL: The treatment of liver injuries. Surg Gynecol Obstet. 134:298-302, 1972.
25. Trollope ML, et al.: The mechanism of injury in blunt abdominal trauma. J Trauma 13:962-970, 1973.
26. Frey CF et al.: A fifteen-year experience with automotive hepatic trauma. J Trauma 13:1039-1049, 1973.

Chapter Eight

SMALL BOWEL AND MESENTERY

NORMAN CHRISTENSEN

INTRODUCTION

The discovery of ether anesthesia in 1846 made it possible to perform abdominal surgery, but 70 more years were to pass before exploration of the abdomen for intra-abdominal injury became standard surgical practice. It was not until the later stages of World War I that exploration for presumed intestinal injury was adopted as a surgical principle. There are scattered reports of repair of small bowel injuries before the advent of ether, but since there was no practical way to explore the abdomen, these repairs were apparently done only when the injured bowel had eviscerated through a laceration of the abdominal wall. In 1275, Guillaume de Salicet of Italy described the simple suture of an intestinal wound.[1] The patient recovered. Prior to his death in 1460, Leonard Bertapaglia of Italy discussed the suture of intestinal wounds, declaring that complete transverse section of the bowel was incurable, but if the wound was partial or longitudinal or if it was in the small rather than the large intestine, it should be stitched.[1] In 1720, Sachenus repaired a subparietal rupture of the small bowel and in 1730 Ramdorh successfully sutured a completely divided small bowel.[2]

In the latter half of the nineteenth century and the early part of the twentieth century, there was a vigorous and continuing argument by military surgeons as to whether or not the abdomen should be explored if it was thought that the contents had been injured. In 1881, Marian Sims, the American surgeon, urged laparotomy for gunshot wounds of the abdomen, but the results were poor.[3] Military surgeons were divided into two camps: "the interventionists," who advocated laparotomy for suspected intra-abdominal injury, and "the abstentionists," who favored no operation even if it was known that intra-abdominal injury had occurred. Invertention was practiced in the Sino-Japanese War, the Spanish-American War, and the Tirah campaign, but the results were dismal, and laparotomy for suspected injury was prohibited or ordered stopped by the various medical departments of the involved nations. During the South African War of 1899-1901, laparotomy for suspected perforating wounds of the intestine was tried again, but again results were disastrous and laparotomy was discontinued during the latter stages of the war. The Russians entered the Russo-Japanese War of 1904-1905 with a policy of non-intervention, but changed their policy when it was shown by a woman surgeon, the Princess Gedroitz, that excellent results much superior to those of non-intervention, could be obtained if surgery was performed promptly. Gedroitz operated in a railway carriage unit close enough to the battle front so that casualties could be treated within three to four hours of wounding.[3]

The poor results of laparotomy during the South African War had such a powerful effect on the British that they entered World War I with a policy of not operating on combat casualties with wounds of the abdomen even when it was apparent that intra-abdominal injury had occurred. Bailey describes the mortality during the first phase of the War as "appalling." By 1915, it had become recognized that prompt surgical intervention was necessary and measures were taken to provide the organization and facilities so that this could be done.[3] But, despite the knowledge that abdominal injuries should be operated upon promptly, operation was still not the general rule when the war ended, according to Major General S.B. Hays, former Surgeon General of the United States Army.[4]

The statistics show that small intestinal injuries were very lethal in World War I. In British troops, the fatality rate when injury was restricted to the small intestine was 65.9 percent. A similar fatality rate of between 70 percent and 80 percent was found in American troops with the same injury. Lessons learned in World War I and in the Spanish Civil War of 1936-1938, plus the accumulation of civilian experience, resulted in the policy of operating as promptly as possible on patients with abdominal injuries in World War II. In World War II, the mortality rate of U.S. soldiers with univisceral jejuno-ileal injuries was 13.9 percent. For multivisceral injuries, the mortality rate was 36.3 percent. Better anesthesia, improved facilities, prompt evacuation, an enhanced understanding of the nature of traumatic shock, and a program for resuscitation of the injured patient were some of the factors leading to improvement in outcome. During the Korean and Vietnam conflicts, the overall mortality rate for combat injuries was less than for World War II but specific figures for small intestine injuries are not available.[3,4]

Exploratory laparotomy to treat injury of the intestinal tract is now considered mandatory. There is some controversy, however, regarding the management of patients with penetrating wounds who do not show evidence of visceral injury. This matter is discussed elsewhere in this book. The central point is that prompt recognition of small intestinal injury is necessary to reduce morbidity and mortality. The peritoneal cavity can handle even gross contamination, provided the contamination is not continuous or repeated. Primary mortality from small bowel and mesentery injury alone comes only when there is undue delay in recognition, which allows established peritonitis to develop or gangrene to supervene because of damage to the blood supply. It is probable that when small bowel injuries are treated promptly, the mortality from isolated injury is minimal and related to divitalization of the impaired bowel or missed associated bowel laceration or other injuries.

Injuries to the small bowel and mesentery, if suspected, are generally easy to recognize and straightforward to treat. Thus, the high morbidity and mortality that follow large bowel injuries are not seen with injury of the small bowel. Leakage from suture lines is unusual. In World War II, the leakage rate in 1168 patients was 1.02 percent.[4] The rate in civilian practice is not known but should be exceedingly low.

The small intestine may be injured by either penetrating or blunt trauma. Because much of the volume of the abdominal cavity is occupied by the small bowel, it is the author's policy to assume, until proven otherwise, that the small bowel has been damaged in cases of penetrating trauma. The mechanism of injury in blunt trauma are more varied and sometimes less obvious. They include:

1. crushing or lacerating the bowel between the spine and a firm object such as a seat belt, steering wheel, boot, or hoof;
2. application of a shearing force at fixed points by sudden deceleration so that the bowel may be torn from its attachment or the mesentery avulsed from its attachment or the mesentery avulsed from its root or from the bowel;
3. rupture of the bowel owing to a sudden increase in intra-abdominal pressure.

Laboratory investigations have shown that rupture of the bowel rarely occurs as a result of increase in intraluminal pressure alone.[5] It is probably necessary that the bowel be obstructed at two places so as to produce a closed loop if rupture is to follow a sudden increase in pressure.

Underwater blast injuries were noted during World War II. Multiple blowout injuries of both the large and small bowel were seen in sailors who were in the water near their sinking ships when depth charges exploded near them.[6]

It is clear that seat belts have decreased the incidence of all types of injury, including abdominal injuries. Nevertheless, deceleration injuries are still seen with lap-type belts. Intestinal injuries are rarely seen with the three-point fixation seat belts. Seat belt injuries are usually due to an improperly placed belt (Figure 8-1). When the belt is worn across the abdomen, rather than across the pelvis, loops of the bowel and mesentery may be crushed against the vertebral column when sudden deceleration occurs. If the belt is applied loosely, the patient may slip beneath the belt at the time of accident and force is thus applied to the abdomen. Combined vertebral and visceral injuries occur with lap-type seat belts. Delay in making a diagnosis of visceral injury in these instances is common. A review of 37 cases showed that diagnosis of visceral injury was delayed 24 or more hours in 50 percent of patients.[7] Delays for as long as 44 and 65 days between injury and definitive surgical treatment of small bowel injuries have been reported.[8] Delay in making a diagnosis may occur because signs of peritoneal irritation and ileus are attributed to the spinal injury rather than to the intra-abdominal injury.

ANATOMY

The small bowel distal to the duodenum consists of the jejunum and the ileum with a combined length of about 260 cm, about 1 ½ times body height. The jejunum is approximately 105 cm long. The mesentery is fan-shaped, with its dorsal root attached to the posterior abdominal wall from the duodenal-jejunal junction to the right sacro-iliac joint. It crosses the third portion of the duodenum, the aorta, the inferior vena cava, the right gonadal vessels, and the right ureter. Although typical ileum can be distinguished from typical jejunum, there is no clear cut dividing line between the two (Figure 8-2). The jejunum is thicker, owing to more prominent mucosal folds, and has a larger diameter than the ileum. The mesenteric circulation of the jejunum is less complex and contains fewer arcades and longer vasa recti than the ileum. The vasa recti are the vertical vessels that lead from the arcades to the bowel. There is more fat in the ileomesentery so that the spaces between the vasa recti and the arcades are less translucent than they are in the jejunum. The arterial supply to both is provided by the superior mesenteric artery which emerges from under the pancreas, runs over the uncinate process of the pancreas to enter the root

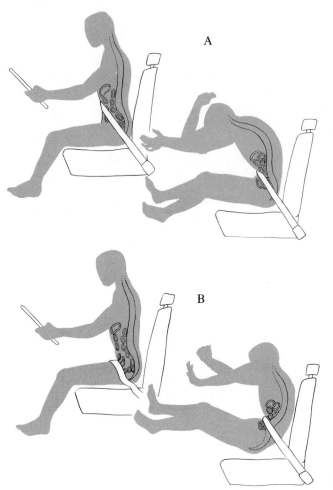

Figure 8–1. Abdominal injuries resulting from improperly used seat belts.

of the mesentery, and ends in the ileo-colic branch (Figure 8-3). In its course, it gives off the right colic and middle colic branches and numerous intestinal branches. The intestinal branches form loops or arcades within the mesentery and assure excellent collateral blood supply.

The superior mesenteric vein corresponds to the superior mesenteric artery and receives branches from the colon and small intestine before passing under the pancreas to join the inferior mesenteric vein and splenic vein to form the portal vein. Additional components of the mesentery, besides the fat, are the lymphatics (which run parallel to the arteries), the veins, and the lymph nodes. There are no major blood vessels communicating between the root of the mesentery and the retroperitoneum, thus making it possible to mobilize the entire small bowel and right colon mesentery up to the inferior surface of the pancreas.

ASSESSMENT

Although it is often obvious that intra-abdominal injury has occurred, clinical findings following both penetrating and blunt trauma to the small intestine may be

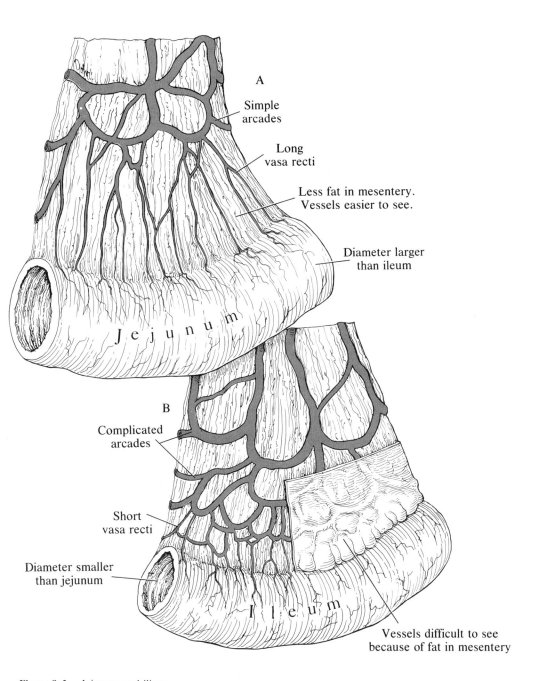

Figure 8–2. Jejunum and ilium.

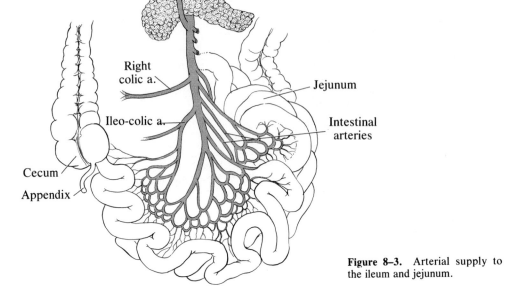

Figure 8–3. Arterial supply to the ileum and jejunum.

minimal at first. This is because much of the small bowel content has an almost neutral pH and is relatively sterile, resulting in a minimal inflammatory response.[9,10] If all penetrating wounds of the abdomen are treated by exploration, a perforating wound of the intestine should not be overlooked.

Perforations of the small bowel may be recognized by signs of peritoneal irritation: tenderness, rebound tenderness, guarding, and a reluctance of the patient to change position.

Small bowel injury following blunt trauma may be difficult to diagnose and must be considered, even if initial signs of intra-abdominal injury are absent. In patients wearing lap-type seat belts, combined visceral and lumber spine injuries may occur and the resultant peritoneal signs may be erroneously ascribed to the lumbar spine injury.[7]

Signs of pure mesenteric injury, if initially present, will be those associated with blood loss and intra-abdominal bleeding: hypotension, abdominal distention and tenderness, shoulder pain, and a falling hematocrit. At times, peritoneal blood will not cause much in the way of signs or symptoms. If there is evidence of bleeding somewhere and the site is not obvious, the most likely place is in the abdominal cavity.

If devascularization of the small bowel occurs as a result of mesenteric injury it may be recognized by increasing tenderness, pain, and manifestations of obstruction in the devascularized segment. In very rare instances, a traumatic laceration of the mesentery may be the site of internal herniation of small bowel with obstruction.

Laboratory work will provide little direct help in making a diagnosis, but a progressive increase in the white blood count after abdominal injury, in the absence of other reasons for its increase, is indirect evidence of intestinal injury.

In evaluating blunt trauma, films of the abdomen should include supine, lateral decubitus, and upright views and should be examined for free air and small bowel ileus (Figure 8-4). Peritoneal lavage may be used, but should usually be reserved for patients with multiple injuries, patients with head injuries who are unconscious or obtunded, or patients in whom, for one reason or another, physical examination of the abdomen is unreliable. In small bowel injury, the returning fluid after lavage may or may not be bloody. Nonbloody, turbid fluid or bile-stained fluid indicates a bowel perforation. Laboratory examination of the fluid may show an elevated white count or elevated amylase content.

PRE-OPERATIVE PREPARATION

In the emergency room, intravenous fluid support should be initiated, a nasogastric tube passed, a Foley catheter inserted, and a broad-spectrum antibiotic administered intravenously before surgery. Currently, the antibiotic of choice is a second generation cephalosporin.

OPERATIVE EXPLORATION

Exploration should be rapid and systematic. The first priority is to locate and control hemorrhage. The second is to locate any colon injury so that fecal contamination can be controlled until definitive therapy is carried out. The third priority is to identify injuries to the small bowel, including duodenum, stomach, pancreas, extrahepatic biliary tract, and the urinary tract. A thorough examination of all organs should be routine, so as to avoid overlooking an injury remote from where the surgeon expects to find it. The assessment and treatment of injuries to organs other than the small intestine are discussed elsewhere in this book.

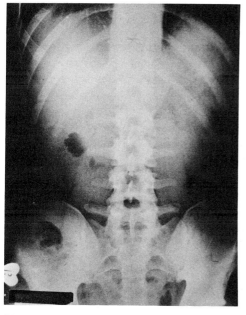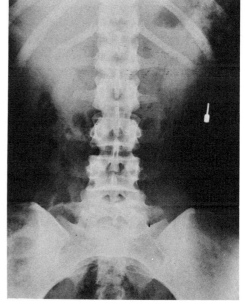

Figure 8–4. Diagnostic films of the abdomen.

The abdomen should be opened through a generous midline incision extending from the xiphoid to below the umbilicus. After control of hemorrhage and a thorough examination of the large bowel with control of fecal spillage, if it is present, the small intestine should be eviscerated onto the abdominal wall, the mesentery spread out, and the bowel and its mesentery examined in their entirety from the ligament of Treitz to the ileocecal junction, first on one side and then on the other. The surgeon should count the number of perforations. When one perforation is found in a penetrating injury, the presumption is that there is a second. An odd number of perforations must be explained; failure to do so may mean missing another perforation. Usually the missed perforation will lie on the mesenteric side of the bowel. Any hemorrhage in the mesentery adjacent to the bowel implies a perforation. The mesentery should be cleared away sufficiently to establish whether or not perforation has occurred. When, because of multiple injuries or vigorous intraperitoneal bleeding, the initial exploration has been done in haste, small perforations may easily be missed. Therefore, prior to closure of the abdomen, a final careful examination of the bowel should be made from the ligament of Treitz to the ileocecal junction.

OPERATIVE TREATMENT

Simple perforations and relatively short lacerations of the small bowel may be closed with a single layer of seromuscular nonabsorbable sutures. It makes no difference whether lacerations of the bowel are closed transversely or longitudinally as long as the lumen is not narrowed. Larger wounds, multiple perforations in short segments of the bowel, and devascularized segments of the bowel are indications for resection and anastomosis.

Resection and anastomosis should be done when the length of a laceration equals or exceeds 50 percent of the bowel diameter or when the total length of multiple lacerations in a short segment of bowel equals or exceeds 50 percent of the bowel diameter.

All damaged or marginally damaged bowel should be removed. Ragged wounds or wounds made by high velocity missiles must be thoroughly debrided. Often by the time debridement is completed, the defect in the bowel will be so large that resection and anastomosis are necessary. Time can be saved if the surgeon appreciates the extent of injury and goes directly to resection and anastomosis of the injured segment, omitting debridement.

Evidence of compromise of the blood supply to the bowel from an associated mesenteric laceration is a clear indication for performing resection and anastomosis since resection is well tolerated and failure to recognize devitalized bowel can lead to perforation and death. If the bowel has a normal appearance and responds to pinching with peristalsis, it is viable. The mucosa is much more active metabolically than the rest of the bowel. Therefore, if the bowel is dusky on the outside, the mucosa is probably dead or dying and resection is indicated. Hypovolemia causes poor perfusion, and it is important to restore blood volume when trying to determine viability of the bowel. Pulsations in the small vessels of the arcade should be felt for, since their presence indicates the bowel is probably viable. If there is any question about viability, the segment of bowel should be resected.

For practical purposes, all but 50 cm of the small bowel may be removed with minimal resultant disability. If resection is required, it should be carried back to where the bowel wall, including the mucosa, bleeds. Depending upon the surgeon's preference, the anastomosis can be performed using an open or closed technique with a single or double layer closure or with staples. Open anastomosis has the advantage of allowing inspection of the mucosa to determine viability. Noncrushing clamps may be applied proximal and distal to the anastomosis to prevent further contamination through leakage of intestinal content during the anastomosis. A single layer anastomosis is adequate since there is no evidence to indicate that a two-layer heals better than a one-layer anastomosis. Although bleeding from the suture line in small-intestinal anastomosis is rare, if the patient is hypotensive at the time of anastomosis or disseminated intravascular clotting, a twolayer anastomosis should be considered, using the continuous inner layer for hemostasis. This can prevent bleeding at the suture line as blood pressure later rises. A double layer open anastomosis is performed by laying a continuous suture of fine absorbable material followed by an outer layer of fine interrupted seromuscular nonabsorbable sutures (Figure 8-5). A single layer anastomosis is performed with interrupted seromuscular, nonabsorbable sutures (Figure 8-6). A closed one-layer anastomosis can be carried out by placing Lembert sutures over the occluding clamps and pulling up on the sutures as the clamps are removed, so as to avoid leakage. With tension maintained on the sutures, they are then tied serially (Figure 8-7). Lacerations and hematomas in the mesentery should be investigated (Figure 8-8). Meticulous hemostasis is obtained by clamping the ends of the divided vessels in such a manner that additional vessels are not injured. Large hematomas should be explored, since the superior mesenteric artery or one of its major branches may be involved. To facilitate exposure of the superior mesenteric artery and veins, as well as the dorsal side of the small bowel mesentery, the right colon is mobilized by incising its lateral attachments, and

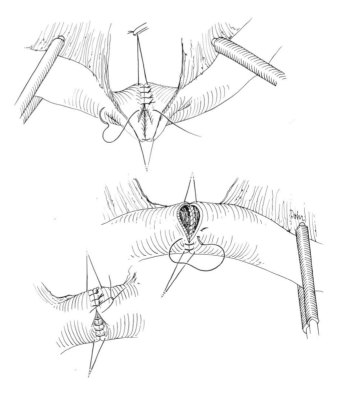

Figure 8–5. A double layer open anastomosis.

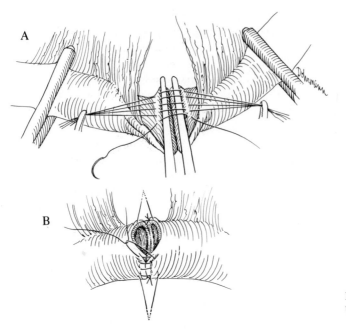

Figure 8–6. A single layer anastomosis.

then the right colon and small bowel mesentery containing the superior mesenteric vessels are raised (Figure 8-9). This exposes the mesenteric vessels as they pass over not only the uncinate process of the pancreas but also the third and fourth portions of the duodenum and the head of the pancreas.[11] Hemorrhage can generally be controlled by pressure. After evacuating a hematoma, small bleeding vessels may be ligated. Therefore, bleeding vessels should not be crushed and ligated before they are fully identified. If there is a major injury to the proximal portion of the superior mesenteric artery or vein, meticulous debridement and repair are indicated. A segment of inferior mesenteric vein or saphenous vein may be used as a patch when a portion of the wall of either the superior mesenteric artery or vein is missing. When the injury involves the distal portion of the mesenteric artery or vein and the viability of the bowel is questionable, the bowel should be resected and anastomosed and the injured artery or vein ligated rather than repaired. To avoid further injury to blood vessels, defects of the mesentery should be closed by continuous or interrupted sutures placed with care through the peritoneal covering of the mesentery alone. Following completion of mesenteric closure, viability of the adjacent small bowel should once again be verified. If there has been contamination of the peritoneal cavity by small bowel contents, the peritoneal cavity may be irrigated with an antibiotic solution of 0.5 gm of kanamycin and 50,000 units of bacitracin in one liter of saline. This same solution is used to irrigate the abdominal wall wound. If contamination is extensive, the skin and subcutaneous tissue should be left open, to be closed at a later date, whereas if contamination is minimal, the skin and subcutaneous tissue may be closed.

POSTOPERATIVE CARE

When there is doubt about hemostasis or viability of the bowel, re-exploration within 24 hours is mandatory (Figure 8-10). Patients can tolerate repeated laparotomy

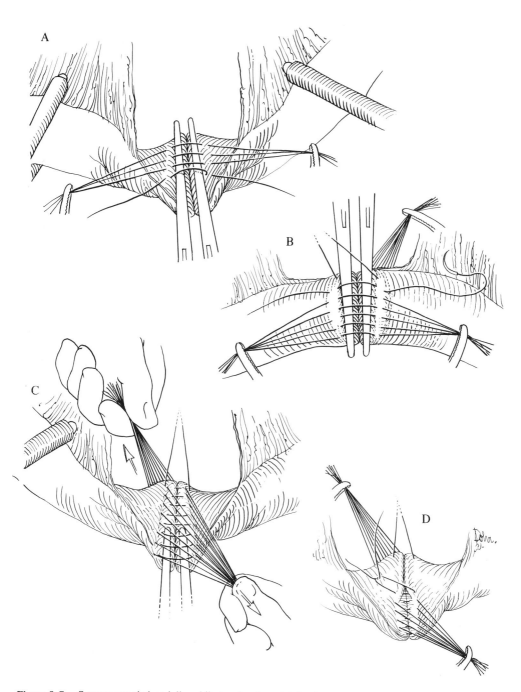

Figure 8–7. Sutures are tied serially while tension is maintained.

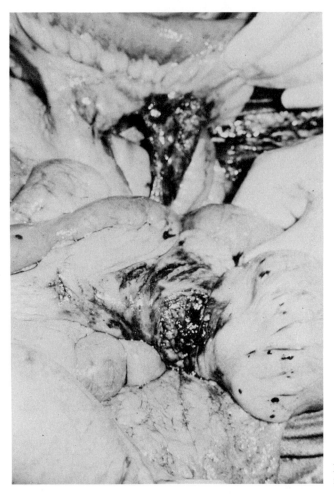

Figure 8–8. Lacerations and hematomas in the mesentery.

well but they do not tolerate bowel disruption or leakage since these complications invariably lead to a fatal outcome. If the status of the repair of the mesenteric vessels is questionable, thrombosis is a possibility. A second look permits removal of any residual peritoneal blood and resection of marginal-appearing segments of the bowel back to bleeding mucosa. This allows for a maximal amount of bowel to be salvaged and minimizes the risk of leakage, disruption, or fistula formation.

If penetration of the intestine has occurred and established infection has not developed, the antibiotic started preoperatively is continued for two to three doses postoperatively. Longer doses of antibiotics do not reduce the incidence of either peritoneal or wound infection.[12] Intravenous fluids are continued for several days until there is evidence of return of bowel function. Nasogastric suction should be used liberally. The hematocrit should be maintained at approximately 30.

COMPLICATIONS

Complications include postoperative bleeding, wound and intraperitoneal infections, suture line leaks, fistula formation, and ischemia of the bowel leading to obstruction or progressing to necrosis with perforation.

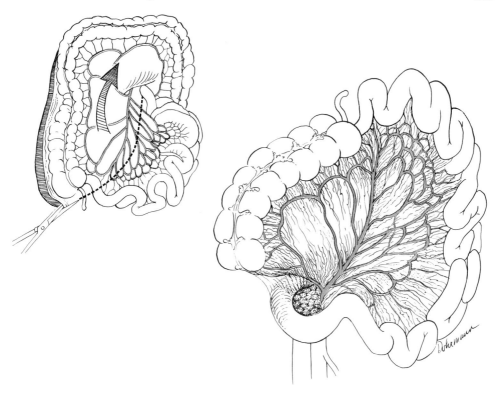

Figure 8–9. The right colon is mobilized, and the right colon and small bowel mesentery are raised.

Postoperative bleeding may occur into the peritoneal cavity or into the bowel lumen from the suture line. If signs of hypovolemia develop, with or without an initial fall in the hematocrit, bleeding must be suspected, and if stabilization does not occur promptly, reoperation should be performed. If the bleeding is found to be into the gastrointestinal tract, the anastomosis and the small areas of intestinal closure should be taken down and inspected for bleeding.

Infection of contaminated wounds may often be avoided by closing the fascia but leaving the skin and subcutaneous tissue open. If it looks healthy, the wound may then be closed four or more days later with plastic tape strips or sutures, (so-called delayed primary closure). Wound infections usually are not evident until the fourth or fifth postoperative day and usually require that the closed wound be opened widely. If peritoneal toilet has been good and hemostasis maintained, intraperitoneal infection is rare unless leakage develops. If postoperative peritoneal bleeding occurs, contamination may result with development of intra-abdominal abscesses in the pelvis, subphrenic or subhepatic spaces, either lateral gutter, or between loops of bowel.

Leakage of the anastomosis is usually catastrophic, leading to either prolonged morbidity or death from sepsis. The peritoneal cavity can handle contamination if the source of contamination is controlled, but it handles continued contamination poorly. Reoperation is mandatory when acute leakage from the anastomosis is suspected. When detected acutely, the anastomosis should be exteriorized or converted to a proximal "ostomy" and distal mucous fistula. A chronic leak may manifest itself by systemic signs of infection, abscess formation, or fistula formation through

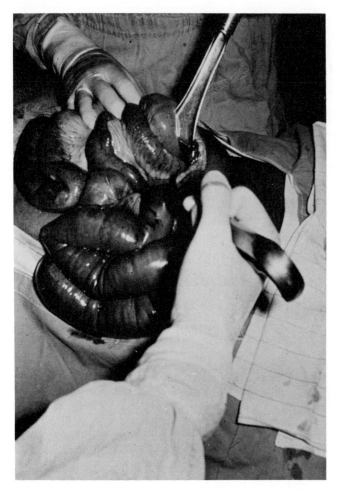

Figure 8–10. Re-explosion within 24 hours. Bowel necrosis is evident.

the wound. If a fistula develops, it is generally best handled conservatively while the patient is proximally decompressed and nourished intravenously with total parenteral nutrition (TPN). An abscess is best treated by dependent drainage, and a fistula accepted. Generalized peritonitis with no localization of the infection requires exteriorization of the leaking bowel.

Intra-abdominal sepsis, whether due to initial contamination or to secondary infection from an anastomotic leak, generally becomes manifest sometime between the third and tenth postoperative day. Often, obvious clinical findings may not be present initially and the only clues may be a slowly rising temperature, an increase in pulse rate, and an increase in white count. Diagnosis may be difficult, even for the most careful surgeon. The patient should receive frequent examinations, since the change in findings may be much more helpful in reaching a correct diagnosis than are the findings at any single examination. If the patient has received antibiotics for longer than one or two days after surgery, the antibiotics may mask the signs of developing sepsis.

Ischemia of the bowel is difficult to diagnose and usually, when it is recognized, the patient has reached the point of clinical catastrophe (Figure 8-10). A high index of suspicion with early reoperation is the key to avoiding serious consequences.

Ischemia may be suspected when there is unremitting severe abdominal pain, abdominal distention, a rising temperature, a rising white count, or signs of systemic sepsis. The patient appears toxic and seems sick out of proportion to the local findings. Signs of ischemia may be similar to those seen in intra-abdominal sepsis. An ischemic segment of bowel releases products of devitalized tissue into the mesentery, which initiate venous thrombosis and extension of the ischemic process to involve previously viable loops of adjacent bowel. Delay in recognition of a major ischemic loop can be associated with death of most of the bowel.

REFERENCES

1. Malgaine JF: Surgery and Ambrose Pare, Hamby, WB (ed.) University of Oklahoma Press: Norman, Oklahoma, 1965.
2. Cerise EJ, Scully JH Jr: Blunt trauma to the small intestine. J Trauma 10:46-50, 1970.
3. Bailey H: Surgery of Modern Warfare, Vol. II, 3rd Ed, Williams and Wilkins, Baltimore, Maryland 1944.
4. Surgery in World War II, Vol. II, General Surgery, Office of the Surgeon General, Department of the Army, Washington, D.C., 1955.
5. Williams RD, Sargent FT: The mechanism of intestinal injury in trauma. J Trauma 3:288-294, 1963.
6. Mathewson C Jr, Chief of Surgery, 59th Evacuation Hospital, U.S. Army: personal communication.
7. Ritchie WP, Ersek WB, Simmons RL: Combined visceral and vertebral injuries from lap-type belts. Surg Gynecol Obstet 131:432-435, 1970.
8. Zacheis HG, Condon RE: Seat belts and intra-abdominal trauma: Report of two unusual cases. J Trauma 12:8590, 1972.
9. Thadepalli H, Lou MA, Bach VT, Matsui TK, Mandal AK: Microflora of the human small intestine. Am J Surg 138:845-849, 1979.
10. Drasar BS, Shiner M, McLeod GM: Studies on the intestinal flora. The bacterial flora of the gastrointestinal tract in healthy and achlorhydric persons. Gastroenterology 56:71-79, 1969.
11. Gattell RB, Braasch JW: A technique for the exposure of the third and fourth portions of the duodenum. Surg Gynecol Obstet 111:379, 1960.
12. Stone HH, Haney BB, Kolb LD, Geheber CE, Hooper CA: Prophylactic and preventative antibiotic therapy. Ann Surg 189:691-699, 1979.

Chapter Nine

TRAUMA TO THE COLON AND RECTUM

THEODORE R. SCHROCK

INTRODUCTION

The large intestine is among the most lethal sites of abdominal injury. Trauma to the colon and rectum is not fatal immediately, but death occurs later as a result of sepsis and, even among survivors, the complication rate is high. Most of the deaths and many of the complications are preventable by following a few basic principles of management.

Military conflicts provided most of the early experience with wounds of the large intestine (Table 9-1). Prior to World War I, treatment was expectant, and death was the usual result; in the American Civil War for example, 90 percent of soldiers with penetrating abdominal wounds died.[26] Early in World War I, however, a few bold surgeons began to operate on these casualties.[8] Wangensteen has recounted a study in which the mortality rate was 95 percent in non-operated patients with wounds of the large bowel compared with only 44 percent in patients treated by prompt operation.[33] The overall mortality rate from colorectal trauma in World War I was about 60 percent; delayed evacuation and lack of resuscitative and antibiotic resources are reflected in this record, even though aggressive surgical treatment had been introduced. [9]

Table 9–1 MORTALITY FROM COLON INJURIES

Civil War	90%
Spanish American War	65%
W. W. I	60%
W. W. II	30%
Korea	15%
Vietnam	13%

(Modified from Haygood FD, Polk HC Jr: Gunshot wounds of the colon: A review of 100 consecutive patients, with emphasis on complications and their causes. Am J Surg 131:213, 1976.)

The mortality rate from trauma to the large intestine was 30 percent in World War II and 15 percent in the Korean conflict.[15] Many factors contributed to this improvement, including changes in surgical management. One important surgical development was recognition of the need for exteriorization or fecal diversion in every case of colonic or rectal trauma.[5] However, when military surgeons returned

165

to civilian practice and encountered less severe penetrating injuries, those caused by stab wounds and low velocity missiles, many felt that the conservative war time approach was unnecessary, and a policy of primary closure of colonic wounds was adopted in selected cases.[7,34] Controversy continues today over the relative merits of primary closure and the older, more conservative methods.

Civilian injuries to the colon and rectum are penetrating in 96 percent of patients.[15,16,19,28] Wounding agents vary according to regional preferences for methods of inflicting harm upon fellow human beings; generally, stabbing is responsible for about 25 percent and firearms account for about 75 percent of cases.[35] The firearms category includes occasional high velocity missiles, and shotgun wounds comprise 5 percent to 15 percent of the total; the majority, however, are low velocity missiles.[15] Foreign bodies introduced for erotic purposes are frequent causes of rectal perforation.[32] Iatrogenic perforation of the colon by colonoscopy, enema, or barium enema is relatively uncommon. [29]

Blunt trauma to the colon occurs from motor vehicle accidents (seat belt, steering wheel), pedestrian accidents, assault (kicks, blows), and falls. Most of these wounds are contusions rather than full thickness tears, although delayed rupture of the colonic wall is a potential threat and occasionally occurs.[16] Rectal lacerations associated with compound pelvic fractures are particularly dangerous because they are often overlooked (see Chapter 14).[13,16,20,32]

The mobile segments of the colon (transverse and sigmoid) are most vulnerable to blunt trauma, and the transverse colon is also the most frequent site of penetrating injury; from 33 percent to 47 percent of penetrating wounds occur in this region.[14,15,16,19,21,28,29,35] Perforation involves the right colon (cecum and ascending) in 20 percent to 30 percent of patients, and the left colon (descending and sigmoid) is affected in about 30 percent of cases. Rectal injuries comprise approximately 10 percent of cases of trauma to the large intestine. Multiple colonic or rectal sites are perforated in about 10 percent of patients.[35]

Only 15 percent to 25 percent of patients have isolated wounds of the colon or rectum; the majority have associated injuries of other abdominal or thoracic organs.[15,19,28,29,35] The small bowel is by far the most common site of associated injury, affecting nearly 50 percent of patients. [15] Stomach, liver, and kidney each are involved in 15 percent of patients; other organs that may be injured include spleen, thorax, major vessels, and pancreas.[15,19] The number and severity of associated injuries is the most important determinant of survival in patients with trauma to the colon or rectum.[19]

ANATOMY

Knowledge of anatomic relationships allows one to estimate the likelihood of injury to the colon from a penetrating wound and to predict which other organs may be injured also. This exercise is fallible, however, since knife and missile tracks sometimes course in unexpected directions.

The large intestine is divided into colon, rectum, and anal canal, and the colon in turn can be subdivided by embryonic origin into the *right colon* (cecum, ascending colon, hepatic flexure, and proximal transverse colon) and the *left colon* (distal transverse colon, splenic flexure, descending colon, sigmoid colon, and rectosigmoid) (Figure 9-1). It is common practice, however, to consider the transverse colon

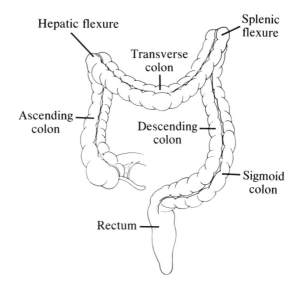

Hepatic flexure

Splenic flexure

Transverse colon

Ascending colon

Descending colon

Sigmoid colon

Rectum

Figure 9–1. Anatomy of the large bowel.

separately in discussions of colonic trauma; the right colon in this convention includes just the cecum and ascending portions, and the left colon is comprised of the descending, sigmoid, and rectosigmoid.

The cecum occupies the iliac fossa, and the ascending colon extends cephalad in the posterior axillary line. The posterior one-third of the cecum and ascending colon usually are retroperitoneal but, in some individuals, the right colon is incompletely fixed and remains quite mobile on a long mesocolon, so that most of the bowel's circumference is intraperitoneal. The third part of the duodenum and the ureter lie posterior to the ascending colon and its mesocolon.

At the hepatic flexure, the colon is fixed just below the right lobe of the liver adjacent to the gallbladder. The right kidney, inferior vena cava, and duodenum lie behind the colon in this region.

The transverse colon is suspended in the peritoneal cavity on a long mesocolon, and the omentum is draped over and attached to the superior surface of the bowel. The stomach is a few centimeters cephalad, and the pancreas also lies cephalad to the transverse mesocolon just behind the stomach.

The splenic flexure usually extends high into the upper quadrant and has ligmentous attachments to the diaphragm and to the lower pole of the spleen. It is in immediate proximity to the tail of the pancreas and the left kidney, both of which lie posterior.

The descending colon is retroperitoneal around half to two-thirds of its circumference, and it lies anterior to the left kidney and ureter. It extends inferiorly in the posterior axillary line to the left iliac fossa. At this point, the descending-sigmoid junction, it curves anteriorly into the peritoneal cavity to become the sigmoid colon.

The sigmoid colon is suspended on its mesocolon. The length and mobility of this segment of bowel are variable; in some people, a redundant sigmoid colon extends well into the upper abdomen and, in others, the sigmoid is short and fixed. The left common iliac vessels and the left ureter lie behind.

The rectosigmoid junction is a zone several centimeters long. In this region, just above the sacral promontory, the taeniae coli spread to form a complete longitudinal muscular layer which encircles the rectum.

The rectum, the lower portion of the large bowel, is 12 to 15 cm long. The upper rectum is invested by peritoneum anteriorly and laterally, but the posterior wall is retroperitoneal from the rectosigmoid junction downward. The anterior pelvic peritoneal reflection is approximately 7 cm above the anal verge; a perforating injury of the anterior or lateral rectum above this point is intraperitoneal.

The rectum passes through the levator ani muscles to fuse with the anal canal. This structure is approximately 3 cm long, lined by stratified squamous epithelium (anoderm), and innervated somatically.

The arterial blood supply to the right colon, from the ileocecal junction to the midtransverse colon, is from the superior mesenteric artery through its ileocolic, right colic, and middle colic branches (Figure 9-2). The middle colic artery is a proximal branch of the superior mesenteric artery as it emerges from the inferior border of the pancreas, and it passes ventrally in the transverse mesocolon to form arcades communicating with the right colic and the left colic arteries.

The inferior mesenteric artery arises from the abdominal aorta at the level of the fourth lumbar vertebra, and it divides into the left colic artery and the superior hemorrhoidal artery. The left colic artery courses towards the left upper quadrant to supply the descending colon, splenic flexure, and transverse colon, and it anastomoses with branches from the middle colic artery. The superior hemorrhoidal gives off sigmoidal branches and then passes inferiorly in the base of the mesocolon to supply the rectum.

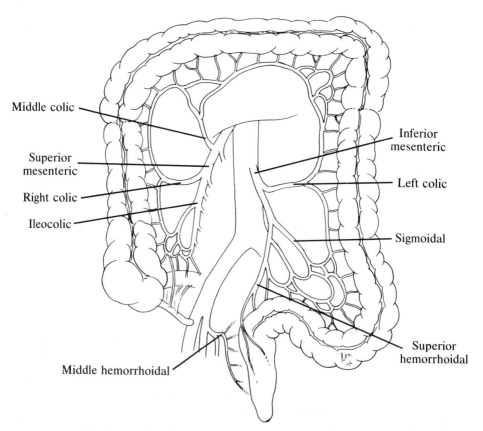

Figure 9–2. Arterial supply of the colon.

The rectum obtains additional blood from the internal iliac (hypogastric) arteries by way of the middle hemorrhoidal arteries; these vessels extend medially to the rectum in the lateral ligaments above the levators. The inferior hemorrhoidal arteries derive from the internal pudendal branches of the hypogastrics, which pass though the ischiorectal fossa to reach the bowel. There is extensive collateral circulation available among these networks of vessels supplying the rectum and anus.

Venous blood from the colon accompanies the corresponding arteries and drains into the liver through the portal vein. Blood from the right colon enters the superior mesenteric vein, and blood from the left colon empties into the inferior mesenteric vein, which enters the splenic vein just proximal to its junction with the superior mesenteric vein. Some venous blood from the rectum drains upward into the portal vein, and some enters the systemic circulation directly by way of the middle hemorrhoidal and inferior hemorrhoidal veins.

ASSESSMENT

Patients with possible injury to the large bowel should undergo the same thorough evaluation that is applied to all patients with abdominal trauma.[31] If possible, details of the traumatic incident should be elicited: the nature of the wounding agent, proximity of the patient to the weapon, and the position of the patient at the time of injury. Unfortunately, these historical items are not always available, and they are often unreliable. The time of the last meal and any alcohol or drug intake are important points to note. Also inquire about previous tetanus prophylaxis, illness, and operations.

The abdomen, both flanks, back, buttocks, perineum, and genitalia should be inspected for external evidence of trauma, and wounds should be carefully described. Conscious patients may indicate the presence of pain, and palpation may disclose abdominal tenderness or muscular rigidity. It is essential to perform digital rectal examination in every patient with abdominal trauma, and if blood is present on the examining finger or if there is other suggestions of rectal injury, anoscopy and sigmoidoscopy should be done. Speculum examination of the vagina is indicated if involvement of that structure is suspected. Neurologic examination should include assessment of anal sphincter tone. A careful search should be made for urologic injury.

Injuries of the large bowel may be manifested by hemodynamic signs of blood loss (usually from associated injuries) or by peritoneal irritation from blood or feces. After several hours, there will be symptoms and signs of invasive infection if there was much fecal contamination. Abdominal pain and tenderness, fever, and leukocytosis are typical of this development. One goal of surgical therapy is control of the fecal contamination before infection becomes established, so early recognition of injury and prompt operation are essential. It is our policy to explore most patients with penetrating abdominal trauma and, therefore, injury to the colon is usually detected early. Authorities generally agree that laparotomy is always indicated in patients with gunshot wounds but, in many centers, stab wounds are managed selectively. If fecal contamination is minimal, early signs of colonic perforation may be absent, and extensive infection may develop by the time the diagnosis is made. We recommend at least local exploration of stab wounds; if the tract of the sharp instrument penetrates the fascia anterior to the posterior axillary line, there is potential for intra-abdominal injury, and laparotomy should be performed. Stab wounds behind the posterior axillary line have a lower incidence of significant trauma to hollow viscera, and some of these wounds may be managed expectantly. The location of the ascending and descending colon in the posterior axillary line should be kept in mind and the possibility of a retroperitoneal laceration of the colon considered.

Blunt trauma to the colon or mesocolon may produce obvious peritoneal signs that dictate immediate laparotomy, but in many cases the diagnosis of major trauma to hollow viscera is difficult and delayed.[16] In addition to the physical examination, x-rays of chest and abdomen should be obtained. Free air, disappearance of the psoas shadow, loss of the retroperitoneal fat line, or small loculated air bubbles may suggest colonic injury. X-rays are helpful in patients with rectal injuries, either blunt or penetrating. Barium enema x-rays are contraindicated in patients with suspected colonic or rectal perforation, but water-soluble contrast medium can be administered per rectum with minimal risk of serious consequences if the material enters the peritoneal cavity. Since these x-rays may be falsely negative, however, laparotomy is the appropriate diagnostic maneuver in patients with suspected colonic injury.

PRE-OPERATIVE PREPARATION

Standard pre-operative measures include intravenous fluids, typing and cross-matching of blood, and insertion of a urinary catheter and a nasogastric tube. Bacterial contamination of the peritoneum becomes an invasive infection 6 to 8 hours after wounding, and antibiotics help prevent or at least minimize this development.[23] Therefore, intravenous broad spectrum antibiotics should be started before operation. A combination of antibiotics such as clindamycin (600 mg I.V. q 6h) and an aminoglycoside is recommended (e.g., gentamicin 80 mg I.M. q 8h).[23]

No attempt should be made to prepare the gastrointestinal tract with laxatives or enemas in the trauma victim requiring emergency operation; these measures may aggravate the spillage of stool through colonic or rectal perforations.

OPERATIVE EXPOSURE AND EVALUATION

A midline incision is used in most patients. Control of hemorrhage takes first priority upon entry into the peritoneal cavity, and then leakage of feces from large colonic rents should be controlled temporarily with sutures or intestinal clamps. Gross fecal material is removed by irrigation and aspiration. When these maneuvers have been completed, the abdominal cavity is thoroughly explored, all injuries are identified, and a treatment plan is formulated.

Examination of the large intestine should proceed systemically, usually from proximal to distal. The small intestine is retracted to the left when examining the right colon and to the right when examining the left colon; it is usually best to eviscerate the small bowel to facilitate exposure.

The cecum and appendix are examined in the right lower quadrant. The lateral peritoneal reflection can be incised to permit mobilization of the right colon and mesocolon, thus bringing the posterior surface of the colon, the duodenum, and the right ureter into view (Figure 9-3). The hepatic flexure also can be taken down for

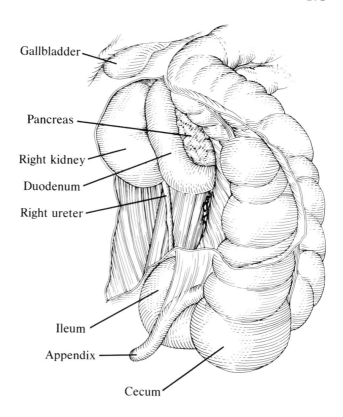

Gallbladder

Pancreas

Right kidney

Duodenum

Right ureter

Ileum

Figure 9-3. Mobilization of the right colon is readily performed by severing the lateral peritoneal attachment. This exposes the duodenum and right kidney.

Appendix

Cecum

inspection. These steps are unnecessary if there is no reason to suspect a retroperitoneal wound and if there is no hematoma or ecchymosis in the soft tissues adjacent to the colon. Injury to the anterior portion of the right colon is an intraperitoneal wound; mobilization is not required to identify this lesion, although it is usually necessary to rule out through-and-through penetration and for treatment of the injury.

The transverse colon is easily examined in most patients. It may be necessary to detach the omentum from the transverse colon by dividing the avascular plane of fusion. The appendices epiploicae receive blood supply from the colon, and they are a source of hemorrhage during this maneuver if the correct plane is not followed. Omental fat often is granular and appendiceal fat is smoother; there are color differences as well.

The splenic flexure is by far the most difficult area to examine because it is situated high under the left diaphragm. If there is no reason to suspect injury in this region, simple inspection for hemorrhage and fecal leakage is all that is necessary. Blood in the left upper quadrant or an external wound in this region requires that the splenic flexure be taken down (Figure 9-4). This is done by first mobilizing the proximal descending colon and bluntly separating the colon and mesocolon from the anterior surface of Gerota's fascia behind. Attachments of the colon to diaphragm and spleen are brought into view for division, and the attachments of omentum to the colon in the splenic flexure can be sharply separated in the avascular plane. It is possible in this way to mobilize the splenic flexure without dividing and ligating any large vessels, a procedure that is required if the omentum is cut through instead of just detached from the colon.

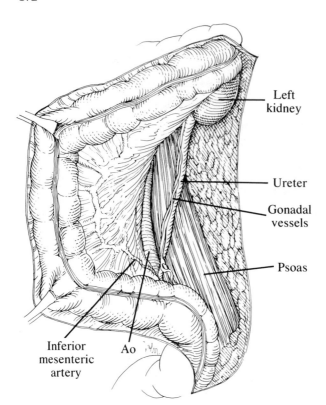

Left
kidney

Ureter

Gonadal
vessels

Psoas

Inferior   Ao
mesenteric
artery

Figure 9–4. Left colon is mobilized by severing the lateral peritoneal attachment and developing the areolar plane behind the mesocolon.

The principles of inspection of the descending colon are the same as described for the right colon. Although the sigmoid colon is easily examined when it is normally mobile, many patients have fixation of the sigmoid from pelvic surgery or diverticular disease, and it may be necessary to lyse these adhesions to facilitate exposure.

The rectum is examined with the small bowel retracted through the incision or into the upper abdomen. Wounds of the anterior and lateral intraperitoneal surfaces are readily apparent, but posterior perforations of the rectum may not be so obvious. Pre-operative evaluation of the rectum and intra-operative findings determine whether the rectum should be mobilized to look for such wounds. An overlooked rectal perforation may prove lethal, yet the decision to mobilize the rectum should not be made lightly; sexual function in males is jeopardized if autonomic nerves are injured during rectal mobilization. The pelvic peritoneum is incised to the right of the rectum just below the common iliac artery and medial to the right ureter. The presacral space is entered, and the rectum is bluntly dissected from the sacrum. The lateral ligaments can be divided, but of course this interrupts some of the rectal blood supply and should be done only if it is essential for exposure. Dissection anterior to the rectum below the peritoneal reflection is also required in some cases.

The surgeon should evaluate the colonic and rectal wounds with respect to certain characteristics that help decide the method of management: number of wounds, segments of bowel involved, location around the circumference of the bowel (mesocolic or antimesocolic), size of each perforation, presence of contusion or hematoma in the colonic wall, and amount of fecal contamination. Trauma to soft tissues is severe in wounds from high velocity missiles, and the presence of devitalized or contused tissued adjacent to the intestinal perforation should be noted.

The number and severity of injuries to other organs and the amount of blood in the peritoneal cavity are important factors also.

OPERATIVE TREATMENT

The choice of operative treatment of trauma to the colon and rectum depends on many factors in addition to detailed assessment of the intra-abdominal injuries as described above. Age of the patient, presence of other medical conditions such as diabetes and heart disease, interval from wounding to performances of definitve operation, condition of the patient initially and after resuscitation, and severity and duration of shock must all be considered in the therapeutic decision making.

Types of Operative Treatment

PRIMARY SUTURE. The colonic perforation is sutured primarily in one or two layers, and the colon is replaced into the peritoneal cavity (Figure 9-5a). Primary suture is suitable for small, discrete, clean penetrating wounds without surrounding contusion or hematoma. Many stab wounds and some low-velocity gunshot wounds fit into this category. Other criteria for primary closure include the following: preoperative shock being absent or mild; blood loss less than 20 percent of estimated normal volume; few (probably only 1 or 2) other organ systems injured; minimal fecal contamination; and operation within 6 hours of wounding.[30] Some surgeons exclude elderly patients and those with perforations on the mesocolic border or in the retroperitoneal colon. Inexperience of the surgeon is another factor that weighs against attempting primary repair.

Primary suture was regarded by some surgeons as a dangerously bold maneuver when first introduced, but it has gained favor and now is used in about 50 percent of patients with civilian trauma in many centers.[2,4,14,17,21,25,31] The benefit of primary closure is the avoidance of multiple operative procedures necessitated by exteriorization methods described below; the hazard of primary closure is that the intestinal suture line will leak and thus increase operative morbidity and mortality. The benefits and risks as judged by retrospective studies have been argued in the literature for many years. Recently, however, Stone and Fabian reported the results of a prospective randomized comparison of primary suture and exteriorization; the mortality rate was the same with the two methods, but the morbidity rate was lower with primary closure.[30] Patients in this study met the rigid criteria for primary suture that are listed above.

Primary suture was advocated only for wounds in the right colon initially, because the right colon was believed to heal more predictably than the left colon. Despite a substantial body of literature that documents theoretical and practical differences in healing properies of right and left colon in animals and humans, data on trauma do not support the notion that primary suture is safer on one side than the other.[28] Stone and Fabian treated wounds in either the right or left colon by

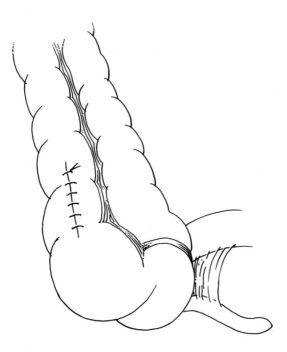

Figure 9–5. Primary suture of the colon.

primary suture if they met the established criteria, and other authors share their view that it makes no difference where the perforation is located provided that the hole is small, fecal contamination is minimal, and so forth.[17,21,24,30] This point is controversial, however, and many surgeons still are reluctant to apply primary suture to wounds of the left colon.

PRIMARY REPAIR AND PROXIMAL FECAL DIVERSION. The intestinal wound is sutured primarily, but the fecal stream is diverted (or the bowel is decompressed) proximally (Figure 9-6). Diversion can be complete (divided colostomy) or partial (loop colostomy), or one can just provide a vent for flatus and liquid stool (tube cecostomy). The evidence suggests that proximal diversion or decompression does not prevent dehiscence of a sutured colonic wound, but if leakage occurs, the consequences are minimized.[28] This method is used most often for wounds of the rectum; the rectal perforation is sutured, and a completely diverting sigmoid colostomy is performed.[20,32] A few surgeons still do tube cecostomy in association with primary closure of colonic wounds, but this method has been replaced by primary suture alone or by one of the exteriorization procedures in most situations.

PRIMARY SUTURE AND EXTERIORIZATION. The colonic perforation is sutured primarily, and the loop of colon containing the suture line is exteriorized through an opening in the anterior abdominal wall (Figure 9-7a). If the suture line heals, the loop is simply replaced into the peritoneal cavity 7 to 10 days later. If the exteriorized loop leaks, no great harm results, and the colonic opening is enlarged to form a colostomy. The method is applicable only to perforations on the antimesocolic border. If a perforation on the mesocolic side is exteriorized, leakage into the subcutaneous or subfascial plane may develop, and severe necrotizing infection

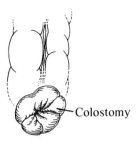

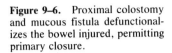

Figure 9–6. Proximal colostomy and mucous fistula defunctionalizes the bowel injured, permitting primary closure.

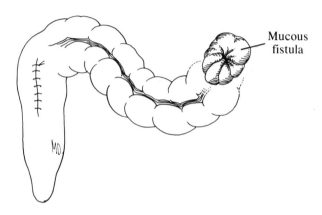

can result. Some surgeons exteriorize the colon over a glass or plastic rod, and others prefer to create a window in the mesocolon near the colonic border and suture the anterior fascia together behind the colon through this window.

This method appears to offer the advantages of primary repair without the risks, especially in patients with high likelihood of intra-abdominal sepsis. Our experience is such that we rarely use this technic because 50 percent of the exteriorized suture lines dehisce, and the loop becomes obstructed at the level of the fascia in other cases. However, other authors have reported excellent results: primary healing in 60 percent to 70 percent of patients and avoidance of colostomy in two-thirds of patients.[3,18,24,25,35] It is possible that in our series the perforations were not closed carefully enough, the blood supply was compromised, or the fascial opening obstructed the distal segment. Certainly, obstruction is easily prevented by making the fascial opening large enough, although too generous an opening risks herniation of small bowel alongside the colonic loop.

At present, primary closure and exteriorization can be recommended for patients whose colonic perforations are suitable for primary closure but in whom some problem with healing is anticipated—either because of the site of colonic injury or because of other intra-abdominal conditions. An example is a patient with combined penetrating wounds of the colon and the liver; allowing a primarily sutured colon to rest against the traumatized liver incurs the risk of colonic dehiscence, and exteriorization of the sutured bowel is a good approach.

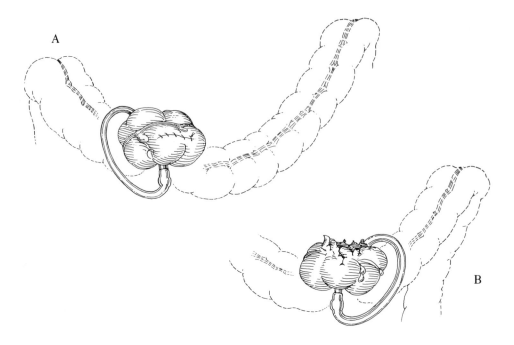

Figure 9–7. Exteriorization of the area of injury is carried out over a glass rod. *A* Demonstrates primary closure.

EXTERIORIZATION. The loop of colon ´containing the perforation is exteriorized with no attempt at definitive suture repair (Figure 9-7b). Some surgeons approximate the edges of the perforation with a few sutures to prevent further contamination and then open the loop to form a colostomy 24 to 48 hours later; others enlarge the perforation to construct a colostomy immediately.[6] Here, too, it is important to prevent leakage of feces into the subcutaneous tissue.

Exteriorization is recommended if local or systemic conditions are unfavorable for primary healing or if the perforation is too large or contused to exteriorize as a sutured loop.[1,30] It is used most often with wounds of the transverse or sigmoid colon; the right colon and the descending colon are difficult to exteriorize and some other method of management is usually preferable.

RESECTION WITH ANASTOMOSIS. Severely damaged colon is resected and a primary, usually end-to-end, anastomosis is performed at the same operation (Figure 9-8a). The patient must be in excellent general condition, and there should be little risk of postoperative intra-abdominal complications from the colonic injury or associated problems.

Primary anastomosis is applied most often after resection of the right colon.[11] The ileum, a structure with excellent healing properties, is anastomosed to the transverse colon. There is little enthusiasm for primary anastomosis of colon to colon (e.g., after left colectomy).[10] Recently it has become clear that the incidence of leakage from ileotransverse colonic anastomosis in trauma and other emergency situations is high, so that even in this "favored" part of the bowel, emergency anastomosis should be undertaken with great caution in carefully selected patients.[11]

RESECTION WITH PRIMARY ANASTOMOSIS AND PROXIMAL DE-COMPRESSION. When the colonic wounds are large or devitalizing, it is necessary to remove the damaged bowel (Figure 9-8b). In these instances, anastomosis and proximal decompression can be added. This is not a common method of management. One variant is resection of the right colon, end-to-side ileotransverse colonic anastomosis, and exteriorization of the proximal stump of ascending or transverse colon as a stoma to provide a vent for gas and stool (Figure 9-8c).[6] Few surgeons espouse this technic because it combines the worst features of anastomosis and colostomy: the anastomosis can still leak, yet the patient has a colostomy, too.

RESECTION WITHOUT ANASTOMOSIS. The colon is resected, the proximal stump of colon (or ileum) is fashioned as an end colostomy (for ileostomy), and the distal stump is oversewn (Hartmann procedure) or brought to the surface as a mucous fistula (Figure 9-6). Mucous fistula is preferable, but in the case of the rectum, the distal stump cannot reach the anterior abdominal wall. This procedure is often the method of choice if badly damaged colon must be resected.

PROXIMAL DIVERSION OR DECOMPRESSION ALONE. A colostomy is constructed proximal to a perforation which is not sutured; a small extraperitoneal rectal wound might be handled in this way. A small cecal perforation could be treated by placing a tube directly through it to form a tube cecostomy.

Management of Wounds in Various Bowel Segments

Methods for managing wounds in various bowel segments are listed in Table 9-2.

CECUM AND ASCENDING COLON. It is difficult to exteriorize this large retroperitoneal structure. Small wounds are treated by primary suture if the previously described criteria are met. Larger wounds are best managed by resection: anastomosis is done if conditions are favorable, otherwise an ileostomy and mucous fistula are constructed. Anastomosis with proximal end vent (the sixth choice above) and primary suture plus tube cecostomy are used occasionally.

Table 9–2 MANAGEMENT OF MAJOR WOUNDS IN VARIOUS BOWEL SEGMENT

	Major Injury	Alternative
Cecum	Resection with ileostomy	Resection with primary anastomosis
Ascending Colon	Resection with ileostomy	Resection with primary anasomosis
Hepatic Flexure	Resection with ileostomy	Resection with primary anastomosis
Transverse Colon	Resection or Exteriorization with colostomy	Exteriorization with closure
Splenic Flexure	Resection or Exteriorization with colostomy	Exteriorization with closure
Descending Colon	Resection or Exteriorization with colostomy	Exteriorization with closure
Sigmoid Colon	Resection or Exteriorization with colostomy	Exteriorization with closure
Rectum	Proximal colostomy and suture irrigation of distal segment	Proximal colostomy, irrigation of distal segment

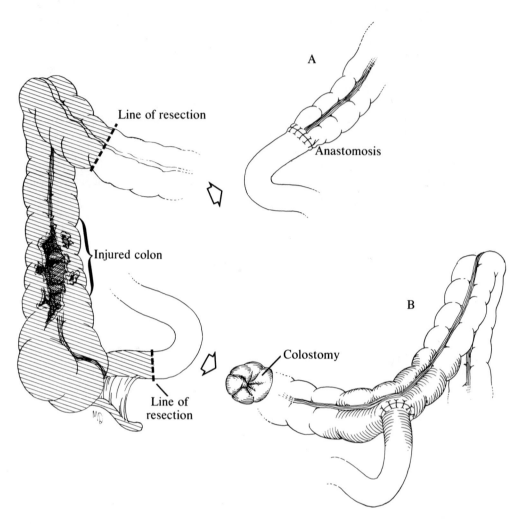

Figure 9–8. Demonstrates a badly lacerated ascending colon—the shaded area representing the area of resection. In *A* an ileocolic anastomosis has been carried out. In *B* an ileocolic anastomosis has been carried out distal to a "venting" colostomy.

HEPATIC FLEXURE. Wounds in this area may be associated with trauma to the liver, kidney, or duodenum and pancreas, and the potential for postoperative intra-abdominal infection with any of these combinations is great. Since the hepatic flexure can be mobilized, exteriorization—with or without primary suture—is preferred to primary suture or anastomosis in cases of associated injury.

TRANSVERSE COLON. The transverse colon is easy to exteriorize, and this method—with primary suture, if possible—is commonly employed. Primary suture alone is used if the situation is appropriate. If resection is necessary, anastomosis is avoided, and the ends are brought out as a colostomy and mucous fistula.

SPLENIC FLEXURE AND DESCENDING COLON. These areas are not readily brought to the abdominal surface, nor are they favored areas for primary suture. Primary suture should be attempted only in highly selected patients, with strict

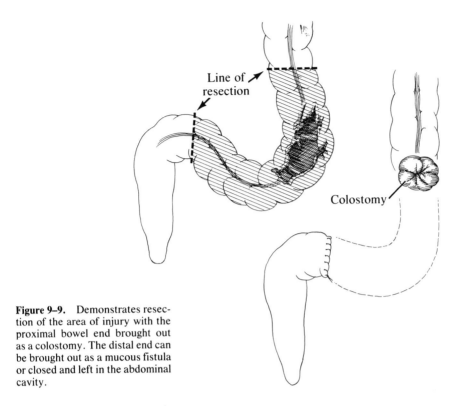

Line of resection

Colostomy

Figure 9–9. Demonstrates resection of the area of injury with the proximal bowel end brought out as a colostomy. The distal end can be brought out as a mucous fistula or closed and left in the abdominal cavity.

strict adherence to the criteria described earlier. Injury to adjacent pancreas, spleen, or kidney contraindicates primary suture. If the bowel can be mobilized sufficiently, exteriorization alone may be used. Resection with end colostomy and mucous fistula is most often the treatment of choice. Primary anastomosis should be avoided.

SIGMOID COLON. Like the transverse colon, sigmoid injuries are best exteriorized with or without primary closure or colostomy. Primary suture alone is reserved for ideal situations, such as colonoscopic perforation in a patient with mechanically prepared bowel, inadvertent trauma during performance of some other operation, or small penetrating wounds with minimal fecal contamination. Anastomosis should not be done primarily after emergency resection of the sigmoid colon for trauma.

RECTUM AND RECTOSIGMOID. Special considerations apply to wounds of the rectum. Minor partial thickness injuries to the rectal wall from within the lumen, such as those caused by foreign bodies, do not require specific treatment. Lacerations or perforations above the levators and below the pelvic peritoneum require transabdominal debridement and repair (if possible), sigmoid colostomy, and external drainage. The colostomy should be completely diverting, and a divided colostomy is the best guarantee of that. Drains have no role in colonic trauma, but in extraperitoneal rectal trauma they are important. Presacral drainage is accomplished by dissection behind the rectum from above and passage of soft rubber drains through a small perineal incision anterior to the coccyx. An alternative used by some surgeons is to place sump drains behind the rectum and bring them out through the anterior abdominal wall.

Another essential feature of management of rectal injuries is irrigation of the rectum with copious quantities of saline to remove feces completely.[20] This is easily done from above at the time of constructing a mucous fistula, or it can be accomplished from below instead. The anal sphincters should be gently dilated to facilitate rectal emptying. Rectal washout is credited with substantial lowering of morbidity and mortality rates.[20]

Perforation of the intraperitoneal rectum is managed by suture and sigmoid colostomy; drains are unnecessary. Extensive destructive trauma by high velocity missiles, blast, shotgun wounds, or crushing injuries is treated by debridement, rectal washout, drainage, and proximal colostomy. Abdominoperineal resection has been reported, but this drastic step is rarely, if ever, required.

ANUS. These wounds are most often the result of blunt trauma and consist of lacerations of varying degrees of severity. Those in continuity with pelvic fractures (compound pelvic fractures) should be treated with proximal diversion with irrigation of the rectal segment until clean. The purpose is to minimize contamination of the large pelvic hematoma which always accompanies these injuries and which carries a high mortality from sepsis.

Other extensive lacerations, particularly when associated with probable rectal injury or perirectal hematomas, should be treated similarly. The anal laceration should be left open in all instances and secondary sphincter reconstruction (which is rarely necessary) should be carried out at a later date, after healing has occurred.

Blunt Trauma

Wounds of the colon from blunt trauma most commonly are hemorrhagic contusions without disruption of serosa. [16] Incomplete laceration, full thickness perforation, and total loss of bowel continuity are seen also. Management of contused but intact bowel requires careful appraisal of the situation. Minor injuries can be reinforced with sutures or left alone altogether, but if viability of the bowel is questionable, resection or exteriorization is advised.

Compound fractures of the pelvis, with or without obvious rectal injury, and closed pelvic fractures with rectal laceration, should be managed as described for penetrating rectal injuries (see also Chapter 14).

Technic of Colostomy

An elective colostomy is usually opened and the bowel is sutured circumferentially to the skin ("matured") at the time it is constructed but, in a trauma case, fecal loading of the colon may make it unwise to mature the colostomy primarily because of the risk of subcutaneous infection adjacent to the stoma. There is a trend toward more frequent primary maturation of colostomies, however, even in emergency circumstances.

The bowel should be brought through the abdominal wall at a convenient location, preferably through the rectus abdominus muscle several centimeters from the midline. The fascia is incised longitudinally, the muscle is split, and the peritoneum is incised to create an opening 3.5 to 4.0 cm or two fingerbreadths in diameter for an end colostomy. The colon should be mobilized sufficiently to reach the skin without tension to avoid retraction into the peritoneal cavity later. A few sutures of absorbable material may be placed between appendices epiploicae or mesocolon and peritoneum, but generally these sutures should not grasp the bowel wall itself. If an end colostomy is not to be primarily matured, a clamp is left on the exteriorized colon; it is removed three or four days later, and the colonic mucosa is sutured to the skin at that time or the colostomy is allowed to mature secondarily. It should be noted that a colostomy clamp will not prevent retraction of a colostomy that is on tension; the clamp crushes the bowel, and the viable colon separates from the necrotic portion as it sinks into the abdomen.

A mucous fistulacan be brought out through the lower end of the abdominal incision or through a separate wound. It is not necessary to mature a mucous fistula primarily; it can be managed as described above with a clamp that is removed in a few days.

Loop colostomy and exteriorization of a sutured perforation are discussed in an earlier section. The bowel is supported by a glass or plastic rod or a fascial bridge. A large abdominal wall opening atleast 2 to 3 fingerbreaths in diameter is required to avoid obstruction of the loop.

MANAGEMENT OF THE ABDOMINAL INCISION

Between 20 percent and 40 percent of primarily closed abdominal incisions become infected in patients with trauma to the colon or rectum.[6,15,28,35] The variable incidence of infection in different reports reflects severity of trauma, extent of fecal contamination, and other factors. If delayed primary closure is used, the rate of infection is much less; therefore, this method is strongly recommended.[6,14,28]

The peritoneum and fascia are sutured, the subcutaneous fat and skin are left open, and moist gauze is packed loosely in the wound. Sterile dressings are maintained and the wound is not inspected for four to five days if there is no reason to suspect an infection. A wound that is clean at this time can be closed with paper tapes, but if there is exudate or other evidence of infection, the wound is allowed to heal by second intention. Some surgeons recommend that moist gauze dressings be changed several times daily beginning immediately after operation. This practice stimulates formation of granulation tissue which converts the wound to secondary healing by the time it is closed. Apposition of these granulating surfaces may permit exudate to accumulate beneath the skin; this is equivalent to a wound infection, and the skin edges need to be reopened.

In circumstances in which there has been minimal contamination and a thin subcutaneous layer, the skin can be loosely approximated with tape sutures. These should be removed at the slightest sign of wound irritation and the wound packed open.

POSTOPERATIVE CARE

Associated injuries pose the greatest threat to the patient during the first few postoperative days. Maintenance of good circulation and oxygenation is important for healing of colonic wounds and prevention of infection, as well as for protection of other organ systems.[12]

Although necrotizing infections can appear within hours of injury, more commonly the development of such infections is delayed for several days. Antibiotics which were started preoperatively should be continued for 24 to 48 hours, and patients should be closely watched for indications of abdominal or incisional infection. Modern radiographic and nuclear medicine imaging technics have greatly improved the success of pinpointing the location of intra-abdominal abscesses for surgical drainage.

Some authorities recommend antibiotic irrigation of the rectum in cases of rectal trauma, but this may increase intrarectal pressure if it is not done carefully, and the efficacy of such irrigation has not been established.

Exteriorized colon should be protected by petrolatum or moist saline dressings. A colostomy is managed by standard methods. If a colostomy has been done, it requires formal surgical closure later. Authorities disagree on the optimal interval from construction to closure of a colostomy, and recommendations vary from 2 weeks to several months.[22,27] It is advisable to wait until the colonic wall is no longer edematous, because edematous colon does not hold sutures and dehiscence is likely. An interval of 6 weeks to 3 months is optimal before attempting closure of a loop colostomy. A few weeks may be enough if the loop is resected and normal colon is anastomosed end-to-end and the patient is young and in good condition. Restoration of continuity in patients with end sigmoid colostomy and a Hartmann closure of the rectum is a major operation that may not be feasible for 3 months or longer.

COMPLICATIONS

The mortality rate from penetrating trauma to the colon and rectum is now below 10 percent, and some authors report a rate under 5 percent.[2,6,15,21,28.29] Death within the first 24 hours is due to hemorrhage, head injuries, or other problems not directly related to the perforated bowel. Later deaths, about half of the total mortality, are most commonly due to septic complications. The main correlation of survival is the number of associated injuries; survivors generally have only one or two organ systems injured, and as the number of involved organs increases, so does the mortality rate. If the liver, pancreas, or kidney is injured along with the large bowel, the mortality rate is as high as 30 percent.[15,19] Shotgun wounds, high velocity missile injuries, and blunt trauma also are fatal more frequently than simple penetrating trauma.

Even among patients who survive trauma to the large bowel, complications are common. The overall morbidity rate is about 50 percent, and many of these patients have more than one complication. In selected groups, such as those with massive rectal trauma, recovery without complication is exceptional.

Infection is the most important complication, affecting about one-third of patients in most reports. Wound infection was discussed in an earlier section; it occurs in 20 to 40 percent of primarily closed wounds and 8 to 20 percent of delayed primary closures. Abdominal abscesses develop in about 20 percent of patients, and numbers much larger and smaller have been reported. The interval from injury to operation influences the incidence of abdominal abscess importantly; abscesses occur in twice as many patients if operation is delayed beyond 6 hours.

Leakage of a primary sutured-perforation or a primary anastomosis is unusual if patients are selected carefully according to the criteria discussed earlier. Recently, colonic suture line dehiscence has been reported in 2-5% of patients.[2,4,14,17,21,25,31] These leaks are all clinically obvious, and the true incidence of leakage must be higher. Fecal fistula develops in approximately 3 percent of patients. When leakage is suspected, prompt operative intervention with exteriorization or resection of the suture line and colostomy or ileostomy is mandatory.

Early colostomy complications include peristomal small bowel herination, necrosis, retraction, and peristomal infection. These problems are serious and often require re-operation. Later complications of colostomy—hernia, stenosis, and prolapse—are usually just inconveniences and are resolved when the temporary colostomy is taken down. Complications of colostomy closure are relatively frequent and include wound infection, anastomotic leakage, and intraperitoneal infection. These complications must be considered in determining total morbidity of trauma of the large bowel.[22,27]

Dehiscence is another serious wound complication; usually it is related to wound infection. Small bowel obstruction and pulmonary, cardiac, and renal complications also occur in these severely injured patients.

REFERENCES

1. Abcarian H, Lowe R: Colon and rectal trauma. Surg Clin N Am 58:519, 1978.
2. Arango A, Baxter CR, Shires GT: Surgical management of traumatic injuries of the right colon. Twenty years of civilian experience. Arch Surg 114:703, 1979.
3. Barwick WJ, Schoffstall RO: Routine exteriorization in the treatment of civilian colon injuries: A reappraisal. Am Surg 44:716, 1978.
4. Beall AC Jr, et al.: Surgical considerations in the management of civilian colon injuries. Ann Surg 173:971, 1971.
5. Biggs TM, et al.: Surgical management of civilian colon injuries. J Trauma 3:484, 1963.
6. Chilimindris C, et al.: A critical review of management of right colon injuries. J Trauma 11:651, 1971.
7. Christensen N, Ignatius J, Mathewson C Jr: Treatment of injuries of the large bowel in civilian practice. Am J Surg 89:753, 1955.
8. Dunphy JE: The cut gut. Am J Surg 119:1, 1970.
9. Fraser J, Drummond H: A clinical and experimental study of three hundred perforating wounds of the abdomen. Brit Med J 1:321, 1917.
10. Ganchrow MI, Lavenson GS Jr, McNamara JJ: Surgical management of traumatic injuries of the colon and rectum. Arch Surg 100:515, 1970.
11. Garrison RN, et al.: Evaluation of management of the emergency right hemicolectomy. J Trauma 19:734, 1979.
12. Gilmour DG, et al.: The effect of hypovolaemia on colonic blood flow in the dog. Br J Surg 67:82, 1980.
13. Haas PA, Fox TA Jr: Civilian injuries of the rectum and anus. Dis Colon Rectum 22:17, 1979.
14. Haygood FD, Polk HC Jr: Gunshot wounds of the colon. A review of 100 consecutive patients, with emphasis on complications and their causes. Am J Surg 131:213, 1976.
15. Haynes CD, Gunn CH, Martin JD Jr: Colon injuries. Arch Surg 96:944, 1968.
16. Howell HS, Bartizal JF, Freeark RJ: Blunt trauma involving the colon and rectum. J Trauma 16:624, 1976.
17. Josen AS, et al.: Primary closure of civilian colorectal wounds. Ann Surg 176:782, 1972.

18. Kirkpatrick JR: Injuries of the colon. Surg Clin N Am 57:67, 1977.

19. Kirkpatrick JR, Rajpal SG: The injured colon: Therapeutic considerations. Am J Surg 129:187, 1975.

20. Lavenson GS Jr, Cohen A: Management of rectal injuries. Am J Surg 122:226, 1971.

21. LoCicero J III, Tajima T, Drapanas T: A half century of experience in the management of colon injuries: Changing concepts. J Trauma 15:575, 1975.

22. Machiedo GW, Casey KF, Blackwood JM: Colostomy closure following trauma. Surg Gynecol Obstet 151: 58, 1980.

23. Martinez O, et al.: Antibiotic prophylaxis in penetrating colorectal injuries: The comparative effectiveness of clindamycin and cephalothin in combination with an aminoglycoside. Am Surgeon 45:378, 1979.

24. Matolo NM, Wolfman EF Jr: Primary repair of colonic injuries. A clinical evaluation. J Trauma 17:554, 1977.

25. Mulherin JL Jr, Sawyers JL: Evaluation of three methods of managing penetrating colon injuries. J Trauma 15:580, 1975.

26. Otis GA: The Medical and Surgical History of the War of the Rebellion, Part II. Washington DC, Goverment Printing Office, 1876, p.205.

27. Samhouri F, Grodsinsky C, Fox T Jr: The management of colonic and rectal injuries. Dis Colon Rectum 21:426, 1978.

28. Schrock TR, Christensen N: Management of perforating injuries of the colon. Surg Gynecol Obstet 135:65, 1972.

29. Steele M, Blaisdell FW: Treatment of colon injuries. J Trauma 17:557, 1977.

30. Stone HH, Fabian TC: Management of perforating colon trauma. Randomization between primary closure and exteriorization. Ann Surg 190:430, 1979.

31. Walt AJ: Emergency treatment of wounds of the colon. Compr Ther 2:60, 1976.

32. Wanebo HJ, Hunt TK, Mathewson C Jr: Rectal injuries. J Trauma 9:712, 1969.

33. Wangensteen OH: Discussion of Stone HH, Fabian TC: Management of perforating colon trauma. Randomization between primary closure and exteriorization. Ann Surg 190:430, 1979.

34. Woodhall JP, Ochsner A: The management of perforating injuries of the colon and rectum in civilian practice. Surgery 29:305, 1951.

35. Yaw PB, Smith RN, Glover JL: Eight years experience with civilian injuries of the colon. Surg Gynecol Obstet 145:203, 1977.

Chapter Ten

SPLEEN

DONALD D. TRUNKEY

INTRODUCTION

Aristotle was the first to state that the spleen was not necessary for existence.[1] This assumption persisted through Roman and Medieval times and was re-emphasized by Malpighi in the fifteenth century.[16] It was difficult for anyone to challenge this assumption since the function of the spleen was not known. Early writers including Pliney and Galen thought that the spleen controlled laughter. However, Halevi, writing in the tenth century, stated, "the spleen is called laughing because of its nature to cleanse the blood and spirit from unclean and obscuring matter." Maimonides supported this concept in the mid-twelfth century but little was done to refute the concept that the spleen was indispensible into modern times.[27] Animal experiments in the eighteenth century added little knowledge to splenic function.

The first experiments relating the spleen to resistance to infection came in 1919 by Morris and Bullock who studied rat plague in splenectomized rats.[19] They showed that the spleen is important in resisting infectious processes in rats and that its removal had a deleterious effect on resistance. Although splenectomy was compatible with survival they concluded "this does not settle the problem as to whether or not a splenectomized person can weather a critical illness." Subsequent papers challenged this very important concept and controversy continued until 1952, when King and Schumaker published their classic paper on increased susceptibility to infection in infants following splenectomy.[2,5,13]

Until recently the spleen has been regarded as little more than a sac of blood with no essential function. As a result, general policy dictated removal should there be any evidence of injury, including minor iatrogenic tears during other surgical procedures. One factor which contributes to the problem is that delayed hemorrhage from the spleen is a well established fact. Although this has been referred to as delayed rupture we do not know of any established case in which a spleen verified to be intact at laparotomy accounted for secondary hemorrhage. A poll conducted at the Western Surgical Association disclosed that no member of that organization could verify delayed rupture.[3] Delayed hemorrhage simply implies that the spleen initially ruptured may not bleed sufficiently to produce clinical signs. Hours, days, or even months later, secondary hemorrhage may occur. This is due to further trauma to the spleen, the expansion of a large hematoma, or to continued ongoing slow hemorrhage. The highest incidence of delayed hemorrhage is within the first 24 hours. The incidence of secondary bleeding decreases in geometric fashion with the passage of time.[20]

ANATOMY

The spleen is an elongated ovoid body located in the left upper quadrant of the abdomen directly beneath the diaphragm, behind and to the left of the stomach. The shape of the spleen varies considerably in different individuals, as does its size. The size is influenced directly by blood pressure and is also increased after meals; the average weight, however, is 250 g. After the age of 60 years a slight involution of the spleen begins.

The hilum of the spleen is in immediate proximity to the tail of the pancreas. The superior and anterior surface of the spleen is in proximity to the greater curvature of the stomach. The anterior inferior portion of the spleen is in intimate relationship to the splenic flexure of the colon. Laterally and posteriorly the spleen lies in contact with the diaphragm. Medially and posteriorly lies the left kidney. The attachments of the spleen consist of the splenophrenic ligament posteriorly, a thin member readily disrupted by blunt traction. In addition, there is the gastrosplenic ligament in which run the short gastric vessels and the splenocolic ligament consisting of the lateral portion of the greater omentum. This may be relatively short, with immediate proximity of the splenic flexure to the hilum of the spleen, or it may be long, with the two separated by four or five cm.

Blood supply to the spleen includes the splenic artery, which runs along the superior surface of the pancreas to the phrenicolienal ligament and the hilus, a varying number of pancreatic branches, and several short branches from the stomach (gastra brevia). The splenic artery can be quite torturous, particularly in older individuals. The main splenic artery usually divides into five or six main branches in the hilum before entering the splenic pulp (Figure 10-1). The splenic vein is likewise formed outside the hilus and courses along the dorsal surface of the pancreas to join the superior mesenteric vein and turning into the portal vein.

Anatomical variants are common in spleens including contour, fetal lobulations, and shape. Equally important is the incidence of accessory spleens which may be found in up to 30 percent of patients. This latter variant may have an obvious important role in function after splenectomy for trauma.

The spleen has a capsule 1 to 2 mm thick, which with the trabeculae enclose the splenic pulp. Lymphoid tissue or malphighian follicles are scattered throughout

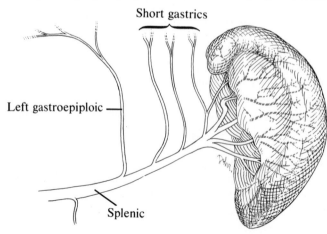

Short gastrics

Left gastroepiploic —

Splenic

Figure 10–1. Arterial supply of the spleen. Five to six branches take origin proximal to and in the hilum providing segmental circulation to the spleen. The most proximal brand of the splenic artery shown here is the left gastroepiploic followed by the short gastric arteries to the proximal portion of the greater curvature of the stomach.

this pulp and constitutes 25 percent of the reticuloendothelial system. The controversy as to whether the splenic circulation is "closed" or "open" is still unsettled. Current theories support that of Knisely which is basically an "open" concept.[15] The main trabecular arteries give off central arteries which in turn divide into many small arterioles that come off at right angles to the central artery. These small arterioles feed the splenic pulp. The blood is collected into venous sinuses ("the splenic sinuses"), then into trabecular veins and eventually into the main splenic veins and the portal circulation. The critical feature of the splenic circulation is the passage of arterial blood into the venous sinuses. In order to do so the blood must pass through the splenic cords, which are a connective tissue network between the splenic sinuses. It is here that the red cells must pass through the basement membrane which have fenestrations as small as 0.5 to 2.5 um much of the "sieving" effect is carried out. Approximately 5 percent of the body's total blood flow passes through the spleen per minute and 90 percent of it passes through these splenic sinuses to be sieved.[3]

FUNCTION

Splenic function can be divided into five broad categories of which four are very important to the trauma patient (Table 10-1).[7] The first function is that of filtering and this includes blood-borne particulate antigens, blood cells, and bacteria. The spleen is a very important source of two opsonins, tuftsin and properdin. The spleen is also important in the production of IgM which is markedly decreased after splenectomy for trauma. It is also an important organ in the regulation of both T and B lymphocytes. The fifth function, hematopoiesis in utero, is relatively unimportant to the trauma patient; this function may assume more importance as fetal surgery increases.

Table 10–1 FUNCTIONS OF THE SPLEEN

1. Filter for particulate matter, old red cells
2. Source of opsonins–tuftsin and properdin
3. Source of immunoglobulin IgM
4. Regulates T and B lymphocytes
5. Source of hematopoiesis in utero

The spleen is the primary defense organ when the host invaded by blood-borne bacteria has little or no pre-existing antibody. This is due to the unique microcirculation of the splenic pulp, in which the arterial blood must pass through the tiny pores between the endothelial cells lining the wall of the venous sinuses in order to enter the venous circulation. This "delays" circulation and allows splenic phagocytes to remove even poorly opsoninized bacteria. Although the liver is the most important organ in removing well opsoninized bacteria from the blood, the spleen, because of this efficient filter, is more effective in removing poorly opsoninized bacteria.

Particulate antigens are similarly cleared in this sieving effect and in addition initiate IgM antibody response in the germinal centers. Red cells are similarly altered or culled out as they pass through this splenic sieve. The spleen is capable of removing surface craters, pits from normal red cells, Howell-Jolly bodies, Heinz bodies or Pappenheimer bodies. As red cells become senescent they lose enzyme activity and the spleen recognizes this, traps the cells and destroys them.

Asplenia leads to subnormal levels of tuftsin and properdin. Tuftsin is a tetra-peptide that coats white cells and promotes phagocytosis of particulate matter, bacteria, and aged blood cells. Properdin is an important component of the alternate pathway of complement activation and subnormal levels will impair the serum opsoninization of encapsulted bacteria, such as meningococci and pneumococci. It is of interest, however, that normal children undergoing splenectomy for trauma have normal pneumococcal serum opsoninizing activity.[29]

ASSESSMENT OF INJURY

Rosoff has divided the clinical manifestations of traumatic rupture of the spleen into two distinct categories: (1) the systemic symptoms of acute hemorrhage and (2) the local symptoms of peritoneal irritation in the region of the spleen.[23] Peritoneal hemorrhage is usually a diagnosis of exclusion, since overt signs are often absent or attenuated. Assessment of any trauma patient should include a chest x-ray, which will eliminate the hemithoraces as a significant source of blood loss. Similarly, clinical assessment of the thighs and lower legs will rule them out as a major source of hemorrhage. By exclusion the abdomen then becomes the primary cavity of suspicion for continued blood loss. This is documented by repeated physical examinations, serial hematocrits, serial white counts, and the use of special adjunctive procedures such as CT scanning and sonography. The latter is particularly useful in detecting free fluid and may be sensitive to as little as 300 of blood. If the patient is unconscious, paralyzed, uncooperative, or lost to physical examination for any reason, peritoneal lavage should be considered (see Chapter 3). Absolute signs for peritoneal exploration include involuntary guarding and unexplained shock.

Though many signs have been described and attributed to peritoneal irritation secondary to splenic rupture, very few have clinical meaning. Blood, per se, may not be irritating to the peritoneum. Clinical signs are usually secondary to diaphragmatic irritation or contusion, chest wall contusion, rib fractures or associated injuries. The Ballance sign "large, fixed dullness in the left flank," Kehr's sign "pain at the top of the left shoulder caused by irritation of the inferior surface of the left diaphragm," and Seagesser's sign, "pain produced in the neck by pressure over the phrenic nerve" have been only of slight help in determining splenic injury.

The enlarged, diseased spleen is easily traumatized and rupture may occur from such mild trauma that it is not remembered by the patient. The spleen is predictably prone to rupture during pregnancy when the splenic capsule may be thinned and the spleen relatively congested. In most instances there is a history of significant trauma to the left upper quadrant or the lower rib cage. Since the hilum of the spleen is centered on the posterior axillary line, with the spleen lying between the eighth and tenth ribs, fractures of the eighth, ninth, and tenth ribs posteriorly risks splenic rupture. In fact, our statistics show that fractures of any one or combination of the eighth, ninth and tenth ribs are associated with a 20 percent chance of splenic rupture. Therefore, assessment of the possibility of splenic rupture begins with assessment of the integrity of the chest wall. If the patient is able to take a deep breath without discomfort, the likelihood of rib fracture is slight. Conversely, if pleuritic type pain occurs with respiration, and this is referred to the lower ribs, fracture can be assumed, despite negative rib x-rays. Palpation will confirm the ribs involved. Current adjunctive measures most useful in evaluation of splenic trauma are sonography, CT scan and arteriography (Figure 10-2). All are capable of detecting defects within the hepatic parenchyma and are capable of detecting free fluid within the posterior gutters of the peritoneum (see Chapter 2). Another diagnostic approach is to utilize splenic scanning. The scintillation scan may reveal an enlarged spleen, displacement of the spleen from the abdominal wall or a cleft in the spleen compatible with fracture. False positives are frequent, as congenital clefts in the spleen may resemble lacerations (Figure 10-3). Abnormal enlargement of the spleen may be interrupted, as injury and fluid collections in the left upper quadrant may result from other injuries.

Chest x-rays may confirm the presence of rib fractures, or reveal a left pleural infusion which may mark irritation below the diaphragm or an elevated diaphragm. A flat film of the abdomen may occasionally be of value, if it shows displacement

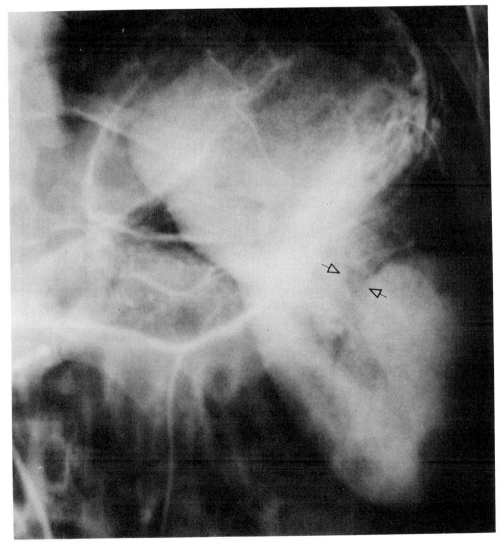

Figure 10–2. Arteriography has been of value in certain acute instances. This study demonstrates a nearly complete splenic fracture (arrows). A bisected spleen was found at the time of exploration.

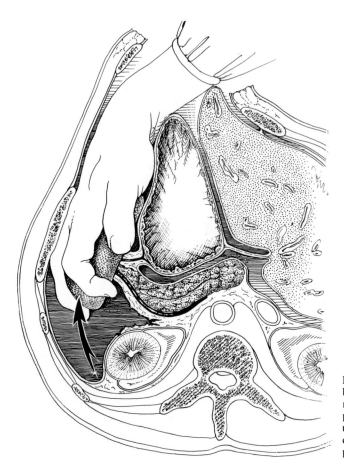

Figure 10–3. The spleen is mobilized by traction upward and medially, developing the plane posterior to the pancreas. This is usually done most quickly by blunt digital dissection of the lateral and posterior splenic attachments.

of the gastric air bubble and apparent enlargement of the spleen or fluid collection between bowel loops. When injury is confined to the abdomen, however, we rarely utilize lavage, but rely on clinical guidelines. In multiply injured patients, when monitoring blood loss is difficult, peritoneal lavage may be indicated and may lead to an earlier diagnosis of splenic injury.

PRE-OPERATIVE PREPARATION

After the initial assessment and resuscitation certain preoperative adjuncts should be considered. Broad spectrum antibiotics should be administered prior to operation when there is suspected associated colon or small bowel injuries. This is particularly appropriate in penetrating wounds of the abdomen. If no colon or small bowel injuries are found at the time of laparotomy these antibiotics can be discontinued. On the other hand, if such injuries are found they should be continued for 24 to 48 hours.

A team approach is often mandatory in the patient with multiple injuries and may include decompression of space occupying intracranial blood by neurosurgeons while general surgeons explore the abdomen. Priorities must be established immediately. In the patients with abdominal injuries and associated widened mediastinum, exploration of the abdomen with repair of the injuries is indicated first. Following laparotomy the patient should be taken to x-ray for an aortogram and possible thoracotomy with repair of the thoracic aorta. If the patient has associated major vascular injuries in the extremities, control of these must be obtained prior to abdominal exploration. If the patient remains unstable, exploratory laparotomy should be carried out before definitive treatment of the vascular injury.

OPERATIVE EXPLORATION AND SPLENIC EVALUATION

For rapid access and wide exposure the midline incision is strongly recommended. Only rarely will transverse or oblique incisions be needed for splenic injuries. The surgeon should always be prepared to extend the midline incision up the sternum or into the left or right chest, if necessary. The chest should, therefore, always be prepped prior to surgery along with the abdomen.

After the initial incision has been made, the surgeon should rule out major vascular injury (Chapters 12 and 13). When the abdomen is entered the patient is rapidly eviscerated and blood aspirated from all quadrants of the abdomen with each quadrant packed to localize bleeding. The presence of clot points to the site of hemorrhage and with splenic rupture clot is usually found in the left upper quadrant surrounding the spleen. In the absence of localizing clot, the spleen should be exposed extremely gently, since the probability of injury is low and in the course of exposing the spleen, the spleen may be inadvertently traumatized.

Once splenic rupture is verified by the presence of clot around the spleen, palpation of the laceration, or visualization of the ongoing hemorrhage, the spleen is mobilized by blunt dissection, severing the splenophrenic ligament posteriorly. With this, the greater curvature of the stomach, the tail of the pancreas, the splenic hilum, and the splenic flexure of the colon can be mobilized medially and into the wound by continued gentle dissection posteriorly (Figure 10-3). Severing the lateral attachments of the colon, sharply if necessary, facilitates the exposure. Care should be taken not to injure the pancreas, or tear the attachments of the splenic hilum to the greater curvature of the stomach. Exposure and control of splenic hemorrhage is best obtained by full mobilization of the spleen into the midline either onto the abdominal wall or such that the spleen is in total view of the surgeon. Attempts should not be made to control the splenic circulation through the lesser sac or at the hilum prior to repair or splenectomy since this may aggravate or add to the bleeding.

Splenic injuries vary from small capsular avulsion injuries to the more extensive fragmenting types of injuries. Attempts have been made to classify the severity of splenic trauma, however, this may or may not be useful.[4] In general, injuries to the costal surface lend themselves to repair more readily then those to the hilar surface. Similarly, horizontal fractures and avulsions of the capsule are easier to control then the larger stellate and fragmenting type of injuries.

Although controversy still exists, there are certain general rules that can now be applied to splenic salvage. It is prudent to salvage all spleens when possible in both adults and children, particularly in the latter group when below the age of five years. Factors which would mitigate against splenic salvage include: uncontrolled hemorrhage from the spleen, major hilar avulsion injuries, severe associated injuries requiring considerable time to repair and fragmenting injuries of such a nature that salvage is impossible.

OPERATIVE TREATMENT

In our experience, about one-third of splenic injuries can be salvaged and two-thirds require splenectomy. The exact rules regarding splenic injury management are still undergoing evaluation and it is our presumption that undue enthusiasm for preserving spleens may render the patient vulnerable to more severe complications than those following splenectomy.

With the spleen exposed, the injury can be treated by observation, by packing with microcrystalline collagen or with omentum, by suture of lacerations, by partial splenectomy, or by complete splenectomy. Control of the hilar vessels can be partially obtained manually, the key being to grasp the tail of the pancreas in the thumb and the forefinger. Division of the short gastric vessels between the greater curvature of the stomach and the hilum of the spleen facilitates control of bleeding at the hilum. If there is room between the tail of the pancreas and the hilum, a soft vascular clamp (Fogarty type) can be applied to give complete hemostasis. This is best facilitated by mobilizing and separating the splenic flexure of the colon from the splenic hilum.

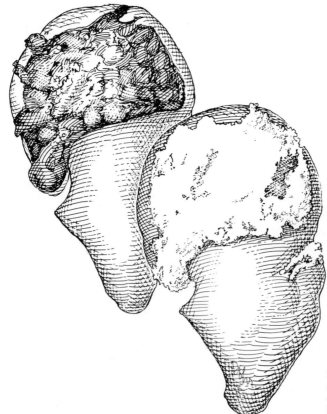

Figure 10–4. Capsular tears or avulsions can be treated with microcrystalline collagen as shown here.

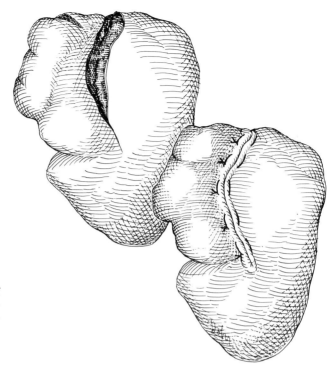

Figure 10-5. Many lacerations of the spleen are amenable to capsular repair utilizing fine monofilament vascular suture.

A small capsular tear may not require treatment. If bleeding has ceased spontaneously, it may be treated with coagulation current or with microcrystalline collagen application. Larger capsular avulsions and superficial lacerations can be treated by packing with microcrystalline collagen (Figure 10-4). This is best applied with a dry sponge, applied firmly over the injured area with pressure maintained for five to ten minutes. This will control most superficial bleeding satisfactorily. For deeper capsular tears, when there is associated hematoma in the splenic pulp, the hematoma should be evacuated. Larger bleeding points should be controlled by suture or by coagulation current, if possible, and the capsular tear approximated with 5-0 or 6-0 Prolene suture as used for blood vessel repair (Figure 10-5). The sutures must be placed meticulously, similar to that utilized for a fragile vein. Control of bleeding digitally or with a vascular clamp at the splenic hilum facilitates the placement of sutures. For deeper lacerations or lacerations bleeding more vigorously, mattress sutures, using a larger needle, and suture, such as polyglycolate or Chromic, tied over Teflon bolsters may be necessary (Figure 10-6).

In some injuries, such as those involving the upper or lower pole of the spleen or even as much as one-half of the spleen, segmental resection of the spleen may be possible (Figure 10-6). Bleeding points on the raw surface of the spleen can be controlled by suture ligature and coagulation current. Further hemostasis is obtained by microcrystalline collagen, by omental patch, or by a free graft of peritoneum.

When bleeding is massive, such as gross disruption of the spleen or extensive injury involving the splenic hilum the most conservative treatment is splenectomy. Depending on the magnitude of the bleeding, the hilar vessels can be cross-clamped and divided, this immediately followed by division of the short gastric vessels. Otherwise the short gastric vessels are divided first, followed by progressive tran-

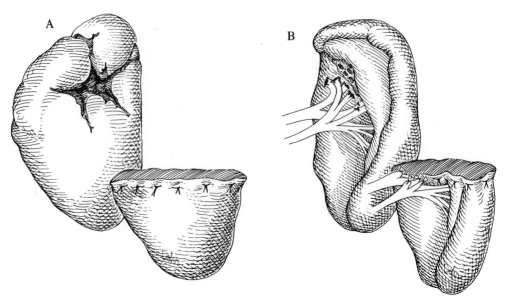

Figure 10–6. Deeper lacerations *(A)* and hilar injuries *(B)* lend themselves to treatment by resection of the injured segment.

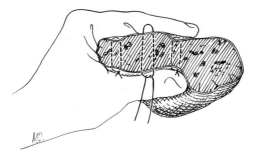

Figure 10–7. Compression of the spleen following segmental resection provides hemostasis, facilitates identification and suturing of bleeding points and the placement of mattress sutures.

section of the splenic hilum between multiple clamps. At the completion of splenectomy, it is necessary to recheck the security of the ligatures. This is best accomplished by locating the tail of the pancreas by palpation and inspecting the vessels and ligatures as the vessels leave the tail of the pancreas. The greater curvature of the stomach should always be inspected, since this area is the most common source of postoperative bleeding. Frequently, one or two unligated short gastric vessels will be detected and securing these with ligature and suture insures adequacy of hemostasis. Devascularization of the greater curvature of the stomach is best avoided by meticulous technique rather than by taking gross bites of tissue. In the absence of pancreatic or other associated injuries the placement of drains is not necessary and may increase the incidence of infection. Irrigation of blood and particulate matter is a useful adjunct. If there is continued blood loss in the postoperative period and the patient's spleen has been repaired, assessment of the spleen as the source of blood loss is best accomplished with CT scans and sonography. Arteriography may also be useful in this assessment.

Areas that remain controversial in the management of splenic trauma include splenic reimplantation, splenosis, and splenic artery ligation. Reimplantation of splenic tissue has been attempted and there is some evidence that partial splenic function may return. [9] The splenic function that returns, however, is associated with its sieving effect of red cells and there is probably little or no return of opsonin production, but opinion on this is divided. [6,21,29] There is also evidence that diffuse peritoneal seeding of splenic tissue or splenosis does not protect the patient from overwhelming infections and at least two deaths have been reported in patients with splenosis after trauma.[22]

The role of splenic artery ligation as an adjunct to splenic salvage is as yet unproven. At least one report in the literature advocates its use; however, experience at our hospital has not supported this, since in both instances ligation of the splenic artery led to splenic necrosis.[12]

POSTOPERATIVE CARE

In patients who have undergone splenectomy, the use of polyvalent pneumococcal vaccine is now accepted treatment. However, this vaccine does not encompass all capsule-containing organisms and therefore does not provide absolute protection against infection. How long prophylaxis should be continued is as yet undetermined, but most reports would indicate that susceptibility to infection and overwhelming sepsis lasts for many years. Therefore in young susceptable patients prophylactic, limited spectrum antibiotics such as oral penicillin have been advocated by some. Nevertheless, the patient should be advised to start oral antibiotics such as ampicillin at the first signs of any upper respiratory illness and to see a physician immediately.

Asplenia increases the risks of other postoperative complications, including wound infection, subphrenic abscess, and thromboembolic phenomena. All of these entail a dramatic increase in the immediate postoperative period. The use of prophylactic antibiotics is probably not warranted in simple noncontaminated injuries, but probably should be utilized for at least 24 to 48 hours following contaminated and complex injuries. Anticoagulants may be of value in selected instances when the injury has been limited to the spleen, but is often contraindicated in more complex trauma cases because of the immediate complications of bleeding. When utilized, low dose heparin is probably not adequate and larger doses are required. This may consist of 75 to 150 units/kg of the initial bolus followed by 15 to 20 u/kg per hour by continuous intravenous infusions.

In those patients where splenic salvage has been accomplished, bed rest and inactivity may be a useful adjunct for periods up to three weeks after the operation. This may reduce the chances of postoperative hemorrhage and hematoma formation.

POSTOPERATIVE COMPLICATIONS

Although the injury may appear relatively trivial, the complications of splenic injury may be lethal (Table 10-2). The most likely initial complication is bleeding. This is either from the short gastric vessels, or from the hilar vessels in the tail of the pancreas. If the patient manifests more than a unit or two of blood loss in the

Table 10–2   COMPLICATIONS OF SPLENECTOMY

1. Persistent intraperitoneal bleeding
2. Postoperative pancreatitis
3. Devascularization of the stomach
   Gastric fistula
   Subphrenic abscess
   Peritonitis
4. Thromoboembolic complications
   Thrombosis suprarenal veins
   Thrombosis of deep veins
   Pulmonary embolism
5. Infection
   Acute postoperative
   Catastrophic late

first 24 hours, reoperation is indicated to control the bleeding point and to evacuate blood and hematoma. We believe in an aggressive approach to postoperative bleeding to prevent subsequent complication, including subphrenic abscess and pulmonary complications related to irritation of the diaphragm.

Trauma to the pancreas from the original injury or inadvertently during splenectomy may result in postoperative pancreatitis. This is manifested by increased fluid requirement, by the presence of an ileus and/or a distended tender abdomen. The serum amylase may be elevated but this is of no significance in itself in the absence of other signs compatible with pancreatic inflammation. If the surgeon is certain that a primary pancreatic ductal division has not been missed, the treatment is conservative, utilizing nasogastric suction, intravenous fluids, and observation.

In rare instances, devascularization of the greater curvature of the stomach as a result of the division of the gastroepiploic and short splenic vessels may result in a gastric leak or fistula. This is usually manifested three or four days following injury by the development of fever, abdominal tenderness, and elevation of the white count. Reoperation is indicated if this injury is suspected. Attempts at direct suture of the stomach will usually be unsuccessful, and the acceptance of a fistula usually necessary. Good posterior drainage should be instituted and combined with nasogastric drainage and delay in oral alimentation.

Thromboembolic complications have been a much feared complication of splenectomy. The exact incidence is disputed and difficult to determine. However, in our series at San Francisco General Hospital, we found that the incidence of thromboembolic complications approached 5 percent.[26] It is manifest by thrombophlebitis in veins receiving intravenous infusions, clotting in leg veins, or pulmonary manifestations of embolism. Tragic deaths in young patients ocasionally have resulted from thromboembolism. In theory, this complication could be prevented by prophylactic anticoagulation, but anticoagulation of the injured postoperative surgical patient is usually contraindicated for at least 24 hours. Mild forms of prophylaxis, which we utilize, consists of antiplatelet-aggregating agents, such as enteric-coated aspirin, low molecular weight dextran or, in high risk patients, heparin anticoagulation.

Another complication is infection, either acute infection, complicating the immediate postoperative period, or late devastating infections related to encapsulated organisms, such as pneumococcus and meningococcus. The risk of the latter is greater in infants and children, but has been documented in young adults. The advent of pneumococcal vaccine appears to prevent many pneumococcal complications but is of no use against other encapsulated organisms.

REFERENCES

1. Aristotle: Parts of animals, Book III. Chap 12. Peck AL (trans). Cambridge, Massachusetts, Harvard University Press, 1955.
2. Bailey H: Traumatic rupture of the normal spleen. Br J Surg 15:40, 1927.
3. Blaisdell FW: personal communication.
4. Buntain WL, Lynn HB: Splenorraphy: Changing concepts for the traumatized spleen. Surgery 86:748, 1979.
5. Connors JF: Splenectomy for trauma. Ann Surg 88: 388, 1928.
6. Constantopoulos A, et al.: Defective phagocytosis due to tuftsin deficiency in splenectomized subjects. Am J Dis Child 125:663, 1973.
7. Eichner ER: Splenic function: Normal, too much, and too little. Am J Med. 66:311, 1979.
8. Ein SH, et al.: The morbidity and mortality of splenectomy in children. Ann Surg 185:307, 1977.
9. Fleming RC, Dickson RE, Harrison EG: Splenosis: Autotransplantation of splenic tissue. Am J Med 61: 414, 1976.
10. Gopal V, Bisno AL: Fulminant pneumococcal infections in "normal" asplenic hosts. Arch Int Med. 137:1576, 1977.
11. Joseph TP, Wyllie GG, Savage JP: The nonoperative management of splenic trauma. Aust NZJ Surg 47:179, 1977.
12. Keramidas DC: The ligation of the splenic artery in the treatment of traumatic rupture of the spleen. Surgery 85:530, 1979.
13. King H, Schumacher HB Jr: Splenic studies. I. Susceptibility to infection after splenectomy performed in infancy. Ann Surg 136:239, 1952.
14. Klaue P, Eckert P, Kern E: Incidental splenectomy: Early and late post-operative complications. Am J Surg 138:296, 1979.
15. Knisely MH: Spleen studies. II: Microscopic observations of the circulatory system of living traumatized spleens and of dying spleens. Anat Rev 65:131, 1936.
16. Malpighi M: DeLiene. In Malpighi M: DeViscerum structura excercitatio anatomica. Golonga, J Monitus 1666, pp 101-150.
17. Meakins JL: Splenectomy for rupture of the spleen: A reappraisal. CMA J 121:11, 1979.
18. Mishalany HG, et al.: Modalities of preservation of the traumatized spleen. Am J Surg 136:697, 1978.
19. Morris DH, Bullock FD: The importance of the spleen in resistance to infection. Ann Surg 70: 513, 1919.
20. Olsen WR, Polley TZ: A second look at delayed splenic rupture. Arch Surg 112:442, 1977.
21. Pearson HA, et al.: The born-again spleen: Return of splenic function after splenectomy for trauma. NEJM 298:1389, 1978.
22. Rice HM, James PD: Ectopic splenic tissue failed to prevent fatal pneumococcal septicemia after splenectomy for trauma. Lancet 1980, 565.
23. Rosoff L, et al.: Injuries of the spleen. Surg Clin N Am 52:667, 1972.
24. Sherman R.: Perspectives in management of trauma to the spleen. J Trauma 20:1, 1980.
25. Strauch GO: Preservation of splenic function in adults and children with injured spleens. Am J Surg 137:478, 1979.
26. Steele M, Lim RC: Advances in management of splenic injuries. Am J Surg 130:159, 1975.
27. Rosner F: The spleen in the Talmud and other early Jewish writing. Bull Hist Med 46:82-85, 1972.
28. Weinstein ME, et al.: Splenorraphy for splenic trauma. J Trauma 19: 692, 1979.
29. Winklestein JA, Lambert GH: Pneumococcal serum opsoninizing activity in splenectomized children. J Pediatr 87:430, 1975.

Chapter Eleven

INJURIES TO THE URINARY SYSTEM

JACK W. McANINCH

INTRODUCTION

Most notable historical information involving urinary system injury relates to bladder trauma and the earliest known record is found in the Pope's translation of "The Iliad of Homer" where the "spear of Merion" caused fatal injury.[24] Hippocrates and Golen alleged to have noted patients with fatal bladder injuries. Urinary diversion with a gum elastic catheter was first recorded in 1772 by Chopart and proved to be the principal means of salvage in war wounds, although it was not fully accepted until 100 years later.[9] Mortality from intraperitoneal bladder rupture was reported at 100 percent before Evans and Fowler demonstrated that laparotomy, removal of urine, and bladder closure reduced the death rate to 28 percent. Hinman, in 1935, pointed out the importance of suprapubic drainage by way of a large rubber catheter in the extraperitoneal position, and this viewpoint persists today as a basis for therapy in bladder injuries.[22]

Urinary tract injuries occur in approximately 10 to 15 percent of all abdominal injuries.[35] Major problems occur when diagnosis is not reached or even suspected until complications of bleeding, urinary extravasation, infection, and abscess formation become apparent. Early diagnosis thus is of paramount importance in determining initial management and subsequent primary healing of these injuries.

RENAL INJURIES

Injuries to the kidneys are frequent. Although well protected by heavy lumbar muscles, ribs, vertebral bodies, viscera, and retroperitoneum anteriorly, the kidneys have unusual mobility and, in consequence, parenchymal trauma and vascular injuries due to stretch on vessels occur easily. Fractured ribs at times penetrate the fragile kidney and so do vertebral transverse processes.

Traditionally, based on the etiology of the injury, trauma to the kidney has been separated into blunt and penetrating trauma. *Blunt trauma* accounts for 70 to 80 percent of all renal injuries—from motor vehicle accidents, fights, falls, and contact sports.[45] Rapid deceleration injuries are more likely to cause major renal vascular injuries. *Penetrating renal trauma* is found in approximately 8 percent of abdominal wounds, gunshot and knife wounds being the most common.[1] In 80 percent of these cases there is associated abdominal visceral injury.[14]

Surgical Anatomy

The importance of anatomic relationships and surgical anatomy cannot be over-stressed to the surgeon planning renal exploration for trauma. Massive hematomas and urinomas often obscure and alter the normal relationships, thus thorough knowl-edge of all basic anatomic details are essential.

The kidneys lie retroperitoneally between the 12th thoracic and second lumbar vertebrae. The renal fossa is bounded by the psoas muscle medially, the quadratus lumborum muscle posteriorly, the abdominal muscles laterally, and the diaphragm superiorly. The adrenal glands lie on the superior medial aspect. The anterior re-lationships of the right kidney include the right lobe of the liver superiorly and the hepatic flexure of the right colon inferiorly. The medial anterior aspect of the right kidney is covered by the second portion of the duodenum. Mobilization of the duodenum is required when the right renal pedicle has to be exposed. The anterior relationships of the left kidney include the stomach, spleen, pancreas, splenic flexure of the left colon, and jejunum.

The renal parenchyma is surrounded by a strong fibrous capsule closely adherent to the surface. During renal exploration, careful attention to the capsule after renal repair restores anatomy, aids in hemostasis, and prevents urinary extravasation. Outside the renal capsule and surrounding the kidney is perirenal fat which is confined by Gerota's fascia. Gerota's fascia has the ability to confine hematomas surrounding the kidney. Gerota's fascia fuses anteriorly so that a perirenal hematoma cannot dissect across the midline. It is attached to the diaphragm superiorly and envelops the adrenal gland in a separate compartment. Its lower aspect becomes attenuated and disappears along the lumbar ureter.

Anatomy of the renal vessels has perhaps the greatest significance when renal exploration for trauma is anticipated. Renal pedicle and vascular control by way of a transabdominal approach before the kidney is exposed has rendered nephrectomy rates significantly lower than with the flank approaches previously used. Twenty percent of cardiac output goes to the kidneys and, without arterial control before a renal hematoma is entered, massive hemorrhage can occur, making nephrectomy unavoidable.

The renal artery arises from the aorta as a single vessel in 85 percent of humans whereas multiple vessels are found in 15 percent. The right renal artery is longer, coursing behind the vena cava and arising slightly higher on the aorta than the left renal artery. In the renal hilum, the main artery branches into four or five major segmental vessels. Ligation and control of individual segmental vessels allows partial nephrectomy while preserving the remaining vessels. The renal artery and its branches course anterior to the renal pelvis and posterior to the renal veins. Renal arteries are end arteries and little collateral blood supply exists. Injured or throm-bosed arteries must be repaired and non-viable parenchyma must be excised.

The number and distribution of renal veins is similar to those of renal arteries. The right renal vein is short and broad, draining directly into the vena cava. It lies anterior to the renal artery and usually has no tributaries other than vessels for renal drainage. The right renal vein can cause major problems if lacerated, because it is short and quickly retracts, leaving the vena cava as a major bleeding site. The left renal vein is long, coursing anteriorly over the aorta. Three branches are common, the left gonadal branch inferiorly, the left adrenal branch superiorly, and a renal lumbar branch posteriorly. These branches must be kept in mind as the left renal vein is exposed; individual ligation of these vessels can be done without adverse sequelae. In contrast to the situation existing in renal arteries, segmental renal veins can be ligated without causing renal damage, because of a well developed collateral system.

The left renal vein becomes a prime anatomic landmark in renal explorations for trauma (Figure 11-1). Dissection up the aorta superior to the inferior mesenteric artery encounters, as the first major vessel, the left renal vein crossing anteriorly over the aorta. Even if a hematoma covers the entire aorta, the surgeon can continue the superior dissection with confidence until the left renal vein is exposed. The consistency of this vessel allows one to identify and isolate the main renal arteries quickly.

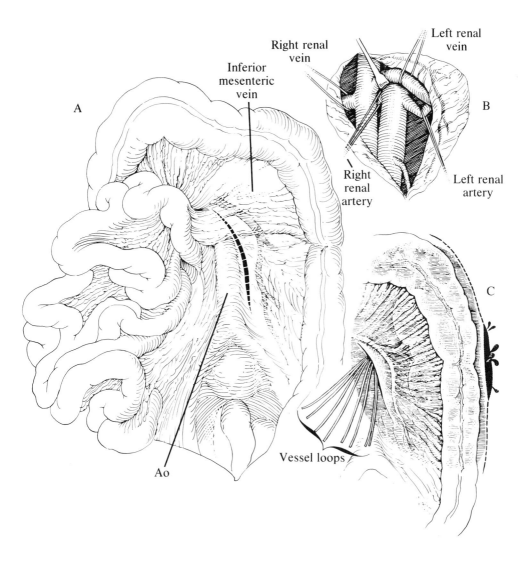

Figure 11–1.   Renal surgical anatomy and exploration technique.

Assessment of Injury

Any patient seen in the emergency room with trauma to the back, abdomen, or lower chest may have renal injury, whether or not symptoms are apparent. Fractures of lower ribs make renal injury more likely. Any stab or gunshot wound of the flank or upper abdomen signifies potential renal injury.

In this age of high-speed locomotion, collisions of vehicles result in major trauma from rapid deceleration. Blunt trauma to the flank, severe enough to cause skin contusions, raises the possibility of renal injury. In circumstances of violent injury, the renal pedicles are particularly susceptible to injury and excretory urography (IVP) is indicated, regardless of findings on physical examination and urinalysis. [49]

HEMATURIA. Generally, hematuria is the initial sign of renal injury.[39-52] Thus, the technique of urine collection is important by way of a clean catch if the patient can void, or by atraumatic catheter passage. Gross hematuria or microscopic hematuria (more than 5 red blood cells per high power field) demand radiographic study to establish whether renal injury is present.[21] No correlation exists between the degree of injury and the degree of hematuria.[35] Many minor renal injuries are associated with gross hematuria and normal results of excretory urography. On the other hand, injuries to the renal pedicle may be associated with mild microhematuria.[16,31,56] Hematuria may be totally absent in 20 to 25 percent of patients having serious renal injuries.[15,31,35]

STAGING. Staging of renal injuries allows one to approach these problems in a systematic fashion. Adequate studies help define extent of injury and concomitantly, appropriate management. For example, blunt trauma to the upper abdomen associated with microhematuria and normal readings of IVP requires no additional renal studies. However, if the kidney was not visualized on the IVP, arteriography would be immediately indicated to define the injury and investigate possible damage to the renal pedicle.[24]

Staging begins with excretory urography in the trauma suite. Other major injuries may be present and, as resuscitation begins with intravenous lines in place, 150 cc of contrast material should be injected intravenously.[29] Once the patient is hemodynamically stable and ready for abdominal radiography, the kidneys and collecting systems should be well visualized. Although this technique avoids the delay of a kidney-ureter-bladder (KUB) radiogram before injection of the contrast medium, the latter does not obscure information usually obtained from the KUB, that is, bony fractures, free air, and displaced bowel. The excretory urogram should (1) establish the presence or absence of both kidneys; (2) clearly define the renal outlines and cortical borders; and (3) outline the collecting systems and ureters (Figure 11-2).

Renal tomography is indicated when the excretory urogram provides inadequate information to fully define the extent of injury. Tomograms are of greatest benefit in outlining cortical lacerations, intrarenal hematomas, and poor parenchymal perfusion from arterial injuries (Figure 11-2a). Excretory urography combined with tomography will stage adequately 85 percent of renal injuries.[55]

Arteriography defines major arterial and parenchymal injuries and is indicated when previous studies have not done so (Figure 11-2c,d).[27] Arteriography is the best technique to diagnose arterial thrombosis and renal pedicle avulsion.[16,32,56] Nonvisualization of the kidney on IVP is an absolute indication for selective renal arteriography. Major causes for nonvisualization are (1) arterial thrombosis; (2) total pedicle avulsion; (3) severe contusion causing vascular spasm; (4) absence of kidney, either congenital or from operation.

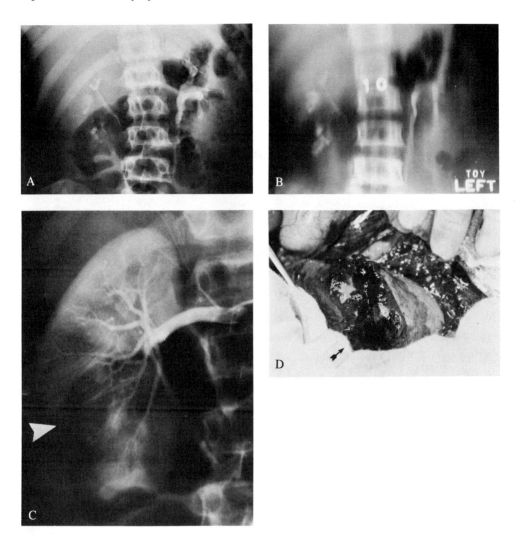

Figure 11–2. *A*, Blunt trauma in 14-year-old boy. IVP shows normal left kidney with poor function in lower pole on right. *B*, Tomograms demonstrate irregular right lower pole calyces and break in cortical margin. *C*, Arteriogram shows poor lower pole perfusion with deep cortical laceration and intrarenal hematoma. *D*, Gross photo of kidney at operation with deep laceration and intrarenal hematoma. Repair resulted in renal salvage.

Computerized axial tomography (CT scan) is used at San Francisco General Hospital to evaluate its effectiveness as a staging tool for renal trauma. Its major advantages are (1) three-dimentional views; (2) noninvasiveness; (3) excellent definition of parenchymal lacerations; (4) clear demonstration of extravasation; (5) outline of nonviable tissue; (6) definition of extent and size of surrounding hematoma; and (7) exploration of surrounding structures. It would appear from early experience in 25 major renal injury cases that CT scan is superior to arteriography in defining these injuries (Figure 11-3). Perhaps one exception is acute renal artery thrombosis, where an arteriogram would be more definitive. For CT scan to be an effective staging tool, 24-hour availability is mandatory.

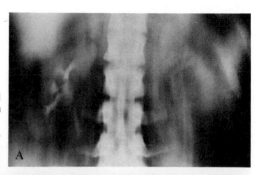

Figure 11–3. *A*. Blunt trauma in a 30-year-old female. Nephrotomogram shows poor visualization of left kidney.
B, CT scan of left kidney shows cortical fractures, extravasation and perirenal hematoma.

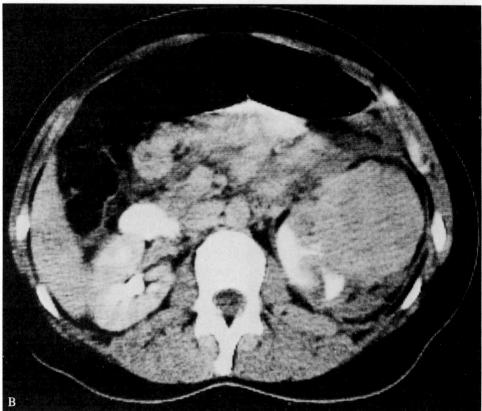

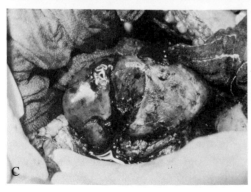

Figure 11-3. *C*. Gross photograph at operation shows deep mid-renal laceration. Kidney was repaired.

Radionucleotide scanning has been utilized in evaluating renal trauma but detects only large lacerations and usually is less effective than nephrotomography, arteriography, or CT scan. It may be of greatest help in patients allergic to contrast medium.[60]

Retrograde pyelography is seldom indicated in renal trauma because it does not outline the parenchyma and therefore cannot define major lacerations. It has the additional disadvantage of introducing infection.

Ultrasonography has proven to be of little benefit in the initial assessment of renal injuries.

In summary, an orderly approach to staging renal trauma is as follows:

1. Excretory urography, combined with tomography;
2. CT scan, if readily available;
3. arteriography, if vascular injury is suspected.

By defining the extent of injury, these studies will allow intelligent, accurate decisions for proper management.

Indications for Operation—Pre-operative Preparation

The need for operation after blunt trauma is based on the severity of injury (Figure 11–4).[7,8] Minor injuries—including superficial cortical lacerations and contusions (Figure 11–4a,b)—usually can be managed non-operatively, with bed rest, until gross hematuria clears. These minor injuries represent 85 percent of blunt renal trauma.[26]

Major parenchymal injuries, representing approximately 10 percent of all blunt renal medulla (Figure 11–4c,d,e). The collecting system may or may not be disrupted. The depth of the laceration causes disruption of large veins and arteries that course through the corticomedullary junction, and causes a high risk for persistent or delayed bleeding.[7]

Definite indications for operation include: (1) persistent retroperitoneal bleeding; (2) urinary extravasation; and (3) evidence of nonviable parenchyma. Aggressive preoperative staging allows to define the injury and to plan exploration when the above conditions exist.

There is controversy in management of these major injuries between operative and non-operative approaches.[7,45,49] Advocates of non-operative management in major injuries fear that an unnecessary nephrectomy could result because of uncontrolled bleeding.[52] This fear is unfounded if, before opening the hematoma, proximal control of the renal vessels has been obtained.[54] At San Francisco General Hospital in the past two years, 100 cases of blunt renal trauma have been seen, 10 percent of which have had operation and renal repair. No nephrectomies were required in this group of patients and no patient had delayed bleeding, urinary extravasation, abscess, or delayed hypertension.

Carlton has noted that non-operative management in this small select group (10 percent of all blunt renal trauma) presents a 50 percent chance of delayed bleeding, urinoma formation, or some other major complication.[4] These problems can be eliminated by early operation and will allow the patient to recover more quickly from the injury.

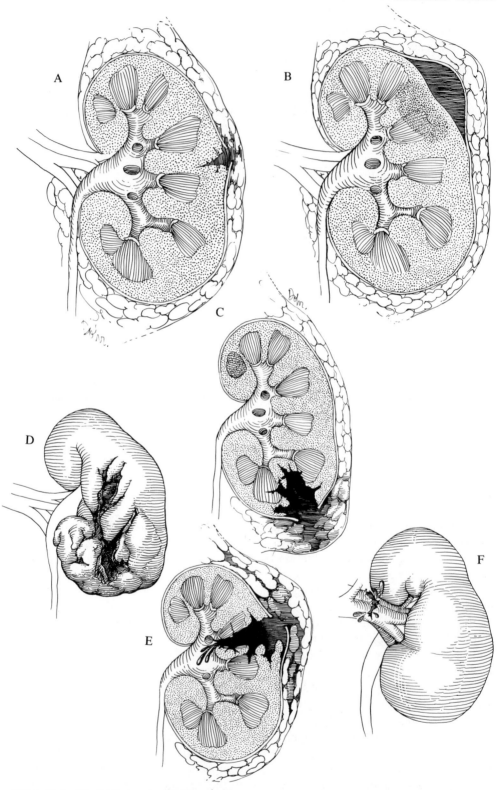

Figure 11–4. Renal injuries classified by severity.
Minor injuries—A and B; Major injuries—C, D, E,
and F.

The massively comminuted kidney from blunt trauma usually requires nephrectomy. In certain patients, consideration should be given to bench repair and autotransplantation of the kidney.

Vascular injury of major renal vessels occurs in 4 to 5 percent of blunt renal trauma (Figure 11–4f). Thrombosis of the main renal artery is the most serious and difficult to diagnose.[16,31,56] Often (30 percent of cases) there is no hematuria, thus the diagnosis cannot be surmised without excretory urography. Nonvisualization of a kidney on IVP then demands renal arteriography (Figure 11-5). Thrombosis of the main renal artery is likely to be seen in patients with major injuries due to rapid deceleration. The kidneys move freely in the retroperitoneum, which results in sudden stretch on the renal artery near its emergence from the aorta. The arterial intima, having little elasticity, tears, which causes thrombus formation (Figure 11-6). Total vascular avulsion can be a result of the same mechanism of injury. Rapid diagnosis and immediate operation can salvage the kidney. Bilateral renal artery thrombosis has also been reported.

Penetrating injuries should be explored surgically.[4,41,49,51] A rare exception to this rule is in a case where staging has been complete, and presenting minor parenchymal injury and no extravasation. In most cases of penetrating injury (80 percent) there is associated organ injury that requires operation; thus renal exploration is only an additional portion of the procedure.[53]

Pre-operative preparation includes adequate resuscitation and staging of the injury. Four to six units of blood should be available for transfusion in all renal explorations. Administration of antibiotics is not required pre-operatively, unless the patient has known infected urine or obvious bowel perforation. Urine outputs should be monitored by catheter bladder drainage.

Operative Exploration and Exposure

A midline transabdominal incision is the preferred approach.[49,53,54] This allows complete exploration of the abdominal contents for associated injury and provides access to both kidneys. In general, associated injury of liver, spleen, bowel, and major vessels should be repaired before renal exploration. However, massive renal bleeding demands immediate attention and control.

The small bowel is lifted to the right and placed in a protective bag. The retroperitoneum along the base of the small bowel mesentery is incised just medial to the inferior mesenteric vein (Figure 11-2). As the incision is carried up to the ligament of Treitz, the small bowel can be easily moved superiorly to expose the aorta. Hematoma may surround the aorta, but once the small bowel is retracted, dissection down to the aorta can be done safely. Once the aorta is identified, dissection on its anterior surface is begun and carried superiorly until the left renal vein is identified and completely exposed.

The left renal artery will lie just superior and posterior to the left renal vein. The right renal artery will be a bit more superior and medial. Careful upward retraction of the left renal vein affords the exposure necessary to isolate either main renal artery. The artery is dissected free and a silicone vessel loop is passed around the vessel for control. The artery need not be occluded at this time unless massive

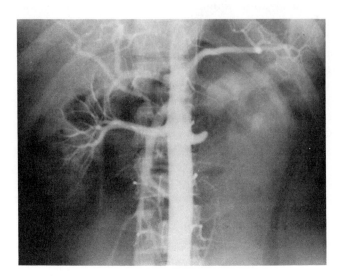

Figure 11–5. Blunt abdominal trauma in 29-year-old man. IVP had non-visualized left kidney. Prompt arteriogram demonstrates acute left renal arterial thrombosis.

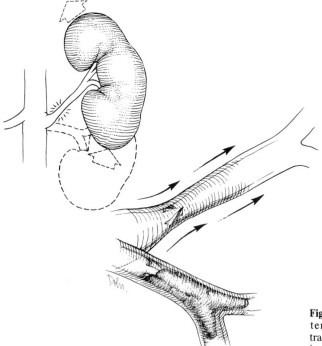

Figure 11–6. Mechanism of arterial thrombosis from blunt trauma. Stretch on vessels results in intimal tear and thrombosis.

hemorrhage is occurring. Artery isolation before the hematoma is entered allows exploration and renal exposure without fear of uncontrollable arterial bleeding.

The peritoneum lateral to the colon is then incised and the colon is reflected medially to expose the entire surrounding hematoma. Gerota's fascia and other landmarks are distorted by blood within the tissues; one should proceed directly through the hematoma to expose the kidney. The entire kidney should be completely exposed and evaluated. If heavy bleeding develops, the main renal artery can be occluded temporarily. Total warm ischemia time should not exceed 60 minutes. Renal cooling with slush ice should be done if longer ischemia is necessary.

Evaluation of Injury

LACERATION. Complete exposure of the kidney is necessary to define the full extent of injury. Large intrarenal hematomas will be present in areas of lacerations and these hematomas must be evacuated to expose venous and arterial bleeding, as well as any opening in the collecting system. Intravenous injection of methylene blue or indigo carmine will provide dark blue urine within 10 minutes and will help detect urinary extravasation. Ureteral occlusion with a vessel loop will cause gentle back pressure in the collecting system and aid in identifying urine leakage. This same technique demonstrates renal pelvis tears.

Ischemic and nonviable tissue will usually be obvious by its dark or totally blanched appearance. On occasion, after removal of intrarenal hematomas, arterial perfusion greatly improves on the laceration margins and more tissue can be salvaged than originally expected.

VASCULAR INJURY. Thrombosis of the main renal artery is obvious when the artery is exposed. A short distance from the aortic take-off the vessel appears contused but intact and will be pulseless distal to the contused area. The contused area represents the site of injury and thrombus formation. Segmental venous and arterial injuries are uncovered as the renal hilum is dissected. The degree of renal ischemia from these injuries must be noted.

Operative Treatment

All nonviable tissue should be debrided and removed. Intrarenal hematomas should be opened and debridement of parenchymal margins should be accomplished. If bleeding becomes heavy, a vascular clamp may be applied to the artery and vein. Individual bleeding vessels should be suture-ligated by figure eight technique, using 4-0 chromic suture on a fine taper needle. The collecting system, if open, should be closed watertight with running chromic sutures. Intravenously injected indigo carmine, when excreted in the urine, will define any areas not completely closed and which require additional sutures.

Persistent vessel oozing is frequently noted after debridement and suture ligature control of bleeding. Application of absorbable gelatin sponge or microfibrillar collagen will provide more complete hemostasis.

Remaining defects in the renal parenchyma need coverage to maintain hemostasis and aid localized wound healing. Ideally, the renal capsule can be approximated over the defect with interrupted chromic sutures. Should the capsule be frayed or or destroyed, a pedicle graft of omentum or free peritoneal patch graft can be used. The omental graft offers viable tissue, rich in lymphatics, which provides an excellent wound healing base. The omentum is most often readily available and can be brought lateral to the colon or through a window in the mesocolon. Interrupted sutures of 4-0 chromic can be used to secure the omentum to the wound edges. The omentum has the capability of assisting hemostasis, sealing small urinary leaks, and its healing capabilities contribute to rapid recovery after trauma. More than 15 cases thus managed at San Francisco General Hospital have had no complications; early ambulation and discharge has been possible.

Retroperitoneal drains should be placed in all cases of injury to the collecting system. They should remain in place until urine no longer extravasates.[8]

In thrombosis of the main renal artery, the injured segment must be totally removed so that circulation may be reestablished. This is best done by interposition of a graft of hypogastric artery or saphenous vein. Autotransplantation is another option.[16,56] Repair of segmental vessels that are lacerated or thrombosed is difficult and may best be managed by ligation. If the area of renal infarction is 20 percent or greater, the nonviable tissue should be surgically removed. Smaller infarcts can be left alone without fear of subsequent complications.

Lacerations of the main renal vein should be surgically repaired with fine vascular suture. Segmental vein lacerations may be ligated since intrarenal collateral circulation is adequate.

Postoperative Care

Assuming no other injuries exist and the patient is managed only for renal injury, postoperative care is very similar to that of any major abdominal procedure. Gastric suction may be discontinued in 3 to 4 days, followed by ambulation. Gross examination of urine usually shows it to be free of blood. Antibiotics are ordinarily unnecessary. Blood pressure and hematocrit levels must be followed closely. The patient ordinarily is allowed to go home in 8 to 10 days.

Complications

Early complications, those occurring within the first 4 weeks, include (1) delayed bleeding; (2) abscess; (3) urine extravasation; (4) sepsis; and (5) fistula formation.[7,8,54] Drainage procedures are indicated on any abscess or accumulation of urine persisting on postoperative IVP. Careful technique and attention to intraoperative details make these problems uncommon in present day management.

Hypertension, hydronephrosis, arteriovenous fistula, calculus formation, and chronic pyelonephritis are important late complications. For major injuries, a follow-up IVP should be obtained within 3 months to detect possible development of late complications.

URETERAL INJURIES

The ureter is rarely injured. A small tubular structure 6 to 8 mm in diameter, running the entire course of the retroperitoneum, the ureter is well protected by muscular and bony structures. Injuries from external violence are mainly from gunshot wounds.[4,5] Blunt trauma of the rapid deceleration type has been reported to avulse the ureter from the renal pelvis; it is a rare injury. Injuries to the ureter from operation (sometimes gynecologic) have been reported to occur in every major procedure involving the retroperitoneum. However, such injuries are more common from extensive pelvic procedures such as radical hysterectomies, vascular procedures, colon and rectal surgery, and radical urologic operations. Radical hysterectomies have a reported incidence of ureteral injuries from 9.0 to 33 percent.[33] Hysterectomy for benign conditions has an incidence of injury less than 2.0 percent.

Anatomy

The ureter leaves the renal pelvis at about the second lumbar vertebrae high in the retroperitoneum, courses inferior on the psoas muscle and passes anteriorly over the common iliac vessels. At this point, it dips posterior into the bony pelvis, lying just medial to the hypogastric artery. It maintains a very posterior and lateral position, finally entering the lower bladder at the trigone.

Blood supply to the ureter comes from branches of the renal artery as they come on to the renal pelvis and then on to the upper ureter. The mid-ureter obtains branches from the common iliac artery. The lower ureter receives branches from the superior and inferior vesical arteries. Its varied blood supply allows the ureter to be mobilized without one being greatly concerned about necrosis. The collateral blood supply from the multiple origins intercommunicate along the submucosa, providing protection from devitalization and allowing the ureter to be transected and reconstructed safely.

Assessment and Pre-operative Preparation

Diagnosis of ureteral injury from external violence is primarily based on suspicion. Urinalysis is most helpful, since approximately 90 percent of cases will show microhematuria. Carlton noted that the number of red blood cells may be small and reported that, in a large series of ureteral injuries from external violence, 10 percent of patients had no hematuria.[5] Excretory urography is indicated in any patient with gunshot or stab wounds over the course of the ureter. Prompt intravenous injection of 150 cc of contrast medium in the process of resuscitation provides visualization of the ureters when the patient's condition has become stable and abdominal radiography can be done. Contrast extravasation is noted but may be only faintly seen and an element of mild hydronephrosis is usually present. It is important to note the presence on films of a normal, well visualized contralateral kidney and ureter. When IVP cannot be obtained immediately because of the seriousness of the injury to abdominal organs, exploration of the ureter should be done at the operating table. Physical examination will usually disclose an entrance or exit wound in the area of the ureter and possibly a palpable abdominal mass from a large hematoma associated with vascular injury.

Signs and symptoms begin to appear in the first seven postoperative days and are generally monitored by persistent ileus, abdominal pain, flank pain, fever and, occasionally, an abdominal mass. The abdominal mass represents urinoma from leakage of partial ureteral tears. Results of urinalysis will be normal.

Diagnosis is made by excretory urography, which demonstrates delayed excretion with hydronephrosis (Figure 11-7). A retrograde ureterogram will define the exact location of injury and defines the presence of extravasation (Figure 11-7). [33] Ultrasonography has proven to be of great help in establishing the presence of retroperitoneal urinoma and hydronephrosis. It is a fine screening procedure for postoperative patients with symptoms suggestive of ureteral injury.

Pre-operative preparation includes complete resuscitation with intravenous fluids and blood. Other intra-abdominal injuries should first have been treated. Pre-operative antibiotics should be given.

Operative Exploration and Exposure

Gunshot wounds and stab wounds should be explored by way of a midline transabdominal approach.[4] Associated organ injury must be suspected and the intraperitoneal contents must be thoroughly inspected. The left ureter is best approached by incising the retroperitoneum lateral to the left colon and mobilizing the colon medially. The ureter is most easily identified in its midportion as it crosses over the common iliac vessels. Once it is identified, the superior or inferior dissection to the area of injury is facilitated. In most instances, it is safer to identify the normal ureter above or below the area of injury, then to dissect carefully into the area of damage. Hematoma and heavy bleeding may complicate exposure and identification of the ureter.

The right ureter is approached by an incision in the retroperitoneum over the common iliac vessels. Identification is most often easy. The principles mentioned above should be used to localize the injury. Should the injury be near the iliac vessels, mobilization of the cecum and right colon medially will expose the ureter.

Delayed recognition of injury may have resulted in urinomas, abscess, and marked hydronephrosis. Surgical exploration must be individualized, but in general should be done by an extraperitoneal approach. Appropriate antibiotic coverage is mandatory before and during the procedure.

Evaluation of Injury

Injuries from external violence must be fully visualized in the area of injury in order to assess the total extent of the damage.[28] Complete transections require a formal repair. Any partial transection must be examined carefully for viability, with aggressive debridement and primary repair when necessary. Blast effect from high velocity injuries must be considered at the operating table when bullets have passed near the ureter.[57] In these cases, there will be delayed leakage after tissue necrosis from the area of injury and a urinoma will develop subsequently. Careful inspection of the ureter at the operating table will often make one suspicious of blast effect injury and allow appropriate resection of nonviable tissue with primary re-anastomosis.[23]

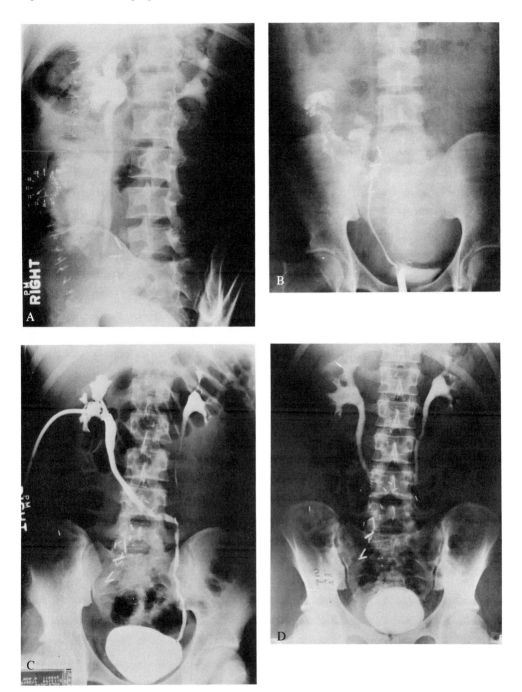

Figure 11–7. *A*, IVP following gunshot wound to right midureter in 20-year-old man. Mild hydronephrosis with extravasation is noted. *B*, Retrograde pyelogram shows site of injury with extravasation. *C*, Ten days after right to left transureteroureterostomy excellent drainage through the anastomosis is seen. *D*, IVP two months after repair shows normal kidneys bilaterally.

Timing is important in evaluation of surgical ureteral injuries. Recognition of injury in the operating room at original operation provides the best opportunity for successful repair. Primary ureteroureterostomy, reimplantation, suture deligation, and transureteroureterostomy offer a variety of techniques in immediate management. If the injury is recognized within 10 to 14 days, and no infection, or abscess, or urinoma exists, immediate re-exploration directly to the injury site with subsequent repair is indicated. With urinoma, abscess or delayed recognition, proximal urinary drainage is indicated by percutaneous or formal nephrostomy, and reconstruction planned for within 6 to 8 weeks.

Operative Treatment

The principles of ureteral repair are (1) adequate debridement; (2) tension-free repair; (3) spatulated anastomosis; (4) watertight closure; (5) ureteral stenting in selected cases; and (6) retroperitoneal drainage.[3]

The procedure of choice in injuries of the lower third of the ureter is reimplantation into the bladder, which may be combined with a psoas hitch procedure to minimize tension on the anastomosis (Figure 11-8).[15] A submucosal tunnel in the bladder will prevent reflux, and spatulation of the ureter allows accurate precise suturing technique. The anastomosis should be as inferior and as near the trigone as possible. Interrupted sutures of 4-0 polyglycolic acid provide an excellent anastomosis. Other options in lower third injuries include primary ureteroureterostomy. When higher injuries have occurred a bladder flap (Boaris) is indicated.

Primary ureteroureterostomy is the best procedure in mid and upper ureteral injuries. Complete debridement should be done back to active bleeding tissue. Spatulation of the distal and proximal ends enlarge the lumen size and allows for contracture during healing (Figure 11-9). A watertight closure should be done by interrupted or running 5-0 polyglycolic acid sutures. Adequate freeing of the ureteral ends provide a tension-free anastomosis.

The anastomosis should be stented if infection, contamination or any of the basic principles of repair are in question. The preferred technique is an internal stent inserted through the anastomosis before closure. These stents are passed over an angiographic guide wire and are double "J"ed so that migration is prevented. After healing in 3 to 4 weeks, the stent can be removed at cystoscopy. The advantages of this stent are (1) maintaining of a straight ureter; (2) maintainance of constant ureteral caliber during early healing; (3) presence of a conduit for urine during healing; (4) prevention of urine extravasation around the anastomosis; and (5) easy removal. Stenting may also be used in uncomplicated ureteral repair but it is not mandatory.

Another technique for stenting is proximal diversion with nephrostomy and a ureteral stent passed from the kidney down through the repair. This allows complete urine diversion and primary healing of the repair. The stent can be removed in 3 weeks, and a nephrostogram obtained to prove adequate drainage through the repair without extravasation.

Transureteroureterostomy can be utilized in cases of loss of long segments of the mid and lower ureter. The opposite ureter is identified and exposed with as little manipulation as possible. A 2 cm ureterotomy is made in the contralateral ureter, while an equal distance spatulation is done on the anastomotic end of the injured ureter (Figure 11-10). Running 5-0 polyglycolic acid sutures provide watertight closure. Retroperitoneal drains should be left in place.

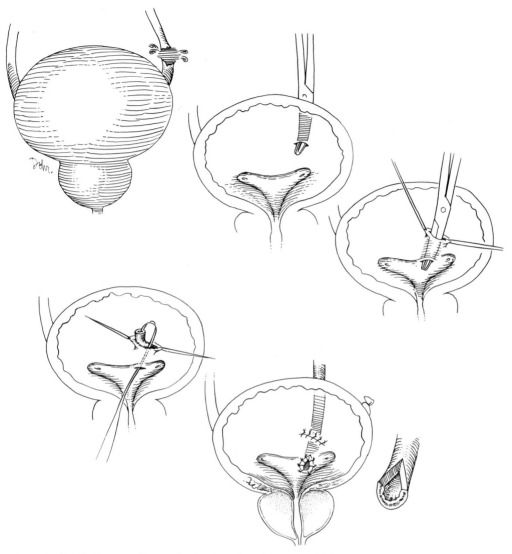

Figure 11–8. Technique of ureteral reimplantation after ureteral injury. Psoas muscle hitch removes tension on anastomosis.

Renal autotransplantation offers a solution for renal salvage when long ureteral segments are lost and previously described techniques are unacceptable. Replacement of the ureter with ileum offers yet another possibility to save the kidney.

Complications

Complications of ureteral injuries may be severe and complex. Stricture formation and resulting hydronephrosis may occur at the site of repair. Urinary extravasation at the repair area may induce retroperitoneal fibrosis sufficient to cause obstruction. This type of fibrosis is generally more severe when the area has not been drained. Urinoma may develop in the retroperitoneum from slow spontaneous

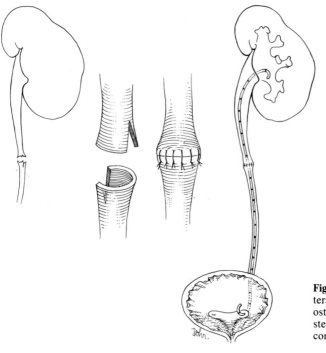

Figure 11–9. Spatulation of ureteral ends prior to ureteroureterostomy over an internal ureteral stent. Watertight closure is accomplished.

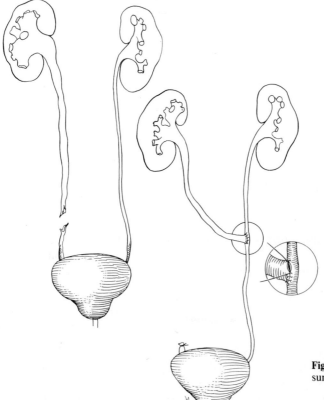

Figure 11–10. Technique of transureteroureterostomy.

extravasations and eventually may develop into very large abdominal masses. Urinomas may cause minimal symptoms when the urine is uninfected; however, if the urine is infected, sepsis sets in rapidly. Pyelonephritis is a potential complication when any degree of obstruction exists. It is important in the follow-up period that urine cultures be carefully monitored and appropriate antibiotics administered to control bacteriuria.

Obstruction following repair may be silent, thus careful follow-up studies are indicated in all cases. Excretory urography 6 weeks to 3 months after injury usually gives adequate information regarding the healing process. A repeat excretory urogram one year after injury should be obtained to be certain that no progressive obstruction develops.

BLADDER INJURIES

Bladder ruptures are most often seen in association with pelvic fractures from blunt trauma.[36] Approximately 15 percent of pelvic fractures (usually from automobile/pedestrian accidents) have concomitant bladder or urethral disruption. Gunshot and stab wounds rarely transect the bladder. Surgical injury to the bladder, if it is unrecognized, may later lead to development of vesicovaginal fistula or pelvic urinomas.

Anatomy

The urinary bladder lies well protected in the lower anterior bony pelvis. Its capacity is 340 to 400 cc. When it is full, its position becomes more intra-abdominal. This position makes injury more likely when a blow strikes the lower abdomen or pelvis. The bladder receives its major blood supply from branches of the hypogastric artery—the superior vesical branch, the middle vesical branch and the inferior vesical branch. Venous drainage corresponds with the arterial supply.

The major mechanism for continence is at the bladder neck and trigone areas. When injured, these areas must be repaired and reconstructed meticulously. On the lateral trigone is the entrance of each ureter, which firmly attaches to the underlying trigonal musculature. Bladder function depends upon nerve supply from the sacral parasympathetic nerves S2, S3, and S4, which course through a plexus along the posterior aspects of the bladder. Extensive dissection in this area can cause nerve interruption and functional problems.

Assessment of Injury

The diagnosis is easily made—assuming the examining physician suspects bladder rupture. The patient often has lower abdominal pain and is unable to void. There may be obvious signs of lower abdominal contusion with, usually, fracture of the pubic rami or symphysis. Gross hematuria is frequent and microhematuria almost always present. Definite diagnosis is made by cystography (Table 11-1). If urethral trauma is suspected in a patient with pelvic injury, a urethrogram should be obtained before urethral catheterization is attempted. If no evidence of urethral injury (blood

Table 11–1   TECHNIQUE FOR CYSTOGRAM AND URETHROGRAM

	Cystogram	Urethrogram
Volume	250 cc	20 cc
Type of Contrast Medium	Cystografic or undiluted contrast material	Undiluted contrast medium
X-ray films	Bladder filled and post-evacuation	With injection
Position	Supine	Oblique

at the meatus) exists, gentle insertion of a Foley catheter may be accomplished with ease. Gravity filling of the bladder with at least 250 cc of contrast material is then done. This volume allows for complete expansion of the bladder and helps to establish all areas of extravasation (Figures 11-11, 11-12). If the initial x-ray film does not demonstrate extravasation, an additional 50 cc of contrast medium may be inserted into the bladder through a syringe. Occasionaly, the bowel adheres to the bladder dome after intraperitoneal rupture: additional injection of contrast material will push away the bowel and extravasation will be noted.

Extraperitoneal ruptures are seen in 75 percent of cases and typically result from penetration of the bladder by bony fragments. The remaining 25 percent of cases show intraperitoneal rupture and may not relate to pelvic fracture. Heavy blood loss and shock may occur from pelvic crush injuries. Resuscitation must be prompt and abundant blood available at operation.

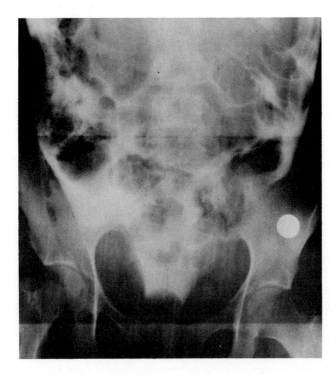

Figure 11–11. Cystogram demonstrates intraperitoneal bladder rupture. Note contrast free in in the abdominal cavity.

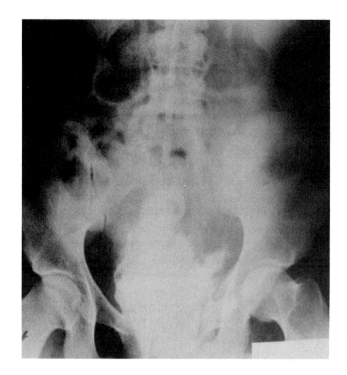

Figure 11–12. Extraperitoneal extravasation from blunt trauma.

Exploration and Exposure

A lower abdominal midline incision allows opening of the peritoneum and, if indicated, exploration for possible visceral injury. A peritoneotomy can be done and, if no free blood is noted, it would seem safe to assume that no major intraperitoneal organ has been injured. Attention is then directed to the bladder. The surgeon should keep the exploration in the midline and not move laterally into the hematoma, where heavy bleeding may ensue. As the bladder wall is exposed, a vertical incision is made well above the bladder neck to expose the bladder lumen.

Operative Evaluation and Repair

Once the bladder lumen is open, the location and extent of damage can be identified from inside the bladder. Extraperitoneal perforations are closed from within the bladder with 3-0 polyglycolic acid sutures. Sutures are single layer and include bladder muscle and mucosa. If the perforation is intraperitoneal, a multi-layered closure is the best choice—closing the bladder mucosa and musculature separately from the peritoneum in three layers.

The ureteral orifices should be carefully observed for efflux of clear urine. Should there be a question of ureteral injury, catheterization and ureteral exploration are indicated.

Occasionally, lacerations extend into the bladder neck: repair in this area should be done with great care to avoid the danger of incontinence or bladder neck contracture. Precise interrupted suturing prevents secondary damage to other structures.

Suprapubic drainage with a 28F Malecot catheter should be done.[41,51] Bladder ruptures often have significant gross bleeding for several days after repair and the large suprapubic catheter offers easy drainage without risk of obstruction by blood clot. Drainage should be maintained for 7 to 14 days, depending upon the extent of injury. The bladder incision is closed in 2 layers by 3-0 polyglycolic acid suture. Penrose drains are left over the area of bladder closure for 48 to 72 hours, then removed. No attempt should be made to drain the pelvic hematomas for fear of inducing infection.

Heavy bleeding from rupture of pelvic vessels may be uncontrollable even though one does not violate the hematoma. Packing the pelvis with laparotomy tapes may control the problem (see Chapter 14). Persistent bleeding may necessitate leaving the tapes in place for 24 hours, and, at re-operation, removing them. Another alternative is embolization of pelvic vessels under angiographic control with absorbable gelatin sponge or skeletal muscle.

Penetrating bladder injuries require special considerations. Since high-velocity gunshot wounds to the bladder may lead to extensive tissue loss, thorough debridement must be done before closure.[51] The ureter must be carefully observed for injury: free efflux into the bladder of blue-stained urine following intravenous injection of indigo carmine suggests an intact ureter. On occasion, bullets pass below the peritoneal reflection and penetrate the rectum and lower sigmoid without creating signs of obvious bowel injury. If rectal injury is suspected, sigmoidoscopy should be done at the time of operation. In such cases missed rectal injuries result in serious morbidity and mortality. When sigmoidoscopy cannot be done and injury to the rectosigmoid is a possibility, a proximal diverting colostomy is recommended.

Surgical injury to the bladder is best managed at the time by closing the defect with interrupted sutures and maintaining catheter drainage for the recommended time. Postoperative catheter irrigations should not be done unless catheter obstruction by clot occurs.

Complications

Once repaired, bladder injuries have remarkable ability to heal. The incidence of dysfunctional voiding, incontinence, and fistulae are extremely low. Vesicovaginal fistulae are perhaps the most common and result from unrecognized injury at operation. Infected pelvic hematomas may require long term care but one can expect an eventual good result.

URETHRAL INJURIES

Urethral trauma is rare. Almost all injuries come from pelvic fractures or straddle type trauma.[10,42] Most injuries to the urethra occur in men. In women they are infrequent.[2,32]

Anatomy

The male urethra can be separated into two broad anatomic divisions. (1) the posterior urethra, consisting of the prostatic and membranous portions and (2) the anterior urethra, consisting of the bulbous and pendulous portions. The proximal urethra, approximately 5.0 cm long, begins at the bladder neck and passes through the prostate; it then becomes the short membranous urethra (2 cm) as it passes through the urogenital diaphragm. The bulbous urethra then begins and remains entirely in the perineum. The entire bulbous and pendulous urethra is surrounded by the corpus spongiosum and is held firmly to the ventral surface of the erectile bodies by Buck's fascia. Buck's fascia is a firm, dense, fascial layer completely surrounding the erectile bodies and corpus spongiosum. It attaches to the deep perineum over the bulbo-cavernous and ischio-cavernous muscles and prevents urine extravasation beyond its limits. In anterior urethral disruptions where Buck's fascia is transected, extravasation of urine can occur with voiding, the only limit being Colles' fascia.[47] Buck's fascia remain intact, extravasation will be confined to the penile shaft.

Arterial blood supply to the posterior urethra comes from branches of the hypogastric artery by way of prostatic vessels. The anterior urethra receives arterial branches from the internal pudendal artery. Venous drainage flows off the anterior urethra posteriorly and enters Santorini's plexus in the deep pelvis lateral and anterior to the prostate. The urethra is endowed with abundant blood supply and devascularization is uncommon. Trauma to the large venous plexus surrounding the prostate and urogenital diaphragm causes massive bleeding, large hematomas and, in acute injuries, make attempts at visual reconstruction largely unsuccessful.

Assessment

Blood at the urethral meatus is the single most reliable sign of urethral disruption.[6,32] Thus it is mandatory to carefully examine the urethral meatus of patients with pelvic fracture. If blood is observed, a urethrogram is indicated before any catheter passage. Attempt to pass a catheter presents risk of infecting the retroperitoneal hematoma and of converting incomplete tears to complete lacerations.

Pelvic fracture will be noted in 90 percent of prostatomembranous disruptions.[11,38] In such instances, patients are unable to void and, on rectal examination, the prostate may not be palpable if it has been lifted from the pelvic floor by a developing hematoma. Rectal examination can be misleading, because tense hematomas may sometimes mimic prostatic tissue. Superior displacement of the prostate does not occur if the puboprostatic ligaments remain intact, attached to the pubis. Partial prostatomembranous disruption (occurring in 10 percent of cases) will not show superior displacement.

Straddle injuries to the perineum result in massive hematomas and bloody urethral discharge.

Once signs and symptoms suggest urethral injury, the diagnosis is confirmed with the help of retrograde urethrography (Table 11-1).[19,20,40] This procedure is best accomplished with an irrigating syringe filled with contrast material (20 cc) injected in a retrograde fashion, the patient being placed in a slightly oblique position. In straddle injuries, extravasation will be seen in the deep bulbous urethra inferior to the urogenital diaphragm (Figure 11-13). In prostatomembranous disruption, the most common injury from blunt trauma, extravasation is visualized in the retropubic space superior to the urogenital diaphragm (Figure 11-14). Should the prostatomembranous urethra be partially transected, small amounts of contrast material enter the prostatic

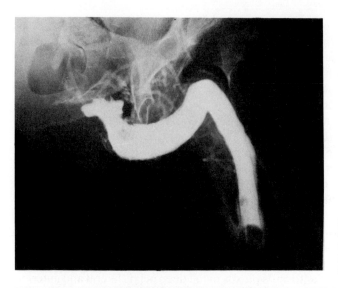

Figure 11–13. Urethrogram following straddle injury to bulbar urethra has extravasation inferior to urogenital diaphragm extending along anterior urethra.

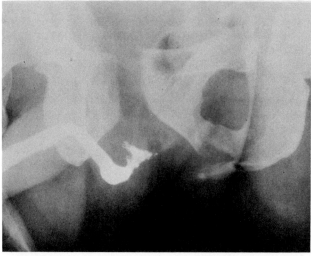

Figure 11–14. Urethrogram in prostatomembranous disruption with extravasation into retropubic space.

urethra and bladder, although significant amounts extravasate at the site of disruption.[20]

Pre-operative Preparation

The patient should be given adequate resuscitation and an additional 4 to 6 units of blood should be available at operation. Preoperative administration of antibiotics should be initiated.

Operative Exploration and Initial Management

The initial procedure for patients with urethral disruption is suprapubic urinary diversion.[32,37] This is best accomplished through a lower abdominal midline incision, which can be extended if necessary for intraperitoneal exploration. Staying in the midline avoids entrance into the pelvic hematoma. Once the bladder is identified, a small incision is made and a 28-Malecot catheter is inserted. The urine is usually clear, unless there is also bladder rupture. In the latter case, the rupture must be repaired. In general, drains are not used in order to avoid any potential infection of the hematoma. The bladder is closed watertight in two layers, using 2-0 polyglycolic acid suture. No attempt should be made to stent the urethra.

Evaluation of Injury

Suprapubic diversion is maintained for 3 months after prostatomembranous disruption. The purpose is to allow resolution of the pelvic hematoma and provide time for the prostate to settle into its usual position. One then must assess the status of the bladder and urethra radiographically to determine length and position of the resulting stricture, which will require repair. Simultaneous cystogram and retrograde urethrogram will provide such information (Figure 11-15).[59] As the bladder is filled with contrast medium, the patient is asked to strain, thereby filling the prostatic urethra: the exact position of the prostate apex and stricture will thus be visualized. Definitive reconstruction can then be planned.

As a rule, patients with partial prostatomembranous urethral disruption can safely void in 3 to 4 weeks after injury and cystostomy. A voiding cystogram will assure that no extravasation or stricture is present, so that the suprapubic catheter can be removed.

Straddle injuries below the urogenital diaphragm will heal with partial stricture following suprapubic cystostomy.[32] A voiding study one month after injury usually reveals no extravasation and incomplete stricture formation. The cystostomy tube can be clamped for 48 hours, allowing the patient to void, and then it can be removed. Should the residual stricture be severely obstructive, the cystostomy can be maintained and reconstruction can be planned.

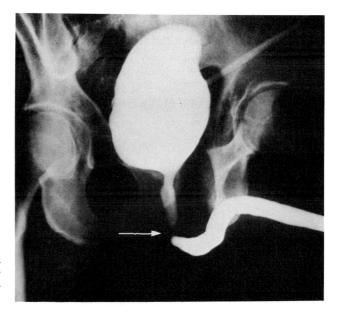

Figure 11–15. Membranous urethral stricture is demonstrated by a simultaneous cystogram and urethrogram.

Operative Treatment

Definitive reconstruction of prostatomembranous disruption should be deferred until approximately 3 months after injury. This period of time will allow resolution of the pelvic hematoma, settling of the prostate into a near normal position, and healing of major wounds. The patient having massive injuries that prevent ambulation should undergo urethral repair later, after walking has been resumed.

In most instances, a 1 to 2 cm stricture will be present after posterior urethral disruption. The repair is best done by a combined perirenal and lower abdominal incision with removal of the pubic symphysis.[1,30,32,59] The patient is placed in a lithotomy position that is not exaggerated. The incision is begun in the lower abdomen and carried down to the penile base. One proceeds to opening of the bladder and excision of the previous suprapubic tract. Attention is directed to the area of the pubis where the entire ventral surface of the symphysis is exposed. The suspensory penile ligament is transected inferiorly. The space of Retzius will be obliterated by fibrous reaction from injury and will be densely adherent to the posterior pubis. The posterior periosteum is sharply dissected inferiorly until the entire posterior symphysis is freed. Gigli saws are passed around the bone so that a wedge of symphysis can be removed. The anterior surface of the prostate is now exposed and a urethral sound passed through the bladder into the prostatic urethra will demonstrate the prostate apex and the stricture. At this time, attention is directed to the perineum, where a midline incision posterior to the scrotum is made, extending back to near the anal verge. The urethra is freed from its attachments to the corpus cavernosum and traced into the deep perineum where the stricture will be noted. At this point in the dissection, the prostate apex is apparent and the stricture is completely excised. All fibrous tissue at the apex must be excised and a 30F urethral sound must pass with ease to avoid heavy bleeding; no attempt should be made to mobilize the prostate. The anterior urethra is then liberally freed distally until a tension-free anastomosis can be done. The anterior urethra should have a 1 cm spatulation on the inferior surface to facilitate a wide caliber anastomosis. The anastomosis is done with 2-0 interrupted chromic or polyglycolic acid sutures. It can be done from above or from the perineum and must be tension-free and watertight. A 16F silicone Foley catheter is passed through the urethra and anastomosis as a stent and left in place for 4 weeks. A suprapubic cystostomy is placed and the bladder is closed. Dead space where the pubis was removed is not filled. Should hemostasis not be perfect, a closed system drain can be placed; care must be taken to avoid infection in this space and the drain should be removed in 24 to 48 hours.

Postoperative Care

In these patients the pelvis is not unstable and pain from pubectomy is minimal. Ambulation is allowed on the fifth postoperative day and by the tenth day most patients are discharged. Antibiotic coverage is maintained up to time of hospital discharge, then discontinued. Four weeks after the procedure, the urethral catheter is removed and a voiding cystourethrogram is obtained through the suprapubic catheter. A patent, open anastomosis is usually noted (Figure 11-16). The cystotomy tube is clamped, permitting the patient to void for 48 hours; it is then removed. Flow rates should be obtained monthly and a repeat urethrogram 3 months after catheter

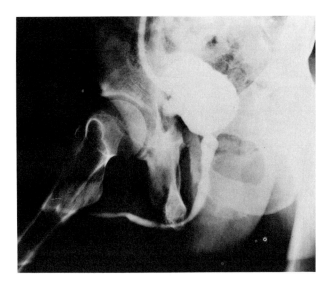

Figure 11–16. Voiding cystourethrogram after repair shows a
patent stricture-free urethra.

removal. Strictures seldom occur with this repair. If they do, they are usually short
and amenable to repair or dilation.

Complications

Posterior urethral injuries create some of the most severe and debilitating complications seen in trauma to the urinary system. Impotence, most devastating in
young men, often occurs if a primary repair has been attempted. Its incidence is
approximately 50 percent.[17,18] Suprapubic drainage with delayed urethral reconstruction as recommended induces a much lower incidence of impotence (10-15 percent).[37,38]

Stricture may develop after repair. Its incidence in transpubic repair is less than
10 percent.[1,30,32,59] Direct vision urethrotomy has proved to be successful in managing
these short fibrous strictures. Dilation represents a temporary measure until more
complete repair can be done.

Incontinence, previously noted in 33 percent of patients having had initial primary repair, is less than 5 percent with the delayed combined perineal transpubic
approach.[14,32,37,38]

REFERENCES

1. Allen TD: Transpubic approach for strictures of the posterior urethra superior to the urogenital diaphragm. Urol Clin N Am 4:95, 1977.
2. Bredael JJ, et al.: Traumatic rupture of the female urethra. J Urol 122:560, 1979.
3. Carlton CE Jr, Guthrie AG, Scott R Jr: Surgical correction of ureteral injury. J Trauma 9:457, 1969.
4. Carlton CE Jr, Scott R Jr, Goldman M: The management of penetrating injuries of the kidney. J Trauma
8:1071, 1968.
5. Carlton CE Jr, Scott R Jr, Guthrie AJ: The initial management of ureteral injuries: Report of 78 cases.
J Urol 105:335, 1971.
6. Cass AS, Godec CJ: Uretheral injury due to external trauma. Urology 11:607, 1978.
7. Cass AS, Ireland GW: Comparison of the conservative and surgical management of the more severe
degrees of renal trauma in multiple injured patients. J Urol 109:8, 1973.

8. Cass AS, Ireland GW: Management of renal injuries in the severely injured patient. J Trauma 12:516, 1972.
9. Chopart M: Traite des malades des vois urinaires. Croullebois, Paris, pp 88-99, 1792.
10. Coffield KS, Weems WL: Experience with management of posterior urethral injury associated with pelvic fracture. J Urol 117:722, 1977.
11. Colapinto V, McCollum RW: Injury to the posterior urethra in fractured pelvis: A new classification. J Urol 188:575, 1977.
12. Cosgrove MD, Mendez R, Morrow JW: Traumatic renal arteriovenous fistula: Report of 12 cases. J Urol 110:627, 1973.
13. Del Villar RG, Ireland GW, Cass AS: Management of bladder and urethral injury in conjunction with immediate surgical treatment of the severe trauma patient. J Urol 108:581, 1972.
14. DeWeerd JH: Immediate realignment of posterior urethral injury. Urol Clin N Am 4:75, 1977.
15. Ehrlich RM, Melman A, Skinner DG: The use of vesicopsoas hitch in urologic surgery. J Urol 119:322, 1978.
16. Fay R, et al.: Renal artery thrombosis: A successful revascularization by autotransplantation. J Urol 111:572, 1974.
17. Gibson GR: Impotence following fractured pelvis and ruptured urethra. Br J Urol 42:86, 1970.
18. Gibson GR: Urologic management and complications of fractured pelvis and ruptured urethra. J Urol 111: 353, 1974.
19. Glassberg KI, et al.: The radiographic approach to injuries of the prostatomembranous urethra in children. J Urol 122:678, 1979.
20. Glassberg KI, et al.: Partial tears of the prostatomembranous urethra in children. Urol 13:500, 1979.
21. Glenn JF, Harvard BM: The injured kidney. JAMA 173:1189, 1960.
22. Hinman F: Principles and practice of urology. WB Saunders, Philadelphia, 398-403, 1938.
23. Holden S, et al.: Gunshot wounds of the ureter: A 15 year review of 63 consecutive cases. J Urol 116:562, 1976.
24. Homer: The Iliad: Translated by Alexander Pope. New York, TY Crowell.
25. Johanson B: Reconstruction of male urethral strictures. Acta Chir Scand, Suppl 176, 1953.
26. Kazman MH, Brosman SA, Cockett ATK: Diagnosis and early management of renal trauma: A study of 120 patients. J Urol 101:783, 1969.
27. Lang EK: Arteriography in assessment of renal trauma. J Trauma 15:553, 1975.
28. Liroff SA, Pontes JE, Pierce JM Jr: Gunshot wounds of the ureter: 5 year experience. J Urol 118:551, 1977.
29. Mahoney SA, Persky L: Intravenous drip nephrotomography as an adjunct in the elevation of renal injury. J Urol 99:513, 1968.
30. Malloy TR, Wein AJ, Carpiniello L: Transpubic urethro 124:359, 1980.
31. McAninch JW: Acute renal artery thrombosis from blunt trauma. Urology 6:74, 1975.
32. McAninch JW: Traumatic urethral injuries. J Trauma 21:291, 1981.
33. McAninch JW, Moore CA: Diagnosis and treatment of urologic complications of gynecologic surgery. Am J Surg 120:542, 1970.
34. McRoberts JW, Ragde H: The severed canine posterior urethra: A strudy of two distinct methods of repair. J Urol 104:724, 1970.
35. Mendez R: Renal trauma. J Urol 118:698, 1977.
36. Montie J: Bladder injuries. Urol Clin N Am 4(1):59, 1977.
37. Morehouse DD, MacKinnon KJ: Management of prostatomembranous urethral disruption: 13 year experience. J Urol 123:173, 1980.
38. Morehouse DD, MacKinnon KJ: Urological injuries associated with pelvic fractures. J Trauma 9:479, 1969.
39. Morrow JW, Mendez R: Renal trauma. J Urol 104: 649, 1970.
40. Moulonguet A: Ruptures traumatiques de l'urethra posteriur. J Urol Nephrol 71:1-96, 1965.
41. Ochsner TC, Busch FM, Clark BG: Urogenital wounds in Vietnam. J Urol 101:224, 1969.
42. Peltier LF: Complications associated with fractures of the pelvis. J Bone Joint Surg (Am), 47:1060, 1965.
43. Persky L: Childhood urethral trauma. Urology 11:603, 1978.
44. Persky L, Forsythe WE: Renal trauma in childhood. JAMA 182:709, 1962.
45. Peters PC, Bright TC III: Blunt renal injuries. Urol Clin N Am 4:17, 1977.
46. Pokorny M, Pontes JE, Pierce JM Jr: Urological injury: Four year experience at Detroit General Hospital. J Urol 120:563, 1978.
47. Pontes JE, Pierce JM Jr: Anterior urethral injury: Four year experience at Detroit General Hospital. J Urol 120:563, 1978.
48. Prather GC: In Campbell MF (ed): Urology, 2nd WB Saunders, Philadelphia, 856-873, 1964.
49. Radwin HM, Fitch WP, Robison JR: A unified concept of renal trauma. J Urol 116:20, 1976.
50. Raffa J, Christensen NM: Compound fractures of the pelvis. Am J Surg 132:282, 1976.
51. Salvatierra O Jr: Vietnam experience in 252 urological war injuries. J Urol 101:615, 1969.

52. Scholl AJ, Nation EF: Injuries of the kidney. In Urology, 3rd ed. Campbell MF, Harrison JH (eds.): WB Saunders, Philadelphia, vol 1, Ch 20, p. 785, 1970.
53. Scott R Jr, Carlton CE Jr, Goldman M: Penetrating injuries of the kidney: An analysis of 181 patients. J Urol 101:247, 1969.
54. Scott R Jr, Selzman HM: Complications of nephrectomy: Review of 450 patients and a description of a modification of the transperitoneal approach. J Urol 95:307, 1966.
55. Schencker B: Drip infusion pyelography: Indications and applications in urological roentgen diagnosis. Radiology, 83:12, 1964.
56. Skinner DG: Traumatic renal artery thrombosis: A successful thrombectomy and revascularization. Ann Surg 177:264, 1973.
57. Stutzman RE: Ballistics and the management of ureteral injuries from high velocity missiles. J Urol 118: 947, 1977.
58. Trunkey DD, et al.: Management of pelvic fractures in blunt traumatic injury. J Trauma 14:912, 1974.
59. Waterhouse K, Laugani G, Patil U: The surgical repair of membranous urethral strictures: Experience with 105 consecutive cases. J Urol 123:500, 1980.
60. Woodruff JF Jr, et al.: Radiologic aspects of renal trauma with emphasis on arteriography and renal isotope scanning. J Urol 97:184, 1967.

Chapter Twelve

ABDOMINAL ARTERIAL TRAUMA

JAMES W. HOLCROFT

INTRODUCTION

The history of arterial injuries in general and of abdominal arterial injuries in particular is well covered in the monograph on vascular trauma by Rich and Spencer.[12] The first successful repair of a stab wound to the abdominal aorta was by Wildegans in 1926 but it has only been in the last 20 years that patients with injuries to large abdominal arteries have had any appreciable chance for survival.[13]

In DeBakey's series of 2471 arterial injuries incurred by Allied Forces in the Mediterranean Theater during World War II, only three patients with injuries to major abdominal arteries survived to reach medical attention.[3] During the Korean Conflict, arterial injuries to the extremities were reconstructed but almost all patients with injuries to major abdominal arteries died.[5]

During the Vietnam Conflict, however, helicopter evacuation allowed some patients with injured abdominal arteries to survive long enough to be taken to the operating room in time to permit definitive treatment. Modern methods of reconstruction were available and consistently applied. As a result, Bill and colleagues were able to report l4 survivors out of 33 patients with abdominal aortic trauma, and recent civilian experience with injuries to major abdominal arteries has been similarly encouraging.[1,2,7,8,9]

The incidence of injuries to major abdominal arteries is unknown since most patients with such injuries die at the scene of the accident and post-mortem examinations are unlikely to list the precise injury beyond the general statement of exsanguination due to abdominal hemorrhage. In a recent series of arterial injuries in patients who survived to reach the hospital, approximately three percent of the cases involved injuries to abdominal arteries; 97 percent involved injuries to vessels in the extremities, neck or chest.[11]

MECHANISMS OF INJURY AND PATHOLOGY

Abdominal arteries can be transected, lacerated, contused, or avulsed as the result of either penetrating or blunt trauma (Figure 12-1). These injuries can lead to massive hemorrhage or thrombosis; they can also lead to the formation of a false aneurysm or an arteriovenous fistula.

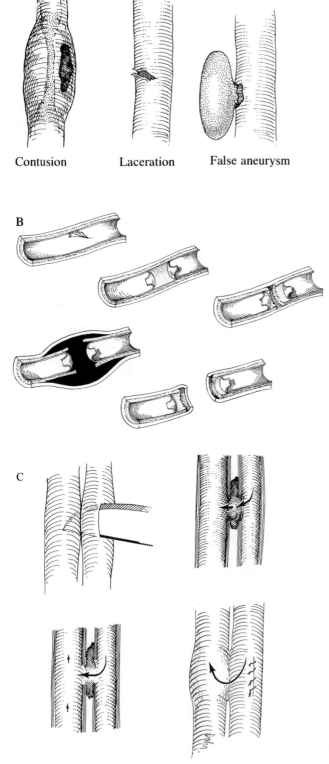

A

Contusion   Laceration   False aneurysm

B

C

Figure 12–1. Nature of arterial injuries.

A, Demonstrates contusion - hemorrhage into the arterial wall, laceration and false aneurysm.

B, Demonstrates the avulsion injury in which the artery is stretched. This may result in partial or complete intimal disruption or complete intimal or medial disruption with or without pseudoaneurysm formation and complete separation of all layers of the vessel wall.

C, Demonstrates the mechanism of the development of an arteriovenous fistula.

Cleanly *transected* arteries, even large arteries, often stop bleeding spontaneously, because the transected intima curls inward and the divided media contracts, pulling the adventitia over the end of the vessel. In contrast, *partially lacerated* arteries seldom stop bleeding spontaneously because this mechanism cannot come into play.[4]

With either a transection or a partial laceration, a hematoma contained by the surrounding tissue may form and lead to the formation of a false aneurysm. If both an artery and an adjacent vein are lacerated, an *arteriovenous fistula* may result.

Contusion varies from an insignificant disruption of the arterial adventitia with some minor periarterial hemorrhage to disruption of all layers of the arterial wall (Figure 12-1b). Although contusion can be caused by the shock wave generated by a high velocity missile, it is usually caused by blunt trauma with the damaging force applied directly to the artery itself. Contusion secondary to severe stretching of an artery typically damages the intima first, the media second, and the adventitia third. Contusion with disruption of the intima may result in partial obstruction of the artery—often misinterpreted as spasm and can result in delayed thrombosis. The thrombus can not only occlude the artery, but it can also break off and embolize to occlude distal vessels. In addition, a disrupted intima can lead to a subintimal dissection of hematoma with the intima prolapsing into the lumen of the artery and occluding the vessel.[10]

Avulsion of the abdominal arteries occurs most frequently with trauma to the renal pedicle or to the root of the mesentery. With sudden deceleration, the kidney or the small intestine as the case may be, can lurch forward and the renal or superior mesenteric artery can be torn off of the aorta.

False aneurysms are aneurysms which result from disruption of all layers of the arterial wall with organization of the resulting periarterial hematoma. The outer layer of the aneurysm is organized fibrous tissue; the inner layer is organized thrombus. The wall of the aneurysms contains neither intima, media, nor adventitia. The aneurysms may rupture or thrombose at any time. Material from inside the aneurysm may also break off and embolize distally.

Arteriovenous fistulae result from decompression of blood from an arterial laceration through a laceration in an adjacent vein (Figure 12-lc). Since veins and arteries tend to lie next to one another, and since decompression, once it begins, precludes effective tamponade, traumatic arteriovenous fistulae occur more often than would be anticipated. The fistula may develop shortly after the injury or it may take months or years to manifest itself. Some fistulae, such as some of those confined to vessels within the hepatic parenchyma, may be well tolerated or may even close spontaneously. Others, such as those involving somatic vessels, usually enlarge with time and can encroach upon adjoining structures or even leak enough blood into the venous system to cause heart failure.

The concept of *spasm* is mentioned only to be dismissed if spasm is defined as severe constriction of the media in an otherwise undamaged large artery. Constriction of large arteries, demonstrated either by physical examination, arteriography, or by operative exposure, almost always suggests trauma to the artery and its intima. The surgeon must prove that the intima is intact in the presence of such severe constriction either by obtaining a definitive arteriogram or by opening the artery at the site of presumed injury and inspecting the intima.

ANATOMY

The thoracic aorta passes through the aortic hiatus of the diaphragm at the T12-L1 level to become the abdominal aorta. The abdominal aorta extends distally to the fourth lumbar vertebra where it bifurcates into the common iliac arteries. The common iliac arteries bifurcate into the internal iliac arteries and the external iliac arteries. The external iliac arteries pass under the inguinal ligaments to become the common femoral arteries (Figure 12-2).

The main branches of the abdominal aorta are the celiac axis, the superior mesenteric artery, the renal arteries and the inferior mesenteric artery. There are several smaller branches which include the paired phrenic arteries, the paired middle adrenal arteries, the gonadal arteries, the lumbar arteries, and the middle sacral artery. The phrenic arteries usually arise from the lateral aspect of the aorta between the origins of the celiac axis and the superior mesenteric artery. The middle adrenal arteries arise from the lateral aspect of the aorta near the origin of the superior mesenteric artery. The gonadal arteries arise from the anterior surface of the aorta distal to the origins of the renal arteries. The lumbar arteries, corresponding to the L1 through L4 vertebrae, arise from the posterior aspect of the aorta and run directly

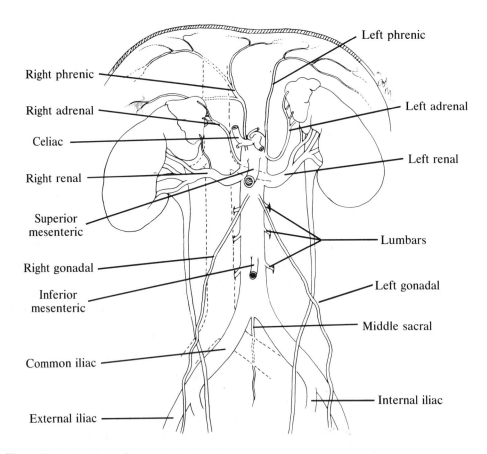

Figure 12–2. Anatomy of the abdominal aorta.

backward to lie on either side of the vertebral column. The small middle sacral artery arises from the posterior aspect of the distal abdominal aorta and runs down the anterior aspect of the sacrum.

The celiac axis, the first major branch of the abdominal aorta, arises approximately 1 cm distal to the diaphragmatic aortic hiatus over the distal body of T12. It branches immediately into the left gastric artery, the splenic artery, and the common hepatic artery. The left gastric artery supplies the proximal portion of the lesser curvature of the stomach. The splenic artery joins the pancreas at the junction of the head and body and runs along the superior surface of the pancreas and gives off pancreatic vessels. Just proximal to the splenic hilum it gives off the left gastroepiploic artery and the short gastric arteries. At the splenic hilum, it divides into its splenic vessels. The hepatic artery courses horizontally in the retroperitoneum in the right upper quadrant. It gives off a branch, the right gastric artery, to the lesser curvature of the stomach at approximately the level of the pylorus. Just distal to this, the largest branch of the hepatic artery, the gastroduodenal artery, takes origin. It passes under the duodenum to enter the head of the pancreas. The hepatic artery curves upward in the portal triad to the left of the bile duct and anterior to the portal vein to reach the hilum of the liver. The hepatic artery branches just proximal to the hilum into the right and left hepatic arteries. The cystic artery usually takes origin from the proximal portion of the right hepatic artery but occasionally arises from the proper hepatic artery (that portion of the hepatic artery between the gastroduodenal artery and the bifurcation into the right and left lobar branches). The hepatic artery may on occasion take origin from the superior mesenteric artery, running upward under the pancreas along the course of the gastroduodenal artery and to the liver hilum. Alternatively, the hepatic artery may supply the left lobe, with the right lobe being supplied from a branch from the superior mesenteric artery (see the liver anatomy in Chapter 7).

The superior mesenteric artery, the second major branch of the abdominal aorta, takes origin from the aorta under the midportion of the pancreas, at the Ll vertebral level, passes under the junction of the body and tail of the pancreas and anterior to the uncinate process. It then passes over the fourth portion of the duodenum and into the root of the small bowel mesentery. Just as it emerges from under the pancreas it gives off the inferior pancreaticoduodenal artery and the middle colic artery. It passes downward in the root of the mesentery and provides intestinal, ileocolic, and right colic branches.

The renal arteries, the third of the major branches of the abdominal aorta, arise from the lateral aspect of the aorta about one cm distal to the origin of the superior mesenteric artery and approximately opposite the upper portion of the L2 lumbar vertebra. These go directly to supply the kidneys as end arteries. They are sometimes multiple, with accessory branches arising from points further distal on the aorta; they also give rise to the inferior adrenal arteries.

The inferior mesenteric artery, the fourth and last of the major branches of the abdominal aorta, takes origin from the abdominal aorta at the L3 - L4 level, 2 to 3 cm above its bifurcation. It curves to the left and then, approximately 2 to 5 cm distal to its origin, branches into the left colic artery and the superior hemorrhoidal artery. The latter gives origin to sigmoidal branches as it passes downward and posterior to the rectum. It divides into two branches which run on either side of the rectum and anastomose with branches of the middle hemorrhoidal arteries at the level of the levators. The left colic artery curves upward, joining branches of the middle colic artery. The middle colic artery curves in the transverse mesocolon to join the right colic artery to form the marginal arcade of Drummond.

The relationships of the abdominal aorta and its branches are as follows: the proximal abdominal aorta is supported laterally by the right and left crura of the diaphragm with the proximal 1 cm of the abdominal aorta surrounded anteriorly by the right crura of the diaphragm. The esophagus lies just to the right of the abdominal aorta and the aorta itself lies on the left side of the vertebral column.

The celiac axis is surrounded by a dense plexus of sympathetic nerves and splanchnic ganglia. The branches of the celiac axis emerge from the retroperitoneum superior to the superior part of the pancreas.

The origin of the superior mesenteric artery, like the origin of the celiac axis, is also surrounded by a dense plexus of nerves. The superior mesenteric artery runs posterior to the body of the pancreas and then emerges from beneath the inferior border of the pancreas to run on the anterior surface of the duodenum and into the mesentery of the small intestine.

The left renal artery runs posterior to the left renal vein to enter the renal parenchyma. The right renal artery runs posterior to both the inferior vena cava and the right renal vein to enter the right kidney.

The inferior mesenteric artery courses to the left directly into the mesentery of the left colon.

The right common iliac artery passes over both common iliac veins along the superior brim of the pelvis for 3 to 4 cm before giving off any significant branches. It then divides into the external and internal iliac arteries. The anatomy of the veins is described in Chapter 13.

The right external iliac artery lies just to the lateral side of the right external iliac vein. The vein remains to the medial side of the artery as it courses proximally. At the aortic bifurcation, the vein passes posteriorly to form the inferior vena cava with the left common iliac vein.

The left common iliac artery passes downward along the brim of the pelvis lateral to the common iliac vein and bifurcates as on the right.

The left external iliac artery lies just lateral to the left external iliac vein. The left external iliac vein remains to the medial side of the iliac artery as it courses proximally until it reaches the aortic bifurcation. At the bifurcation, the vein passes posteriorly to join the right common iliac vein to form the inferior vena cava.

The right ureter courses over the right common iliac artery at variable positions but usually near its bifurcation into the internal and external iliac arteries. It then dives into the pelvis to enter the posterior portion of the bladder. The left ureter runs a similar course. As it passes over the iliac artery, it is usually directly beneath the mesentery of the sigmoid colon.

PRE-OPERATIVE ASSESSMENT OF VASCULAR INJURIES

Any patient with trauma to the lower chest or abdomen can sustain an injury to a major abdominal artery, but some clinical presentations particularly suggest such an injury. Patients in severe shock of rapid onset but with no obvious source of blood loss are usually bleeding intra-abdominally from the laceration of a major abdominal artery. Shock due to bleeding from injuries to the head, neck, or extremities will present with either obvious active external bleeding or an easily detectable hematoma. Shock due to bleeding into the chest will be detected with the placement of chest tubes or with a chest x-ray. Thus, shock in a patient with no external bleeding, no large hematomas, and a normal chest x-ray must be due to intra-abdominal hemorrhage. If the shock is severe and manifests itself shortly after the injury, then the injury is probably to the aorta or one of its major branches rather than to the spleen, liver, pancreas, intestine, or the great veins. These organs, when injured, usually bleed slowly enough so that it takes 30 minutes or more to produce shock.

Gunshot wounds produce most of the lacerations of major abdominal arteries. To assess gunshot injuries, sites of penetration—entrance and exit wounds—should be matched up. If time permits, and if there is an odd number of penetration sites, the missle should be located by radiography of the abdomen and chest. When obtaining x-rays the sites of penetration should be marked with paper clips or some other radiopaque object so that the path of the missle or missles can be assessed as accurately as possible. Even if there are an even number of penetration sites, x-rays should be obtained when possible because there may have been an even number of wounds and all of the missles may lie within the body. If the missle, or missles, are not accounted for, and if they are not seen on x-rays of the abdomen or chest, one should obtain x-rays of the rest of the body to search for those which may have embolized (Figure 12-3). Bullets can embolize anywhere and if time permits every

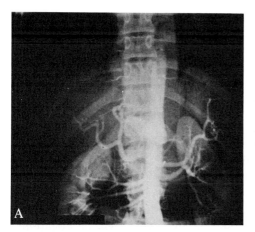
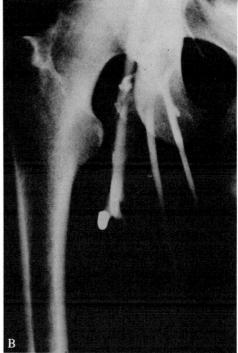

Figure 12–3. Gunshot wound or aorta with bullet embolism.
A, Aortagram discloses defect in aorta just above the celiac axis with dye extravasation.
B, Demonstrates bullet in the profunda femoral artery.

effort should be made to find them. X-rays of the abdomen in patients with gunshot wounds can also be of value because if the bullet strikes a bone it may break into fragments and leave behind a trail that allows one to determine the course of the missle.

Blunt trauma may manifest its damage by occluding major abdominal arteries. Some occlusions will be obvious in the preoperative assessment while others will be silent. Occlusion of the abdominal aorta or of the iliac arteries will present with absent femoral pulses. Other occlusions will be less obvious. Occlusion of one renal artery may present with hematuria or it may not. When there is the possibility of injury to the renal vascular pedicle, an intravenous pyelogram is necessary to assure that the blood flow to both kidneys is intact. Occlusion of the superior mesenteric artery will lead to ischemia of the small intestine and, eventually, signs of peritoneal irritation but the patient may be initially asymptomatic. Occlusion of the celiac axis or inferior mesenteric artery may also be asymptomatic.

Arteriograms can be helpful in selected patients with suspected abdominal arterial injuries. They can pinpoint sites of occlusion, demonstrate extent of vascular injuries in organs which may not manifest their injuries acutely and delineate unusual lesions such as arteriovenous fistulae or bullet embolism.

PRE-OPERATIVE MANAGEMENT

Most patients with injured major abdominal arteries will present with obvious signs of blood volume loss and the majority will present in shock. Once the airway and ventilation are secure, one should begin volume replacement rapidly by administering fluid through the largest cannula possible into the largest available vein. The easiest vein to isolate and cannulate is the greater saphenous vein at the ankle. The vein lies in the subcutaneous tissue along the groove in front of the medial malleolus. There are no important structures in the vicinity of the vein and cutdowns in this vein can be done safely and quickly. Most adult patients will have saphenous veins large enough to admit the end of cut-off intravenous tubing so that administered fluids can run directly into the vascular system with no added resistance other than that due to the intravenous tubing itself.

Superficial veins in the upper extremity can also be used for volume replacement. A cutdown on the medial antecubital vein permits the insertion of a large bore catheter, such as a 5 mm diameter infant feeding tube, into the basilic vein. Another alternative is to cut down directly over the basilic vein itself on the medial aspect of the distal arm. The catheter can sometimes be threaded into the superior vena cava and thus, give a measure of central venous pressure as well as providing a means of administering large amounts of fluid directly into the intravascular space.

In addition, percutaneous lines can be placed in the forearms with large plastic catheters. Resistance to flow through a catheter increases as the catheter is lengthened so short catheters should be used.

We prefer not to use percutaneously placed subclavian or internal jugular catheters for resuscitating patients from major injuries. It is difficult to place such lines in patients with depleted vascular volume because their veins will be collapsed. Patients with multiple injuries are also difficult to position and frequently do not lie still while lines are being placed. Both the subclavian and internal jugular veins are near important structures and misplacement of a line can jeopardize the patient's life. Even when a percutaneous subclavian or internal jugular catheter has been placed, it is not always certain that the line truly is within the vascular space unless a chest x-ray confirms the position of the catheter and, finally, even if a percutaneous subclavian or internal jugular line is placed successfully without complications, it is difficult to infuse fluids rapidly enough through the catheter to resuscitate and maintain resuscitation of a major vascular injury.

For initial resuscitation, we use a balanced salt solution such as Ringer's lactate or Ringer's acetate. We do not use dextrose solution in the initial resuscitation unless there is a question of hypoglycemia. The infusion of large amounts of dextrose can lead to an osmotic diuresis which can deplete the patient's intravascular volume and, at the same time, give the surgeon a false sense of security that renal perfusion is adequate.

If the infusion of 3 liters of fluid resuscitates the adult to an awake, alert state with good vital signs, good peripheral perfusion, and a urine output of 30 ml/hr, time is available for further diagnostic studies. If, on the other hand, the infusion of 3 liters of fluid does not adequately resuscitate the patient, and if the patient's neck veins are flat or the central venous pressure is low, it should be assumed that there is an injury to a major artery with continuing bleeding and the patient should be operated upon immediately.

Once the patient is in the operating room, his entire chest, abdomen, and both groins should be prepped and draped. If the patient is hemodynamically unstable, the prepping and draping should be done before anesthesia is induced. Induction of anesthesia with the initiation of positive pressure ventilation in the hypovolemic patient can cause cardiovascular collapse. If the patient does deteriorate markedly with induction of anesthesia, exposure and control of the intra-adbominal hemorrhage should be obtained rapidly. If the patient is extremely unstable, it is best to open the left chest and control intra-abdominal hemorrhage by compressing the descending thoracic aorta and then finding the specific bleeding site at laparotomy.[6] If the patient is stable with induction of anesthesia, one can proceed more deliberately.

Assuming that operating rooms are immediately available, blood should not be used in the initial resuscitation. It should usually be possible to maintain the patient's hemodynamic status with balanced salt solution until the bleeding is controlled at surgery. Young patients with good hearts and adequately replenished blood volumes can maintain satisfactory cardiopulmonary dynamics with hematocrits as low as ten percent. If it is necessary to give blood before controlling bleeding, both the transfused blood as well as the patient's own blood may be lost. If transfusion can be delayed until bleeding is controlled then the patient will require less bank blood and should develop fewer complications of the sort associated with massive transfusions.

If it is necessary to give blood on an emergency basis, type-specific uncrossmatched blood may be utilized. The typing of blood, as opposed to crossmatching of blood, should take but a few minutes. O negative blood is reserved for patients with rare blood types.

If the administration of three liters of balanced salt solution to the patient in shock does not adequately resuscitate the patient, but the patient's neck veins become distended or the patient's central venous pressure becomes elevated, the patient has either a tension pneumothorax or a pericardial tamponade. If the patient's cardiovascular status is critical, one should insert bilateral chest tubes as both a diagnostic and therapeutic manuever. If insertion of the chest tube does not resuscitate the patient then one should either perform a pericardiocentesis or open the left chest to treat pericardial tamponade.

Finally, broad spectrum antibiotics should be started as early in the hospital course as possible in any patient with a penetrating injury of the abdomen or lower chest. If no intra-abdominal viscus is entered with the injury, the antibiotics can be stopped during the operation. If there is contamination of the peritoneal cavity with bowel contents, antibiotics should be continued intra-operatively and postoperatively.

INITIAL OPERATIVE MANAGEMENT

A midline incision should be made from the xiphoid to below the umbilicus. If there is any trouble with exposure, the incision should be carried down to the pubis and up along the xiphoid and, if necessary, into the chest, if bleeding appears to be from the vicinity of the proximal abdominal aorta (Figure 12-4).

It can be difficult to locate the source of bleeding expecially in the presence of massive hemorrhage. Dry packs should be used to evacuate free intraperitoneal blood. Suction is less effective, as suction tubing often becomes occluded by clots. One should thus look for blood clots which are adherent to any of the intra-abdominal organs or to the parietal peritoneum. Blood clots tend to accumulate near the source of hemorrhage; thus, they can help locate the primary site of bleeding. Free non-clotted blood tells nothing about the source of hemorrhage. As an example, free blood frequently accumulates in the pelvis because of its dependent position even though there may be no primary bleeding in the pelvis itself.

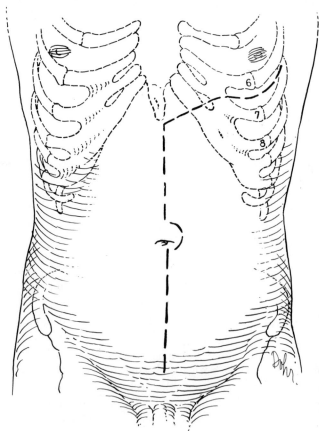

Figure 12–4. Shows incisions used to expose abdominal arteries. The midline abdominal incision can be carried across the costal margin and the seventh costal cartilage to enter the sixth intercostal space if additional exposure in the upper abdomen is necessary.

One should not mistake the first found source of hemorrhage as necessarily the main source. As an example, the mesentery of the small intestine, an area which is easily observed when the abdomen is opened, is frequently the site of bleeding but is infrequently the source of major hemorrhage. The spleen and the liver are also· easily observed and are also frequently injured. Injuries of this sort, however, should not preclude the search for injuries to other less easily observed structures, such as the retroperitoneal vascular structures.

Once a source of hemorrhage has been found, it can usually be controlled by packing and applying pressure while the remainder of the abdomen is quickly examined. This will allow the anesthesiologist to stabilize the patient. The packs can then be removed and definitive control can be obtained of the major bleeding site or sites.

Palpation for pulses and thrills can help in the assessment of arterial injuries. The celiac axis normally has a thrill and can be palpated in a thin patient through the gastrohepatic ligament. When the gastrocolic ligament has been divided, it can be palpated with a hand in the lesser sac. The midportion of the superior mesentery artery can be grasped between the fingers and thumb of the right hand around the mesentery to the small intestine. The artery will usually have a strong pulse and will be easy to feel. Pulses in non-exposed renal arteries are difficult to feel, even in thin patients, but occasionally in trauma it will be possible to feel a thrill in a damaged renal artery. The aorta and common iliac arteries are easy to palpate at the base of the small intestine mesentery with the small intestine eviscerated to the patient's right. The right external iliac artery can be felt as it nears the inguinal ligament just to the left of the cecum. The left external iliac artery is best felt by reflecting the sigmoid colon to the patient's right and palpating for the artery just before it disappears underneath the inguinal ligament. Most major arterial injuries will have large retroperitoneal hematomas associated with them. These hematomas can make exposure of the damaged vessel difficult. Generally, control of the potentially bleeding artery should be obtained before exposing the area of injury. The surgeon must make a decision about how far away from the suspected injury to gain exposure. On the one hand, if the patient has a simple stab wound to the common iliac artery, it would be a mistake to routinely expose the supraceliac abdominal aorta in order to obtain proximal control of bleeding; on the other hand, if the patient has a penetrating injury to the aorta at the level of the celiac axis with an extensive hematoma that extends from diaphragm to pelvis, it would be a mistake to limit the exposure to the abdomen while obtaining initial proximal control.

Usually, it will be necessary to expose the damaged vessel at the time of the original exploration of the abdomen. On occasion, it may be wise to defer exposure of injured vessels, the bleeding of which has been tamponaded by overlying tissue and obtain arteriograms before attempting exposure and definitive repair. Injuries to the suprarenal abdominal aorta can be a case in point. If the hematoma around the suprarenal aorta is non-expanding and non-pulsatile and if it is possible to obtain arteriography quickly, it may be best to defer exposure. An operative arteriogram may be satisfactory in some instances or the abdomen can be closed quickly and the patient taken to the arteriography suite. The patient can then be returned to the operating room and definitive repair carried out. Arteriography should be utilized only when it is unlikely that the delay would decrease the patient's chances for survival. This may be appropriate in certain proximal visceral arterial injuries and arteriovenous communications when the precise location and extent of the injury is uncertain (Figure 12-5).[2]

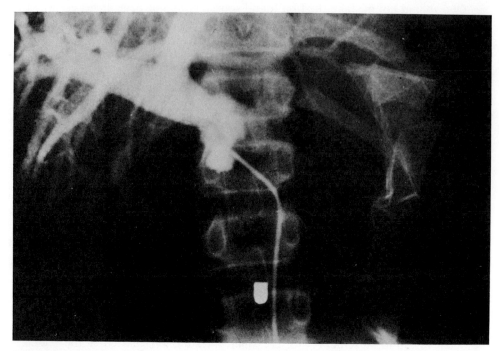

Figure 12–5. Aorto-renal portal vein fistula. This patient was found at laparotomy to have a large hematoma centering on the ligament of Treitz area. A palpable thrill was present. The abdomen was closed, arteriography carried out, and the lesion identified and successfully repaired.

EXPOSURE AND TREATMENT OF INJURIES TO INDIVIDUAL ARTERIES

Suprarenal Aorta

If, after opening the abdomen and assessing the injury, there is a large hematoma surrounding the suprarenal aorta, the chest should be opened through a separate anterolateral thoracotomy in the sixth intercostal space or through the midline incision extended as a thoracoabdominal incision and control obtained of the distal thoracic aorta. The spleen, tail of the pancreas, stomach, left kidney, and left colon are then reflected to the right. The left hemidiaphragm is then detached from the chest wall leaving a cuff of tissue to facilitate later closure. To facilitate exposure the incision can be carried posteriorly to the crura of the diaphragm, which are then cut. This will expose the abdominal aorta from the diaphragmatic hiatus to its bifurcation. The only major branches of the abdominal aorta which will not be exposed by this maneuver will be the right renal artery and right iliac arteries (Figure 12-6). If the injury is to the dorsal surface of the aorta, the exposure described in the first paragraph should be sufficient. If the injury is to the ventral surface of the aorta, more dissection will be required. The left kidney should be left in its normal position, rather than reflecting it to the right with the viscera. The dense plexus of nerves that enmeshes the origins of the celiac axis, the superior mesenteric artery, and the

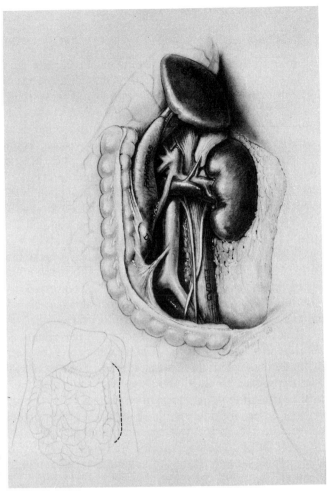

Figure 12–6. Exposure of the upper abdominal aorta, celiac axis, superior mesenteric artery, and left renal vein. The descending colon is severed from its lateral attachments and the spleen, tail of pancreas, and colon mobilized upward to the right.

renal arteries should be dissected free. This dissection can be difficult in a blood-covered field. The safest approach is to dissect the nerves on the left lateral aspect of the aorta first, since both the celiac axis and superior mesenteric axis come off anteriorly. Once the lateral wall of the aorta is identified, dissection of the rest of the suprarenal aorta, including its ventral aspect, can be carried out more rapidly.

If the injury is to the ventral surface of the aorta near the origins of the renal arteries, the left renal vein may hinder exposure. The vein can be either mobilized or transected. If the decision is made to mobilize the vein, the adrenal, gonadal and lumbar veins can be divided. This will allow movement of the vein cephalad and caudad and permit exposure of the ventral aorta at that level along with all of the left renal artery, and some of the right renal artery.

The vein can also be transected and ligated at its entrance into the inferior vena cava. This too will provide exposure of the ventral aorta at that level along with the renal arteries, but it carries with it the disadvantage that any venous bleeding in the hilum of the left kidney will be accentuated by the venous hypertension created by the ligation. The venous hypertension will be particularly pronounced if the collateral branches of the vein are ligated prior to ligating the vein itself.

Celiac Axis and its Branches

Injuries to the celiac axis can be managed with the same exposure that one uses for the suprarenal aorta. There will usually be a large hematoma around the abdominal aorta as it comes through the diaphragm and, as with injuries to the suprarenal aorta, it is best to control the descending thoracic aorta before entering the hematoma. The difficult part in management of the injured celiac axis is the exposure. Once the injury is exposed, the treatment is usually simple, since the celiac axis can be ligated without sequelae so long as its branches and the superior mesenteric artery are intact. Reconstruction of a damaged celiac artery is difficult because the artery is thin-walled and it branches early, so that mobilization for reconstruction is difficult. If one attempts reconstruction of the celiac axis and damages its branches during mobilization, the blood supply to the upper abdominal viscera will be compromised should the reconstruction fail. Thus, it is best, with most injuries of the celiac axis, to ligate the artery and maintain its branches so as to insure adequate collateral flow. On occasion, if there is some question as to the viability of upper abdominal organs following ligation, the splenic artery can be dissected from its bed, transected distally and then anastamosed to the infrarenal aorta so as to provide flow in a retrograde manner from the infrarenal aorta to the celiac axis.

Injuries to the left gastric artery and the splenic artery can also be exposed as described for injuries of the suprarenal aorta. However, if the limited nature of the injury is recognized, this sort of extensive exposure will not be necessary. The most direct approach to both the left gastric artery and the splenic artery is through the lesser sac after dividing the gastrocolic ligament. The left gastric artery can be ligated without compromising the blood supply to the stomach. The splenic artery can be ligated and the spleen will remain viable so long as the short gastric arteries are intact. If the short gastric arteries are taken, however, it is best to remove the spleen if it is necessary to ligate the splenic artery to avoid the possibility of splenic infarction.

The common hepatic artery is best exposed through the gastrohepatic ligament. It too can be ligated if necessary. The proper hepatic artery should be repaired, if possible, but if necessary, it can usually be ligated with minimal subsequent effect on liver function (see Chapter 7).

Superior Mesenteric Artery and its Branches

The origin of the superior mesenteric artery can be exposed as described for the suprarenal aorta. Again, the dissection of the proximal portion of the superior mesenteric artery is difficult because of the dense plexus of nerves surrounding the vessel and care must be taken not to damage the artery, particularly at its origin from the aorta, with the dissection. The superior mesenteric artery, if damaged in its proximal portion, should be repaired, as collateral flow will often be inadequate to maintain viability of the small intestine. Since the proximal 6 cm of the superior mesenteric artery has no branches, once the proper plane is entered and once the nerves around the proximal portion of the artery are cut, the first several centimeters of the artery can be dissected rapidly. Most injuries of the superior mesenteric artery will require patching with a saphenous vein graft or will require an interposition graft using saphenous vein. Attempts to suture a longitudinally oriented laceration of the vessel without benefit of a vein patch will narrow the artery enough so that the small intestine's blood supply will be jeopardized. Alternatively, if the origin of the superior mesenteric artery is avulsed from the aorta, and if one anticipates difficulty in making an interposition graft from the aorta to the superior mesenteric artery with a vein, one can transect the splenic artery and bring it down to the distal superior mesenteric artery with an end-to-end anastamosis. An alternative consists of the use of autogenous internal iliac artery as vascular replacement.

Injuries to the superior mesenteric artery in the mesentery of the small intestine can be patched or the intestine that is affected by ligature of the vessel can be resected.

Renal Arteries

The left renal artery can be exposed as described for injuries of the suprarenal aorta by reflection of the kidney along with the viscera. The left renal artery can also be exposed if the hematoma is small and not particularly troublesome by approaching it through the base of the small bowel mesentery. The fourth portion of the duodenum is reflected off the aorta and retracted to the right and dissection along the anterior portion of the aorta is carried up underneath the inferior portion of the pancreas.

In dissecting out the left renal artery, the left renal vein can be either mobilized or divided as described in the section on injuries to the suprarenal aorta.

The right renal artery can be exposed through the base of the small intestine in much the same way as the left renal artery. A better approach, for most injuries, however, is from the right. The duodenum, head of the pancreas, and right colon are mobilized to the left with a Kocher maneuver, permitting anterior exposure of the origin of the renal artery as it comes off the aorta (Figure 12-7). The inferior vena cava can then be mobilized by ligating and dividing the lumbar veins to expose the entire course of the artery.

If either renal artery is damaged near its origin and if it is necessary to cross-clamp the aorta, it may be necessary to apply the cross-clamp above the origin of the superior mesenteric artery. The superior mesenteric artery comes off a variable distance above the origin of the renal arteries and attempting to place a clamp between the superior mesenteric artery and the renal arteries when the interval is less than 1 to 2 cm will distort the aorta at the level of the renal arteries and make repair difficult.

Injuries to the renal arteries, unless repaired in a transverse manner or unless fairly minor, will require a vein patch in order to assure adequate blood flow to the kidney. In some cases, the splenic artery can be used to make an end-to-end reconstruction. Excessive attempts to repair a renal artery are not warranted, however, assuming that the patient has a functioning kidney on the other side. If the repair requires an undue commitment of time, and especially if there are multiple associated injuries, it is best to remove the kidney. It is optimal prior to doing so that function of the opposite kidney is verified by operative IVP if possible.

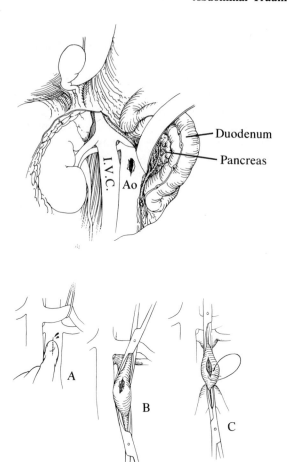

Figure 12–7. Exposure of the right renal artery or the perirenal aorta. The right colon, duodenum and head of pancreas are mobilized upward and to the left. The laceration is controlled to the left. The laceration is controlled digitally, clamps applied and the injury repaired with simple running suture.

Infrarenal Aorta

The infrarenal aorta can be exposed by dividing the parietal peritoneum over the midportion of the vessel in the relatively avascular plane between the mesentery going to the small intestine and the mesentery going to the left colon. As the dissection is carried out in a cephalad manner, the fourth portion of the duodenum should be reflected to the right. The aorta can then be mobilized with care being taken to avoid avulsing the lumbar arteries. When there is a large hematoma, the anatomy may be distorted sufficiently so that the safest maneuver is to mobilize the entire left colon and its mesentery to the right. This removes all important structures but the ureter from in front of the aorta (see Figure 12-6).

Inferior Mesenteric Artery

The inferior mesenteric artery can be exposed with the viscera lying in their normal anatomic position. It may also be exposed by reflecting the left colon to the patient's right. Its origin may be ligated with little risk of damage to the left colon.

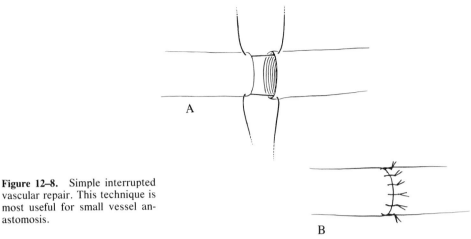

Figure 12–8. Simple interrupted vascular repair. This technique is most useful for small vessel anastomosis.

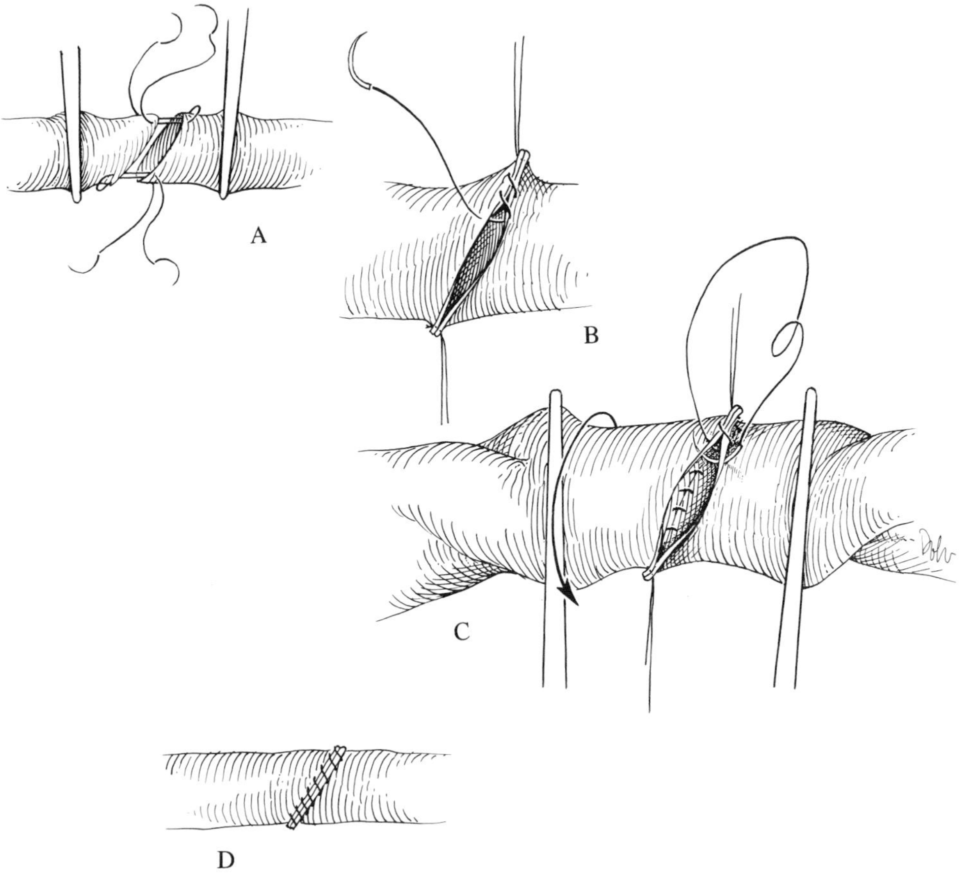

Figure 12–9. Standard technique for repair of medium size (4-6) vessels. Two everting mattress sutures are placed at opposite sides of the proposed repair to initiate arterial eversion. A running suture is placed between. The artery is then rotated to permit running suture of the opposite side.

However, distal ligation at the junction of the descending colic and superior hemorrhoidal arteries (Sudek's critical point) may compromise collateral blood flow to the sigmoid colon. Therefore, the colon should be inspected carefully after ligation has been carried out and, if there is any question of viability, proximal defunctionalizing colostomy with or without colon resection should be carried out.

Iliac Arteries

The common iliac arteries can be exposed with the viscera lying in their normal anatomic position. However, exposure of the right common iliac artery may be facilitated by dividing the lateral and inferior attachments of the cecum and terminal ileum and reflecting these upward and to the left. The distal left common iliac artery can be exposed with the left colon and sigmoid reflected to the right.

The right external iliac artery can be exposed with an incision directly over it as it courses to the left of the cecum. The left external iliac artery is best exposed by reflecting the sigmoid colon to the patient's right.

The hypogastric arteries are best exposed after securing control of both the common iliac and the external iliac arteries. Dissection can then be made down along the course of the hypogastric artery.

TECHNIQUES OF REPAIR

Most major abdominal vascular injuries should be repaired, when possible, by direct suture without using a graft. The best suture material is fine Prolene. Generally, 1 to 2 cm defects of any of the abdominal arteries can be repaired by mobilizing the proximal and distal segments of the artery and bringing the ends together to make a primary anastamosis. Mobilization may require sacrifice of collateral branches. For vessels smaller than 4 mm, interrupted technique is optimal (Figure 12-8). For 4 to 6 mm vessels, interrupted everting sutures at the ends with running sutures in between is most often used (Figure 12-9).

When a large vessel is encountered, narrowing of the anastamosis is not a problem and a continuous running suture may be utilized. The posterior wall can be placed from within if branches prohibit rotation of the vessel (Figure 12-10).

When primary repair would result in marked narrowing of an artery, a graft should be used either as a patch or as an interposition graft. Most major abdominal arterial injuries will be associated with contamination of the peritoneal cavity, since most of the major vascular injuries will be due to penetrating trauma. One should not put prosthetic material into a contaminated field if there is any reasonable alternative and every effort should be made to use autogenous tissue. The saphenous vein makes an excellent graft. The vein from the lower leg is thicker than the vein from the thigh and is easier to handle. The vein from the lower leg is smaller than the vein from the thigh, however, and its small size may make it unsatisfactory for any but a replacement graft of a small artery. If the saphenous vein from the thigh is also too small, one can make a composite graft in which two segments of vein are sutured together to expand the cross-sectional area of the graft (see Chapter 13, Venous Injury).

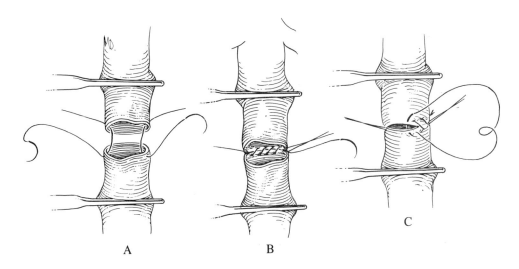

Figure 12–10. Large vessel anastomosis. A running suture can be utilized for the entire anastomosis or the anastomosis initiated with two interrupted sutures at opposite sides of the vessel. The back row can be placed from within the vessel if it is technically easier.

Arteries taken from other areas can also be used as a graft. The first choice would be the internal iliac, since no replacement is necessary. The next choice would be the common femoral artery (Figure 12-11). If one of the groins is not contaminated, the femoral artery from that groin can be replaced with a prosthetic graft and the artery used in the contaminated abdominal field.

In elective cases, the external iliac artery can make the ideal arterial graft since it is large and long and has no large branches. Replacement of the artery is well tolerated with few complications such as infection, false aneurysm formation, or thrombosis, perhaps because the prosthesis lies in a protected, non-stressed location. It is only rarely possible to use the external iliac artery in trauma cases, however, because if the peritoneal cavity is contaminated, it will be hard to obtain the external iliac artery without contaminating its bed. In some cases, the splenic artery can be used to vascularize a critical organ. It can be divided in its distal portion and its proximal end anastomosed to damaged arteries which lie near it, such as the superior mesenteric artery or either of the renal arteries. It is not large enough to revascularize the abdominal aorta and not long enough to reach the iliac arteries.

If, by chance, an artery is injured and the peritoneum is not contaminated, then one can use prosthetic material for reconstruction. Even under this circumstance, however, it is best to use autogenous material if obtaining of the autogenous material does not add too much to operative time.

As mentioned in the section on exposure and treatment of injuries to individual arteries, many of the major abdominal arteries can be ligated without ill effect and ligation should be used if the alternative is to attempt repair in a contaminated field. The celiac axis can be ligated, so long as its major branches are intact. Any of the branches of the celiac axis such as the splenic artery, the left gastric artery, or the proximal common hepatic artery can also be ligated, so long as the celiac axis itself is intact. A renal artery can be ligated and the kidney removed if need be. The inferior mesentery artery can be ligated. The infrarenal abdominal aorta or either of

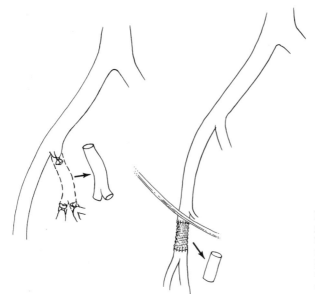

Figure 12–11. Sources for autogenous artery. Either the common femoral, superficial femoral or internal iliac artery can be utilized. In the former two instances the vessel must be replaced with a vascular graft.

the common iliac arteries can be ligated, but ligation will usually cause severe ischemia of the lower extremities. Nonetheless, in an emergency, ligation can be carried out and the patient systemically anticoagulated with heparin. After the abdomen is closed, the extremities can be examined. If they are ischemic, flow can be re-established through a heterotopic (or "extra-anatomic") bypass graft using the axillofemoral or femorofemoral route. Prosthetic material may be used in this reconstruction, assuming that the groins and the axilla and the space in the tunnel are not contaminated.

POSTOPERATIVE CARE

Most patients with isolated injuries of major abdominal vessels do well postoperatively once the injuries are appropriately treated.

Several aspects of postoperative care need special attention, however. Patients with vascular reconstruction can bleed postoperatively and the patient's volume status should be monitored by following the patient's vital signs, abdominal girth, peripheral perfusion, urine output, and hematocrit. Signs of hemorrhage should prompt re-exploration.

Patients with major vascular injuries with tissue trauma and shock can develop the respiratory distress syndrome of shock and trauma. The severity of respiratory failure may be ameliorated by instituting mechanical ventilation in the early postoperative period. We believe that most of these patients will benefit from the institution of PEEP and that mechanical ventilation should be continued for 24 hours before weaning is initiated.

Antibiotics should be continued in the postoperative period for several days if the peritoneal cavity was contaminated with bowel contents. If there was no contamination, antibiotics should be stopped in the early postoperative period, especially if the injury was associated with severe tissue trauma and shock which could predispose to the respiratory distress syndrome. If antibiotics are given unnecessarily under these conditions, the patient may develop a fatal superimposed pneumonia with an antibiotic-resistant organism.

Anticoagulants are not indicated to attempt to salvage a marginal reconstruction as they rarely save such a reconstruction and they increase the risk of hemorrhagic complications. Certain antithrombotic agents of lesser potency such as low molecular weight dextran can, through antiplatelet aggregating and viscosity lowering effects, provide some protection, however. The dose is 10 to 15 cc/kg in the first 24 hours and 7cc/kg daily subsequently during the initial postoperative period.

COMPLICATIONS

Bleeding can occur either as an early or late complication of any vascular reconstruction. Early bleeding can be secondary to technical inadequacies of the repair or it can be secondary to a bleeding diathesis resulting from the shock, and from extensive damage to soft tissues. Some of the bleeding diathesis may be due to dilution of the patient's own clotting factors with transfused blood. Most patients with a major bleeding diathesis, however, will have a consumption coagulopathy to explain their bleeding abnormalities. This bleeding may begin during the operation. Patients who spontaneously start to bleed from small vessels in the subcutaneous tissue, muscle, or from other areas that were dry usually have at least some degree of disseminated intravascular coagulation. In this circumstance, closing the abdomen will allow tamponade and slowing of the bleeding. The hemodynamic status tends to improve when the abdomen is closed because the hypothermia and cardiac depression associated with an open abdomen and general anesthesia can be reversed. As the patient's hemodynamic status improves, tissue perfusion will improve and the stimulus for intravascular clotting will decrease.

If the abdomen is closed in the face of diffuse bleeding, one should re-explore the abdomen within 24 hours. Sometimes, removal of clotted blood will forestall further bleeding. Removal of blood will also remove culture media for bacteria.

Late bleeding after a major revascularization is usually due to infection at the site of reconstruction. The patient can exsanguinate with such a hemorrhage and the patient should be explored promptly. It is usually necessary to ligate the bleeding, reconstructed artery. Sometimes ligation will be well tolerated; sometimes it will not. In the latter case, reconstruction, as described in the section on exposure and techniques of repair, will be necessary.

Thrombosis can occur after any arterial reconstruction. The thrombosis can be caused by inadequate inflow or inadequate outflow, most commonly due to technical errors in the reconstruction. Postoperative thrombosis in some reconstructed arteries will be obvious, as in the cases of a thrombosed iliac artery. Thrombosis in others may be difficult to detect early such as thrombosis of a reconstructed mesenteric artery. Patients with reconstructions of certain critical arteries which could become silently occluded in the immediate postoperative period should be routinely explored within 24 hours of the initial operation; the decision to re-explore should be made at the time of initial surgery. As an example, if a superior mesenteric artery is reconstructed and the surgeon decides at the time of surgery that re-exploration should be carried out the following day, the patient should be re-explored even if doing well. The purpose of the re-exploration is to find a correctable lesion before it progresses to a fatal issue—the *best* time to explore such a patient is when the patient is doing well. If the patient has already begun to deteriorate clinically, serious complications have probably already begun and it may be too late to do anything about them.

Infection is rarely a problem in noncontaminated vascular injuries. Vascular injuries associated with peritoneal contamination can become infected, however, and the infection can encroach onto the vascular repair, with subsequent breakdown and exsanguination or thrombosis. Intra-abdominal infection may manifest itself with the development of a Hippocratic facies, fever, tachypnea, abdominal or rectal tenderness or fullness, leukocytosis, increasing fluid replacement, glucose intolerance, intravascular coagulation, or progressive failure of the lungs or liver. The seriousness of this situation need hardly be emphasized and the infection should be treated with broad spectrum antibiotics and surgical drainage.

Embolization can result following repair of major vascular injuries. The area of the vascular repair can accumulate platelet aggregates and thrombus which then occlude or embolize distally. Embolization is more likely to occur with aortic injuries than with other injuries. Suspicion of embolization should lead to verification by arteriography and anticoagulant treatment or operative repair of a technical defect.

Venous thrombosis can occur in conjunction with abdominal arterial injuries since most arteries are accompanied by veins and any major arterial injury can either directly or indirectly damage these veins. The greater the number of associated injuries, the more likely the possibility of venous thrombosis. Prophylaxis against venous thrombosis which involve agents that alter the coagulation process are usually contraindicated in the immediate postoperative period. However, 24 hours following surgery, if the patient is considered vulnerable to venous thrombosis, he can be treated with low molecular weight dextran as described previously.

Arteriovenous fistulae can form, as described in the introduction to this chapter, from breakdown of an arterial and adjacent venous repair. If this possibility is suspected, an arteriogram should be obtained and definitive repair carried out.

Distal ischemia secondary to either embolization or irreversible damage done by the initial injury can threaten the patient's life. This can involve abdominal viscera, such as the intestine or liver, or the lower extremities. If there is any doubt about the viability of intra-abdominal structures reoperation within 24 hours should be carried out and ischemic tissue resected. When the lower extremities are found to be ischemic, prompt operative intervention is also indicated. The interface between viable tissue and dead tissue allows noxious humoral products and platelet aggregates to be washed back to the lungs and to the systemic circulation, with resultant multisystem failure. If reconstruction is not feasible, anticoagulation with large doses of heparin may salvage an extremity or move the level of demarcation distally. If a dead extremity is threatening the patient's life it should be amputated promptly above the level of demarcation. The clinical problem is deciding when a leg is irreversibly ischemic. Paralysis, anesthesia, and development of induration of the calf muscles indicate a hopeless situation and ill advised efforts to salvage the leg can cost the patient his life.

Renal failure should be a rare complication of vascular injuries. Renal failure is almost always due to either inadequate fluid resuscitation or to a delay in removing necrotic bowel or ischemic limbs. Renal failure is difficult to treat and carries a high mortality in the trauma setting. It is far better to give too much fluid initially and risk pulmonary edema than it is to allow renal failure to develop. If doubt exists regarding the adequacy of the therapy, a pulmonary artery catheter should be passed and left sided pressures determined. Low pressures indicate more fluid, high pressures the need for cardiotonic agents. As mentioned in the section on leg ischemia, it is far better to amputate early and lose an extremity than it is to allow systemic complications, like renal failure, to develop.

REFERENCES

1. Bill LF, Amato JJ, Rich NM: Aortic injuries in Viet Nam. Surgery 70:385, 1971.
2. Buscaglia LC, Blaisdell FW, Lim RC Jr: Penetrating abdominal vascular injuries. Arch Surg 99:764, 1969.
3. DeBakey MD, Simcone FA: Battle injuries in arteries in World War II: An analysis of 2471 cases. Ann Surg 123:534, 1946.
4. Holman E: War injuries to arteries and their treatment. Surg Gynecol Obstet 75:183, 1942.
5. Hughes CW: Arterial repair during the Korean War. Ann Surg 147:555, 1958.
6. Ledgerwood AM, Kazmers M, Lucas CE: The role of thoracic aortic occlusion for massive hemoperitoneum. J Trauma 16:610, 1976.
7. Lim RC Jr, Trunkey DD, Blaisdell FW: Acute abdominal aortic injury. Arch Surg 109:706, 1974.
8. Morris GC Jr, et al.: Surgical experience with 220 acute arterial injuries in civilian practice. Am J Surg 775, 1960.
9. Perdue GD, Smith RB: Intra-adbominal vascular injury. Surgery 64:562, 1968.
10. Pick TP: On partial rupture of arteries from external violence. St George's Hosp Rep (London) 6:161, 1873.
11. Rich NM, Baugh JH, Hughes CW: Acute arterial injuries in Viet Nam: 1000 cases. J Trauma 10:359, 1970.
12. Rich NM, Spencer FC: Vascular Trauma, Philadelphia, WB Saunders, 1978.
13. Wildegans HL: Verlotzungen der aorta. Dtsh. Med. Wochenschr. 52:1810, 1926.

Chapter Thirteen

ABDOMINAL VENOUS TRAUMA

SEBASTIAN CONTI

HISTORICAL ASPECTS

In 1894, an Italian anarchist shot and mortally wounded the President of the French Republic. The inability of surgeons to repair his portal vein injury prompted Alexis Carrel, then a medical student, to study blood vessel suture techniques. [14] His accomplishments in this area earned him the Nobel Prize for Medicine in 1912 and laid the groundwork for the emergence and development of modern vascular surgery.

Other important milestones in the development of vascular surgery are summarized by Rich and Spencer in their monograph on vascular trauma.[34] Of interest here are the contributions they cite which resulted from the study of venous injuries: Travers is credited with the repair of a small femoral vein wound in 1816. Guthrie, in 1830, using a tenaculum and suture, closed a laceration of the internal jugular vein. The first anastomosis between two blood vessels, the portal vein and the inferior vena cava, was performed in a dog by Eck in 1877. In 1882 Schede reported the first clinical application of a lateral suture in repairing a femoral vein laceration. Seven years later, Kummel performed the first clinical end-to-end anastomosis of a femoral vein. Clermont, in 1901, successfully sutured a transected canine inferior vena cava. Goodman, in 1918, advocated lateral suture repair of venous injuries resulting from war wounds despite Makins' assertion that venous injuries were best treated by ligation, especially if concomitant arterial ligation was necessary. Unfortunately, the practice of ligation treatment for injured veins persisted throughout World War II. The considerable morbidity resulting from routine ligation treatment of venous injuries during the Korean War prompted Hughes and Spencer independently to again begin repairing veins. However, it was during the Vietnam conflict that a concerted effort was made by vascular surgeons to repair venous injuries routinely when possible. Follow-up data have been compiled in the Vietnam Vascular Registry and are periodically updated by Rich and his colleagues. In the initial report there were 194 venous injuries among 718 vascular injuries.[31] There were only 28 isolated injuries of major veins noted. (This relatively low incidence may not be accurate because documentation of venous injury is usually not as complete as for arterial injury.) Lower extremity venous injuries predominated, with popliteal and femoral vein injuries the most common. In the interim report, 1000 arterial injuries with 377 associated venous injuries were reported.[22] Venous repair was performed in 124 injuries and ligation was done in 253. Only 12 abdominal and pelvic venous injuries were included and of these three were repaired. The lessons learned from this vast military experience are (1) that venous repair could reduce the incidence of acute venous hypertension with resulting increased amputation rate, and (2) that long-term stasis problems are frequently associated with chronic venous insufficiency. Contrary to previous notions, thrombophlebitis and pulmonary embolism were not increased after venous repair. The value of attempting repair after venous trauma is that if the repair remains patent for 24 to 72 hours, this may allow for relaxation of the arterial spasm and establishment of venous collaterals. Furthermore, veins that have thrombosed can recannalize, as can thrombosed autogenous vein grafts.

A civilian experience with venous trauma was reported by Gaspar and Treiman in 1960.[18] They concluded that the results after repair were superior to those achieved after ligation and that postoperative thrombophlebitis was not a major problem.

Early reports on the management of inferior vena cava (IVC) injuries stressed the rarity of survival, particularly after suprarenal IVC and associated hepatic vein injuries. The first documented survivor of an IVC injury, from a bomb fragment, was reported in 1916 by Taylor.[42] The first of several large series of vena cava injuries, however, was not published until 1961 by Ochsner and others.[26] Up to that time only 19 survivors of IVC injuries had been documented in the literature, all but three as case reports.[40] In Ochsner's series, 16 of 37 (43 percent) patients admitted alive to the hospital survived surgical treatment.[26] Duke and others, and Quast and others subsequently reported survival rates of 47 and 60 percent respectively.[15,28] Improved resuscitation techniques, better blood bank support, and more aggressive operative intervention all contributed to survival rates reported in more recently published series.[3,5] An important advance was the clinical application by Schrock and colleagues of a technique to isolate the suprarenal vena cava and hepatic veins. Variations were subsequently described by others.[2,5,7,10,43,45]

Of interest is the report by Waltuck and colleagues, describing a case in which suprarenal vena cava ligation was successful in treating an avulsion injury at the level of the renal veins.[47] This was the fourth patient reported to survive suprarenal caval ligation for trauma.

Historical accounts of the management of portal and mesenteric vein injuries stressed the importance of repair rather than ligation because ligation was considered to be incompatible with life, owing to massive visceral congestion and portal hypertension. This dogma was based primarily on the results of canine and other lower animal experiments in which death invariably occurred after portal and superior mesenteric vein ligation.[4,20] However, Robson, as early as 1897 and others subsequently reported cases in which the portal vein or superior mesenteric vein was ligated without adverse sequellae.[12,35,49] Child, observed that acute portal vein ligation was possible in humans because of adequate portal collateral flow.[11] Fish reviewed the literature and summarized the techniques available for portal and mesenteric vein reconstruction including lateral repair, end-to-end anastomosis, portacaval shunting, splenic to mesenteric vein anastomosis and graft interposition.[17]

Survival after abdominal venous injury depends upon the nature of the wounding agent, the presence or absence of shock at the time of hospital admission, the level of injury, and the number and type of associated vascular injuries. More destructive firearms and high speed vehicular accidents are frequent wounding agents. With more efficient ambulance services many patients who would otherwise die at the scene arrive at the hospital for treatment.[3] It is this group of patients presenting in profound shock that accounts for most of the reported mortality. In Bricker's series, the mortality rate was increased by a factor of 14 (72 versus 5 percent) for patients presenting in shock.[5] Suprarenal and intrahepatic vena cava injuries carry a much higher mortality because of the increased difficulty in obtaining vascular control. Allen and Blaisdell reported a mortality rate of 78 percent with these injuries compared to one of 35 with infrarenal injuries.[3] The immediate cause of death in 90 percent of vena cava injuries is exsanguination. Late deaths are usually caused by multi-organ failure owing to sepsis. With associated aortic injury, the reported mortality rate ranges between 57 and 100 percent.[3,5,44]

For portal and mesenteric vein injuries, the mortality rate averages 60 and ranges between 53 and 71.[27] There are frequently multiple associated vascular injuries, and death, as in vena cava injuries, is usually caused by exsanguination or complications of hemorrhagic shock. In a collected review of portal vein injuries, Busuttil and colleagues found that the death rate with lateral repair was 30 percent, while that with ligation treatment was 78 percent.[8] Undoubtedly ligation was used in cases with more extensive trauma and this may account for the increased mortality. Stone reported the survival of 16 of 20 patients who required portal vein ligation for trauma.[41] Portal collateral channels appear to be sufficient in most cases to prevent portal hypertension and splanchnic venous infarction after portal or superior mesenteric vein ligation.[11] Portasystemic shunting has rarely been used as a primary procedure because of the frequent development of encephalopathy in patients with previously normal hepatic blood flow.

MECHANISM OF INJURY AND PATHOPHYSIOLOGY

The mechanism of venous injury is similar to that of arterial injury as described in a previous section. Penetrating trauma is more apt to injure major veins than blunt trauma. However, major venous injury can occur in association with pelvic fractures, particularly unstable types associated with sacroiliac disarticulation or in association with massive liver injuries when major hepatic veins or intrahepatic portions of the vena cava may be lacerated. The vena cava is subject to injury during abdominal operation such as lumbar sympathectomy, nephrectomy, adrenalectomy, and aortic surgery. It can also be injured by trocars introduced for peritoneal dialysis or for the diagnosis of hemoperitoneum. The portal vein may be injured during hepatic, biliary, or pancreatic surgery.

Since the veins constitute a low pressure system, overlying tissues are capable of tamponading major lacerations, and the intact abdominal wall with increasing intra-abdominal pressure following bleeding may result in slowing or cessation of bleeding from major injuries. In instances of major ongoing hemorrhage, they either decompress externally or into a body cavity. Missed venous injuries impede intra-peritoneal bleeding from major injuries. In order for major ongoing hemorrhage to occur, venous injuries must either; decompress externally, into a body cavity or into a cavity produced by injury such as that which occur in association with pelvic fractures. Since soft tissues effectively tamponade venous bleeding, missed venous injuries rarely produce secondary hemorrhage.

Trauma to the great intra-abdominal veins when associated with hemorrhage presents a far more difficult problem then that of corresponding arterial trauma for the following reasons:

1. Proximal control of arterial injuries usually stops hemorrhage, since with shock, distal collateral flow is relatively modest and back-bleeding is not a major problem. Venous injuries conversely require both proximal and distal control since distal pressure is raised, causing veins to bleed vigorously in both directions.
2. While cross-clamping of the artery during shock results in very little change in collateral flow, cross-clamping of veins results in a marked increase in pressure and collateral bleeding is augmented dramatically in all branches entering the injured segment. Proximal and distal control therefore does not necessarily result in control of hemorrhage.
3. Arteries have integrity and hold sutures well. Veins often have the consistency of wet tissue paper and tear with the application of clamps or when sutured under tension.
4. Suture lines in large arteries rarely produce thrombotic problems, whereas suture lines in veins that expose raw surface produce a high risk of local thrombosis and embolism. Moreover, suture lines in veins tend to contract and obstruct flow with the passage of time, whereas this is unusual in arteries.
5. Prosthetic substitutes work relatively well in the arterial system and poorly, or not at all, in the venous system.

In partial compensation for these problems the veins can be ligated with relative impunity as compared to arteries, since collateral flow is much better. The exceptions are perhaps major segments of the mesenteric or portal vein or the suprarenal vena cava where serious consequences may occur if ligation is carried out.

ANATOMY

The external iliac veins originate at the inguinal ligament, pass upward just medial to the corresponding arteries, and course upward along the brim of the true pelvis in the medial margin of the psoas muscle. The internal iliac veins join the external iliac veins halfway between the inguinal ligament and the sacral promontory to form the common iliac veins. The latter course upward to unite and form the vena cava. Branches of the external and common iliac veins are few and small. The internal iliac veins are composed of multiple anastomosing branches originating from deep within the true pelvis. The left common and external iliac veins are covered by the mesosigmoid, the right common iliac veins by the retroperitoneum, and near the junction of the vena cava by the small bowel mesentery. Both are crossed by the ureters in the vicinity of the external iliac junction. The left common iliac vein passes under the aortic bifurcation and/or the common iliac artery, pursuing a longer course than the right iliac vein, which it joins to form the cava along the right anterior portion of the vertebral column. The right common iliac vein passes under the right common iliac artery, joining the common iliac vein to form the inferior vena cava (Figure 13-1).

The inferior vena cava passes upward from the sacral promontory to the L2 level, where it is joined by the left and right renal veins. In the lower portion it lies in intimate contact with the aorta and progressively diverges to the point of the renal veins, where it lies approximately one cm to the right of the aorta. It is joined sequentially by paired lumbar veins, corresponding to the underlying vertebrae, and a number of smaller retroperitoneal collateral veins. Just below the renal veins, the

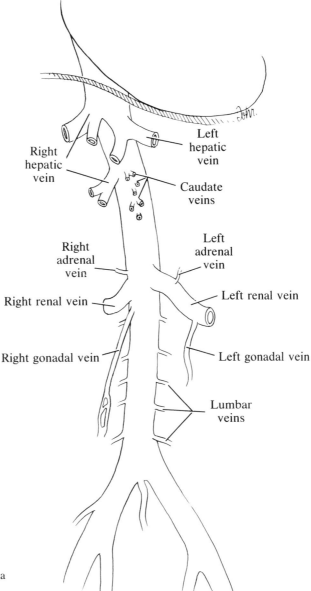

Right hepatic vein

Left hepatic vein

Caudate veins

Right adrenal vein

Left adrenal vein

Right renal vein

Left renal vein

Right gonadal vein

Left gonadal vein

Lumbar veins

Figure 13–1. Anatomy of the vena cava and its tributaries.

vena cava is joined in most instances by the right gonadal vein. The base of the small bowel mesentery overlies the infrarenal vena cava. Just below the renal veins, the fourth portion of the duodenum passes over the cava. The right renal vein is relatively short compared to the left and usually joins the vena cave one cm below that of the left and approximately at the level of L2, L3 vertebral junction. The left renal vein in most instances passes over the aorta as it proceeds from the renal hilum to the cava. The left gonadal vein joins the left renal vein just lateral to the aorta. The left adrenal vein enters the left renal vein just above the gonadal vein. The suprarenal vena cava courses upwards anterior to the L1, L2 vertebral body, passes under the liver in the cava fossa and in some instances is almost entirely surrounded by liver substance as it reaches the caval hiatus in the diaphragm. The cava at or just above the renal veins passes under the second portion of the duodenum, below the portal triad and is covered by the retroperitoneum lining the foramen of Winslow. It is joined by a relatively large right adrenal vein just above the right renal vein, but characteristically no lumbar veins enter this segment of the vena cava.

The only tributaries of the supra renal cava, in addition to the adrenal vein, consist of the hepatic veins, the largest of which, the main right and the left, enter the cava at the superior margin of the liver. There are numerous small hepatic veins that drain directly into the caudate lobe. These are of special significance when the liver is elevated to expose the immediate suprarenal vena cava, as they may tear off the cava, adding to the local hemorrhage. Several small phrenic veins constitute the only other veins entering this caval segment. Approximately two to three cm of cava lie above the diaphragm before the cava enters the right atrium. The supradiaphrag-matic vena cava is surrounded over three-fourths of its surfaces by pericardium, and it lies almost entirely within the pericardial sac. It is therefore easily encircled by appropriate dissection.

The portal venous system is composed of the splenic vein, the inferior and superior mesenteric veins and their tributaries, which join to form the portal vein (Figure 13-2). The inferior mesenteric vein passes upward in the root of the mesocolon just lateral to the aorta and joins the splenic vein just proximal to its junction with the superior mesenteric vein. The splenic vein takes origin at the splenic hilum, passes along the posterior mid-portion of the pancreas to join the superior mesenteric vein forming the portal vein. The superior mesenteric vein receives tributaries from the small bowel and colon and passes upward in the root of the mesentary posterior and to the right of the mesenteric artery, over the uncinate process of the pancreas and under the junction of the body and tail over the second vertebral body to join the splenic vein, forming the portal vein at approximately the inferior margin of the posterior surface of the pancreas. The portal vein passes upward under the junction of the body and head of the pancreas, under the second portion of the duodenum. Here it is joined by the hepatic artery and the bile duct to form the portal triad, which courses anterior to the foramen of Winslow. The portal vein lies posterior and between the common bile duct and the hepatic artery where it enters the liver (see chapter on liver trauma). The only other large vein of consequence in the upper abdomen is the coronary vein, which courses in the gastrohepatic ligament to join the portal vein as it enters the portal triad just above the second portion of the duodenum.

ASSESSMENT

The assessment of the patient for possible major abdominal venous injury is similar to that for a patient with major arterial injury. The possibility of major venous injury exists when any penetrating injury is located in the vicinity of great veins. The patient who presents in shock a short period after injury should be assumed to have a major vascular injury. If the site of penetration corresponds to that of a major vein, there is presumption of major venous injury. Injuries to the great veins are more deceiving than those of the arteries; being a low pressure system there is minimal resistance to blood flow in major channels and tissue resistance and he-matoma formation adjacent to the injury may, for the most part, maintain blood flow

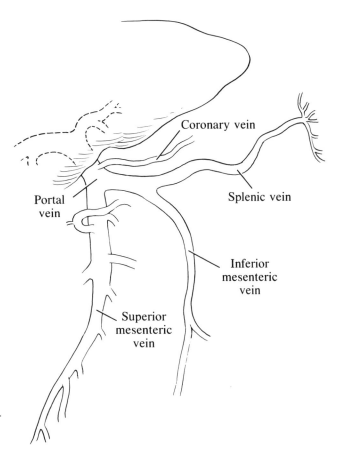

Figure 13–2. Portal venous anatomy.

in the major venous channel. In addition, abdominal pressure serves to prevent exsanguinating hemorrhage, which would certainly occur with arterial injuries of equivalent size. However, once positive pressure ventilation is instituted, central venous pressure in the abdomen is raised and major hemorrhage may ensue. Thus, these patients may "crash" during anesthesia induction. The best way to avoid exsanguination in the initial phases of operation is to assume the possibility of major venous injury with all types of penetrating trauma and provide adequate access to the vascular system via cutdowns and catheters so as to insure the ability to resuscitate the patient should a catastrophe develop.

Several forms of blunt trauma are associated with major venous injury. These include major unstable pelvic fractures, particularly those associated with sacro-iliac disarticulation, in which tearing of pelvic veins frequently occurs. As long as the retroperitoneum is intact, major exsanguinating hemorrhage is unlikely. In some instances, however, the peritoneum is disrupted at the time of pelvic fracture, and exsanguination can occur. Liver injuries, particularly those occurring in falls from heights where victims land on their feet, may result in lacerations of the intrahepatic portion of the vena cava or major hepatic veins, as the liver is literally avulsed from the vena cava. The greater mass of the liver renders the right hepatic veins more vulnerable to these types of tears. Seat belt injuries may result in mesenteric lacerations, with corresponding venous hemorrhage.

PRE-OPERATIVE PREPARATION

As indicated in the previous sections, the intact abdomen and retroperitoneum tissues can tamponade venous bleeding much more readily than arterial bleeding. Thus, a surgeon expecting to deal with a trivial abdominal injury may, on opening the abdomen, instead by confronted with massive venous hemorrhage particularly if the retroperitoneum is exposed. It is for this reason that patients with major trauma, who present with evidence of major blood loss, routinely have at least one cutdown placed during resuscitation in our emergency room. This initial cutdown in reasonably stable patients is best performed in the antecubital fossa. An infant feeding tube approximately five mm in diameter threaded upwards in the basilic vein to an intrathoracic position insures rapid fluid therapy and allows monitoring of central venous pressure. This can be supplemented by whatever percutaneous lines seem appropriate for the administration of drugs or for withdrawal of blood specimens. For the patient presenting in major shock, a second cutdown, usually the initial cutdown of choice, is placed in the saphenous vein at the ankle. This vein is readily accessible, accepts the entire cross-section of intravenous tubing in the average adult male, and permits resuscitation of any patient with reversible vascular injury. Despite the fact that the cava is injured, administration of fluid via the saphenous cutdown is just as effective in resuscitation as that administered through a jugular or subclavian catheter or cutdown, since the venous system constitutes one continuous pool, and raising the pressure in one portion raises the pressure in all portions of the thoracic and abdominal veins. Because of abundant collateral channels in the venous system, effective volume resuscitation can still be carried out with a saphenous cutdown, even with the vena cava clamped. Were this not the case, it would be impossible to cross-clamp the inferior vena cava, and within a few minutes of caval occlusion in the absence of collaterals, the entire blood volume would be theoretically trapped below the occluding clamp.

Pre-operative evaluation should include chest and abdominal films, and if there is any possibility of renal or renal pedicle injury, intravenous pyelography should be performed. A urinary catheter is always indicated in the patient presenting in shock, and a nasogastric tube should be placed for gastric decompression. As is true with most trauma cases, blood should be reserved for administration in the operating room since badly needed reserves can be depleted attempting to resuscitate patients with vascular injury. Patients can tolerate a hematocrit of 10, provided volume is maintained, and it is better to use balanced salt solution rather than red blood cells during resuscitation prior to vascular control. Operative vascular control should be considered part of the resuscitation process.

OPERATIVE EXPLORATION AND EXPOSURE

Abdominal venous injuries, like arterial injuries, are best exposed through a generous midline incision running from ziphoid to pubis. The bowel should be eviscerated, blood evacuated from the abdominal cavity, and areas of major bleeding controlled temporarily with packs while a rapid gross assessment of the abdomen is carried out. Blood should be aspirated from all corners of the abdomen and these areas packed to isolate bleeding. By so doing there is less danger that the patient will exsanguinate from a second injury while the first is being treated. When a venous injury is identified, hemorrhage can in most cases be controlled by the judicious application of pack and pressure. This permits volume restoration before attempts are made to expose the site of injury. The reason for this relates to the fact that attempts to expose the injury result in further hemorrhage and, if the patient is hypovolemic, cardiac arrest may occur. Venous bleeding is also more subtle than arterial bleeding and the surgeon is often less aware of the magnitude of the hemorrhage in venous injury as opposed to that in arterial injury. For this reason, continuous application of suction to the area of injury should not be allowed, since the sucker may remove blood so rapidly that the extent of the hemorrhage may not be appreciated by the surgeon. It is better to have the assistant aspirate for a few seconds, remove the sucker from the field, and then reaspirate.

With the exception of the portal vein, exposure of the great veins is generally easier than that of the corresponding arteries. Local pressure can be used to control bleeding while proximal distal dissection is carried out. In some circumstances temporary intraluminal occlusion by balloon catheters can be used to control hemorrhage. The left external iliac vein is best exposed by severing the lateral attachments of the sigmoid colon and retracting it medially. This permits exposure of the entire left external and common iliac vein. With the exception of the ureter, all critical anatomy, including most importantly the mesenteric circulation of the large intestine, is retracted away.

The most difficult portion of the iliac system to isolate and control is the internal iliac vein or one of its major branches. This is particularly true with multiple injuries to the internal iliac vein that occur in association with major pelvic fractures. For this reason venous hematomas in the vicinity of the pelvis are usually left alone unless there is an associated overlying laceration that results in free intraperitoneal bleeding. The problem with internal iliac vein injuries is that although proximal control is relatively easy, control of internal iliac vein tributaries can be exceedingly difficult, as dissection within the hematoma results in extensive hemorrhage from proximal smaller veins. Since both external iliac and common iliac veins have few, if any, branches the area of injury can be compressed with sponge sticks and direct repair is relatively easily carried out.

The right external, internal, and common iliac veins are readily exposed by severing the overlying peritoneum again, since, with the exception of the ureter, there is no critical overlying anatomy. The vena cava can be exposed from either the left or the right. The optimal method of exposure is to mobilize the ascending colon by severing its lateral attachment and retracting it along with the duodenum upwards and to the left (Figure 13-3). This permits exposure of the entire common iliac vein on the right and the entire length of the vena cava as far as the liver. Also this mobilizes all the mesenteric vessels and moves them upward out of the field so that damage to the circulation of the intestinal tract is avoided. The right renal vein is readily exposed from this approach as is three to five cm of the left renal vein.

Left renal venous injuries can be exposed in the area of the ligament of Treitz or by severing the lateral attachments of the descending colon and mobilizing it upward to the right (see Figure 12-6, Chapter 12). The latter is preferred because injuries near the left renal vein may involve the aorta and the left renal artery as well.

Injuries involving the extrahepatic suprarenal vena cava are readily exposed by a Kocher maneuver, mobilizing the duodenum upward to the left. Proximal control

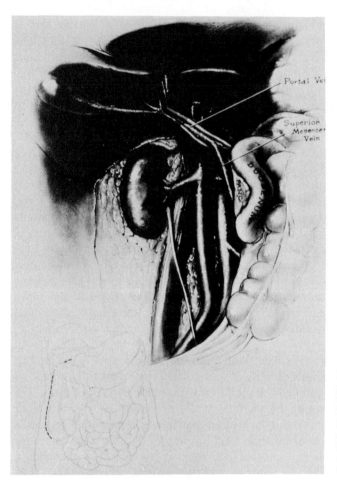

Figure 13–3. Right-sided approach to major vascular structures. Inset shows line of incision in posterior peritoneum. Right colon, duodenum, and head of pancreas are then mobilized upward into the left, exposing intrahepatic vena cava and entire lenght of portal vein.

can be obtained by temporarily trapping the vena cava with a pack or sponge stick at the level of the renal veins. Compression of the liver downward will usually tamponade the vena cava superiorly, thus permitting repair of a laceration, since the only vein entering the segment between the renal veins and the liver is the right adrenal vein, bleeding from which can usually be ignored.

The intrahepatic portion of the vena cava is the most inaccessible portion of the venous system. In most instances the entire anterior surface of the vena cava is surrounded by liver. Multiple large right hepatic veins and the left hepatic vein enter this segment, and attempts to mobilize the liver upward may result in exsanguination before the area of injury can be exposed. For this reason, a technique was developed for isolation of this portion of the vena cava, utilizing an intracaval shunt. Although it is possible to place a shunt from below the liver, this is actually more difficult than placing a shunt from above through the atrium, since excessive bleeding may occur while manipulating the vena cava as the catheter is inserted.

The best way to isolate the liver is to introduce as a shunt, a 34–40 French catheter through the atrial appendage (Figure 13-4). The reason for this is that in the hypovolemic patient, left atrial pressure is low and blood loss is much less since the venous return is not interrupted during placement of the catheter. To accomplish this, the midline abdominal incision is extended up to the sternal notch as a midline

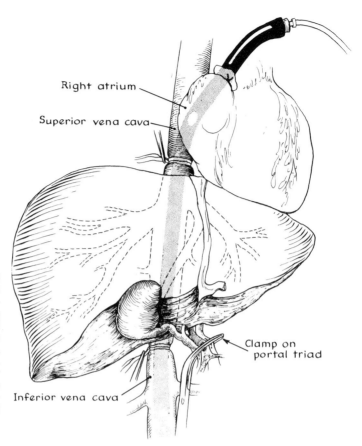

Right atrium

Superior vena cava

Clamp on portal triad

Inferior vena cava

Figure 13–4. View shows a #36 French catheter inserted through right atrial appendage into the inferior vena cava. The tip of the catheter lies just below the level of the renal veins. The side hole of the catheter, 20 cm from the tip, lies at the level of the right atrium. The proximal end of the catheter is connected to an infustion line as depicted. For more rapid infustion, a "Y" connector is provided (see Figure 13–5).

sternoctomy. The pericardium is opened and the right atrial appendage is identified. With a purse-string suture placed around the base of the atrial appendage and an occluding clamp placed across the base of the appendage, the catheter is inserted into the atrium while the intracardiac portion of the vena cava is palpated to insure that the catheter passes into the inferior vena cava rather than the right atrium. The catheter should be manipulated gently since it may pass through a large laceration or may enter the right hepatic vein, which can be 1 1/2 to 2 cm in diameter. Gentle advancement and twisting of the catheter insures its appropriate passage, and palpation at the renal veins verifies the proper location of the catheter. As the tip of the catheter reaches the level of the renal veins, it is cross-clamped at the atrium, and a side hole is cut. It is then advanced into the atrium as the pursestring suture is tightened. This hole provides for egress of blood from the shunt. It is preferable to leave the end of the catheter projecting from the atrium for use in rapidly infusing blood or crystalloid solutions (Figure 13-5). In exsanguinating injuries the author has used the Bentley autotransfusion device, in the pump mode, to infuse crystalloid. With this technique 500 ml/minute can be infused. Crystalloid, balanced salt solution heated to 38' C is used to prevent hypothermia. Umbilical tapes can be placed rapidly around the intrapericardial and suprarenal portions of the vena cava with the catheter in place. When these are pulled up, the caval segment is isolated when simultaneous occlusion of the protal triad by a vascular clamp is carried out.

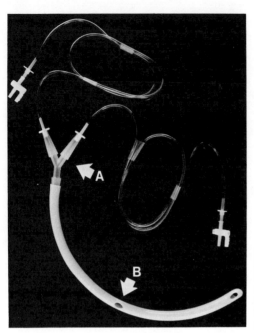

Figure 13–5. Endotracheal tube set-up used for intracaval shunting. *A*, "Y" connector with the femal ends of intravenous tubing attached to allow rapid infusion of crystalloid. Three-way stopcocks are connected to opposite ends of the tubing. *B*, Side hole cut at appropriate level to permit egress of blood into right atrium.

For those not familiar with the transcardiac approach, the abdominal placement of a shunt offers a reasonable alternative (Figure 13-6). In this instance, we have found it better to sacrifice venous return below the renal veins, which constitutes about one-third of cardiac venous return, in order to avoid extensive blood loss. The cava is mobilized just below the renal veins, and the lumbar veins in this segment of the vena cava are clipped. The distal cava is occluded with an umbilical tape, a partial occluding clamp is placed across the vena cava just above the tape, and a 34-36 French endotracheal or similarly sized plastic tube is advanced through a venotomy upward to the atrium. As the tip of the catheter enters the atrium, a side hole is cut in the distal portion of the catheter (which has still not entered the cava) and the catheter is advanced into the vena cava so that the side hole lies at the level of the renal veins, the end of the catheter projecting from the vana cava. Tapes tied around the catheter above the venotomy but below the renal veins and then above the renal veins and the adrenal vein result in diversion of blood through the side hole in the catheter. Another umbilical tape tied around the supradiaphragmatic portion of the vena cava completely isolates the intrahepatic portion of the vena cava, with the exception of that of the phrenic veins, provided the portal triad is cross-clamped and liver inflow is controlled. With the cava thus isolated, the liver can be rolled upward from the right by severing its attachments to the retroperitoneum and the cava can be exposed. Should major hepatic venous drainage of the right or left lobe be involved, lobar hepatectomy may be required. This can be accomplished rapidly in a relatively avascular field when the caval isolation technique is used. Injuries to the intrapericardial portion of the vena cava usually result in intrapericardial hemorrhage with pericardial tamponade. Isolation of this portion of the cava is difficult because of its close proximity to the atrium, but isolation can be obtained as just described for the intrahepatic portion of the vena cava.

It is possible to occlude the inferior vena cava return completely for approximately three to four minutes, provided the patient is reasonably normovolemic prior

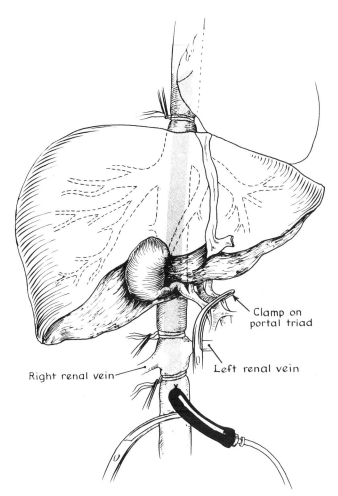

Figure 13–6. Vascular isolation of intrahepatic vena cava and hepatic veins by use of an inferior vena cava shunt inserted from below renal veins.

to interrupting venous flow. Williams and Brenowitz described a technique of sequentially clamping the aorta at the diaphragmatic hiatus and the vena cava within the pericardium to permit repair of a vena cava laceration at the diaphragm.[48] This was done only after adequate volume was restored (Figure 13-7).

The splenic vein can be identified by mobilizing the base of the transverse mesocolon downward from under the inferior portion of the body and tail of the pancreas. This is accomplished by entering the lesser sac, separating the omentum from the transverse and descending colon, and mobilizing the spleen and the tail of the pancreas upward to permit exposure of the posterior surface of the pancreas. Injury to the splenic vein is often associated with injuries to the pancreas. Distal pancreatic resection for treatment of the pancreatic laceration then permits better control of splenic vein bleeding.

The superior mesenteric vein is controlled through the mesentery as it passes over the duodenum and uncinate process of the pancreas and down under the body of the pancreas. Exposure of the subpancreatic portion of the vein requires mobilization of the inferior surface of the pancreas as previously described. Injuries to the junction of the splenic and mesenteric vein and the portal vein can be best exposed by carrying out a generous Kocher maneuver. This is facilitated by mobi-

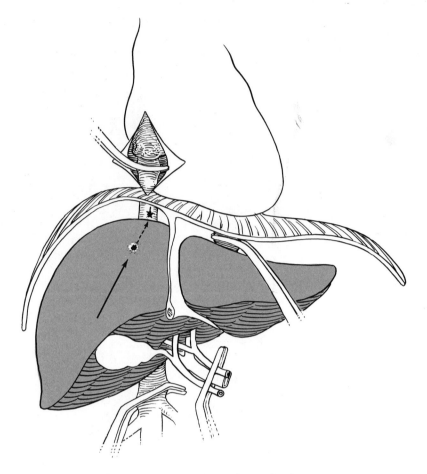

Figure 13–7. Vascular isolation of hepatic circulation for repair of vena cava laceration at diaphragm. This has been achieved by placing occlusive vascular clamps across aorta, porta hepatis, and vena cava above and below liver.

lizing the entire ascending colon along with the duodenum and head of pancreas and the entire base of the small bowel mesentery as necessary. Because the portal vein is a posterior structure in the portal triad, elevation of the head of the pancreas permits exposure of the vein in its posterior location. Injuries to the anterior portion of the portal vein are best repaired through the posterior venotomy if necessary. The portal vein can be trapped by the first assistant's finger, dissected from the pancreas, and isolated for vascular repair. If the integrity of the pancreas has not been compromised, portal venous injuries are often best left untreated, unless free intraperitoneal bleeding is present, since these complex injuries are difficult to expose, more difficult to repair, and can be associated with massive operative blood loss.

TECHNICAL CONSIDERATIONS

The results of anastomoses in the venous system do not parallel the excellent results which are seen almost routinely in the arterial system.[13] Patency of venous anastomoses or grafts is more difficult to achieve for the following reasons:

1. As capacitance vessels, the veins hold seven times more blood than arteries. Since venous return to the heart is identical to aortic outflow, there necessarily has to be a lower blood flow velocity in veins. Thus platelet aggregates which form at the sites of anastomoses or in areas of local turbulance and stasis such as in valve pockets are less likely to be "washed away" by the bloodstream.
2. Veins are thin walled and easily torn, and they collapse and retract when dissected away from supporting tissue. Twisting, buckling, and ridging all predispose to thrombosis.
3. Venous endothelium is more susceptible to damage than arterial endothelium.

In performing venous surgery, a successful outcome depends upon strict attention to technical details and to the use of adjuvant measures to improve patency. The principles formulated by Carrel in 1902 for the construction of a venous anastomosis are still relevant: strict asepsis, gentle handling of veins, use of fine suture materials, and simple continuous suture without tension to avoid narrowing.[9] Because of the lower pressure in veins, less tension is required when using a continuous suture. Leaving the loops of a continuous suture somewhat loose may result in some leakage of blood, but this readily stops with gentle pressure. It is imperative that undue constriction is avoided. Care should be taken not to draw strands of adventitia into the lumen as these will serve as a nidus for thrombosis. For smaller veins the tripartite suture of Carrel (Figure 13-8) permits greater precision in suture placement. Intimal apposition can be assured by using everting mattress sutures. Optimal magnification with operating loupes also permits more accurate suture placement. If grafts are required they should be somewhat longer than the defect to be repaired. Methods of enlarging the ends of veins should be used when possible to prevent anastomotic stenosis. These include diagonal cuts, "fishmouthing" and the use of adjacent branches (Figure 13-9).[30]

The use of an oblique anastomosis may diminish the consequences of vein collapse if it occurs. With a straight anastomosis, compression results in apposition of the entire suture line circumferentially. With an oblique anastomosis, however, apposition of edges occurs only if the suture line is compressed laterally (Figure 13-10). To prevent the collapse and cicatrization of a veno-venous anastomosis, suspension rings and non-suture methods of anastomoses have been used.[12] Mechanical suture techniques can shorten the time required for suturing but the instruments are cumbersome and have not enjoyed widespread popularity. A simple and effective method of stenting an interposition graft or a veno-venous anastomosis is the use of a stainless steel wire spiral.[13] The spiral can be fashioned using #2 wire suture wound about a metal dilator of appropriate size. The vein graft is passed through the spiral and anchored to it with adventitial sutures (Figure 13-11).

When autogenous material is needed for large vein replacement, composite tubular and bifurcation grafts can be constructed (Figure 13-12). The longer suture lines, however, may predispose to thrombosis. In the absence of suitable autogenous tissue, prosthetic grafts may be used to replace large veins, provided adjunctive measures to improve patency are used. These are described later in this chapter. Experimental and clinical studies cited by Scherk and colleagues, indicate that without these adjunctive measures, patency of fabric grafts in the infrarenal vena cava is difficult to achieve.[56] Grafts in the superior vena cava are more likely to remain patent than those in the inferior vena cava. In the superior vena cava, negative thoracic pressure holds the grafts open, whereas positive abdominal pressure causes

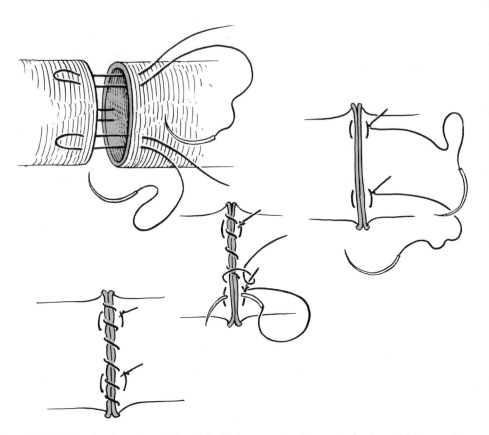

Figure 13–8. The tripartite suture of Carrel facilitates accurate placement of sutures. Mattress sutures ensure intima to intima approximation. Less tension is required in venous anastomosis than in arterial anastomosis.

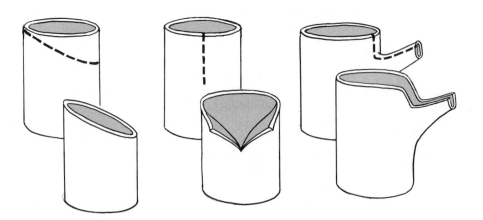

Figure 13–9. Methods of enlarging the ends of veins for anastomosis: oblique end cut, "fish-mouth" cut, and use of an adjacent branch are illustrated.

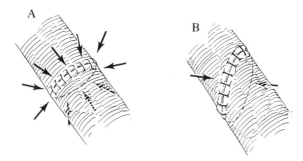

Figure 13–10. *A*, If a vein with a straight anastomosis is compressed, there will be circumferential suture contact. *B*, With an oblique anastomosis suture contact will occur in one plane only.

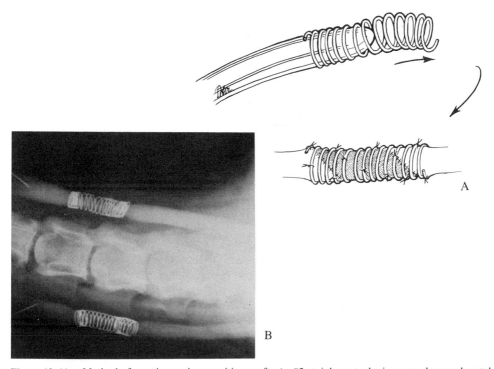

Figure 13–11. Method of stenting an interposition graft: *A*, #2 stainless steel wire wound around metal dilator. *B*, Graft passed through spiral before completion of second anastomosis; vein and graft anchored circumferentially to spiral. *C*, Phlebogram demonstrating stented interposition grafts in sheep jugular veins.

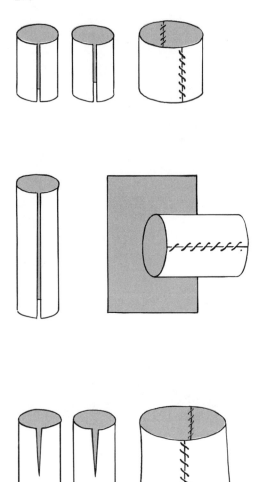

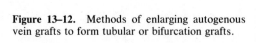

Figure 13–12. Methods of enlarging autogenous vein grafts to form tubular or bifurcation grafts.

graft compression in the inferior vena cava. In addition, superior vena cava flow is isogravitational whereas inferior vena cava flow is antigravitational. An intraluminal fabric graft with rigid ends, developed for use in dissecting thoracic aortic aneurysms, has several theoretical advantages as a large vein replacement: the rigid ends prevent anastomotic compression and narrowing, the luminal surface is devoid of sutures and therefore less thrombogenic, and operating time is shorter. Gore-tex R grafts placed in large caliber veins other than the inferior vena cava (portal, external iliac, thoracic, IVC) have been shown to remain patent in pigs for as long as six months without the use of special adjunctive measures.[38] Vaughn and others, reported the use of Gore-tex R to replace traumatized popliteal, femoral, iliac, and innominate veins with favorable clinical outcomes.[36]

   Adjuvant therapy with antithrombotic agents have been shown to improve patency after experimental venous reconstruction and its clinical use is discussed in the section on postoperative management.[22]

The use of temporary arteriovenous fistulae (AVF) to increase blood flow velocity has been shown to be the most effective way of improving patency rates after venous reconstruction.[21,22,29] Distal H-shaped and K-shaped shunts are associated with generally better results than side-to-side fistulae.[33] To maintain patency of grafts or anastomoses in the iliac veins, a medial branch of the saphenous vein can be connected to the superficial femoral artery. For inferior vena cava grafts, a saphenous vein-superficial femoral artery anastomosis should be used (Figure 13-13).[24] The fistula should be no longer than 5 mm in diameter. A larger fistula risks adverse hemodynamic effects. The arteriovenous anastomosis is marked by a loosely placed suture loop, the ends of which are left long and buried just underneath the skin. This facilitates later closure of the fistula. The recommended time that an AVF should be kept in place is one to two months.[33] Beyond this time venous grafts tend to stay open even with the AVF closed. Adverse effects from a temporary AVF include temporary limb edema and possible venous insufficiency if distal venous valves are rendered incompetent by the elevated venous pressure. There is, of course, the need for a second operation but, theoretically, a temporary AVF might be closed nonoperatively by angiographic catheterization and balloon tamponade.

OPERATIVE TREATMENT

The definitive treatment of injured veins involves lateral repair, ligation, and, on occasion, venous replacement. Isolated injuries of the external, internal, or common iliac veins can be treated with ligation or repair. If the laceration is a simple one, meticulous repair with eversion sutures (utilizing fine monofilament sutures) is usually associated with a good result. However, complex injuries are difficult to repair without producing stenosis of the vein or leaving a raw surface of the vein exposed. This is thrombogenic and may result in complications of thrombosis or, worse yet, embolism. Therefore complex injuries to the iliac veins and the infrarenal vena cava are best treated by ligation of the injured segment. For complex vena cava injuries the distal ligature is best placed at the level of the renal veins and the intervening lumbar veins ligated if necessary, since stasis in the segment above the ligature may be the source of thrombosis and subsequent embolism. If the injury is simple and can be cleanly repaired, this can be accomplished using a partial occluding clamp or by trapping the vein with sponge sticks and packs. Penetrating injuries involving both anterior and posterior walls of the vena cava are best managed by suturing the posterior laceration through a widened anterior hole or, alternatively, rotating the cava for exposure and repair.

Venous injuries may be isolated by pressure or with a vascular clamp. Since the delicate nature of the veins is such that the application of clamps may result in further tearing, we prefer to trap the injured segment of the vein with fingers or a "sponge-stick" above and below and either side to control collaterals (Figure 13-14).

Either renal vein can be ligated but the status of the opposite kidney should first be determined by IVP if possible. The distal 2 or 3 cm of the left renal vein can be ligated with impunity since collateral flow from the adrenal or gonadal veins provides sufficient drainage such that impaired function of the left kidney seldom occurs. Ligation of the right renal vein is not as likely to be associated with recovery of the kidney and a simple laceration should be repaired. Complex injuries may best

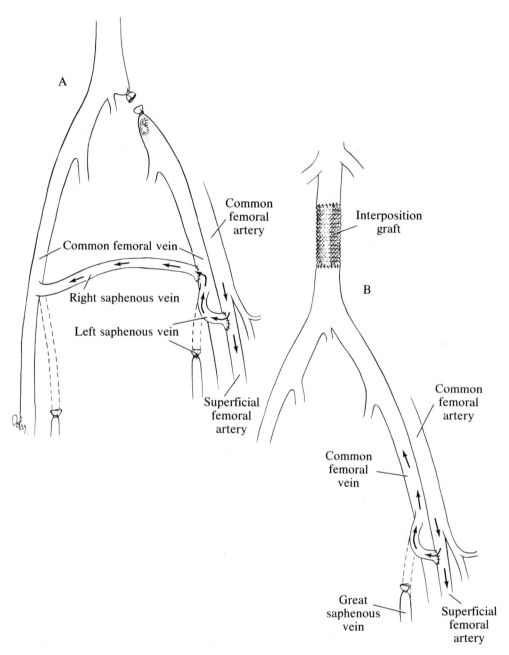

Figure 13–13. Temporary arteriovenous fistula to maintain patency in vein grafts. *A*, Branch of left saphenous vein sewn end-to-side to superficial femoral artery to increase flow velocity through cross-femoral saphenous venovenous bypass graft. *B*, Left saphenous vein sewn end-to-side to superficial femoral artery after inferior vena cava replacement.

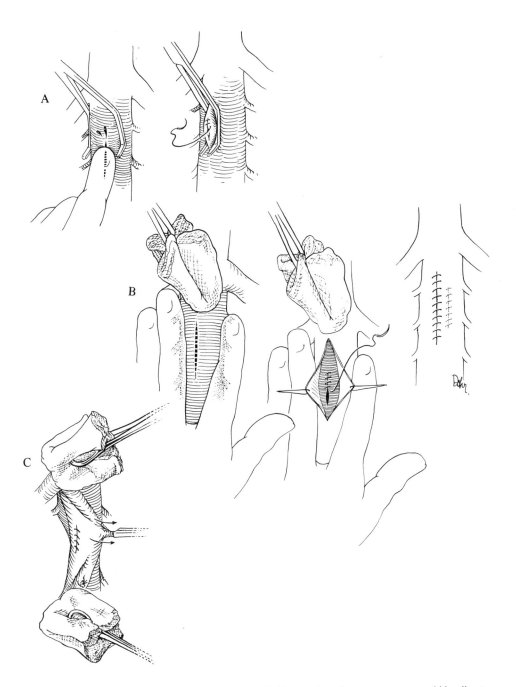

Figure 13–14. Vascular control of vena cava. *A*, Control of hemorrhage from vena cava would by direct pressure, applying partial occluding clamp and suture repair. *B*, Management of through- and-through wound of vena cava. Hemorrhage controlled by direct pressure using sponge forceps proximally and distally and fingers on either side of the cava to compress lumbar veins. The anterior wound is enlarged, the posterior wound is repaired from within and the anterior wound is then trimmed and closed. *C*, Vena cava rotated for repair of a posterior wound. Lumbar veins have been divided and ligated.

be treated by nephrectomy, particularly if there is associated renal artery or renal parenchymal damage.

Ligation of the suprarenal vena cava is usually not compatible with survival, since two-thirds of cardiac venous return is compromised. Therefore this segment should be repaired unless this is absolutely out of the question. Severe injuries to this segment are usually incompatible with survival long enough to reach a point of definitive treatment. The application of an intracaval shunt has permitted isolation of this segment and repair. Prior to the development of this shunt there were no cases of successful repairs of the suprarenal vena cava reported in the literature. Occasionally, if vascular volume has been restored to normal, it may be possible to occlude this segment temporarily for repair as previously described.

There is no technical challenge quite as great as a complex injury of the infrarenal vena cava. There may be massive bleeding from lumbar veins, and as the injury is exposed, collateral bleeding can be such as to result in exsanguination. The assistant should control the vein from above with a sponge stick and roll a pack from above downward, so as to expose a small segment of the laceration, initiate the suture, and then roll the pack further downward as suturing is carried out. As lumbar veins are identified they can be temporarily clipped with silver clips.

Mesenteric vein injuries also constitute a major challenge. When the injury is located well out in the mesentery, ligation can usually be safely carried out. Proximal injuries at the root of the mesentery can often be treated by closing the overlying peritoneum and ignoring the venous injury with planned re-exploration within 12 or 24 hours to assess viability of bowel. Mesenteric vein injuries at the junction with the portal vein or splenic vein injuries at this level may be difficult to manage. The splenic vein can be ligated with impunity; therefore repair of this vein is rarely indicated. Although the superior mesenteric vein can be ligated, thrombosis and loss of viability of bowel may result. Therefore this vein and the portal vein should be repaired if at all possible using techniques illustrated in Figure 13-15. Although severe injuries to the portal vein and the portal triad can be treated with a portacaval shunt, this is often difficult in unstable patients and furthermore is associated with severe morbidity due to protein intolerance. For these reasons ligation is preferred if re-construction is not possible. Injuries to the junction of the portal and mesenteric veins can be treated with a venous patch if the injury is complex or, alternatively, the splenic vein can be divided and used to reconstruct the superior mesenteric vein. The higher pressure portal system tolerates suturing and repair on both an immediate and long term basis better than the lower pressure systemic veins. If an interposition graft is required, a segment of internal jugular vein, internal iliac vein, or external iliac vein is preferred although there has been some limited success using Gore-tex R grafts for interposition.[25]

Abdominal venous trauma carries a high mortality. The victims often present in shock as there are frequently other associated vascular injuries. Inability to obtain vascular control rapidly results in death by exsanguination. Improved results can be expected if operative control of hemorrhage is carried out as part of the resuscitative process. Although repair by lateral suture or grafting is the preferred treatment, in many cases ligation can be used with acceptable results. The main exception may be with injuries to the suprarenal or intrahepatic vena cava, in which case control by means of intracaval shunting is usually necessary to allow repair. However in selected cases, ligation at this level can also be carried out, provided blood volume has been sufficiently restored to insure adequate venous return to the heart.

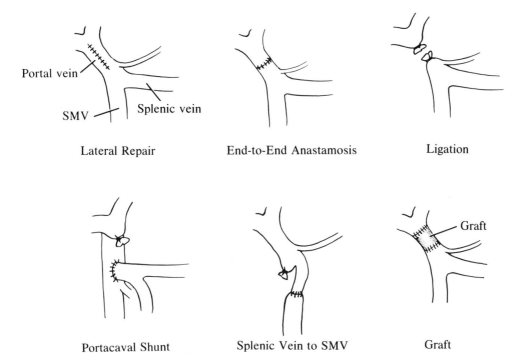

Figure 13–15. Methods used for reconstruction of the portal and superior mesenteric veins.

POSTOPERATIVE CARE

Postoperative management problems presented by venous injuries are relatively mild compared to other types of vascular injury. Once control has been obtained, secondary hemorrhage is unusual. However, because of massive associated blood loss and shock, coagulation defects may develop after multiple transfusions. This is initially a platelet defect which results in persistent oozing from wounds and suture lines. Catastrophic *diffuse hemorrhage* is usually a manifestation of disseminated intravascular clotting with consumption coagulopathy. This can result from a mismatched transfusion, from extensive soft tissue injury in shock or from vital organ damage. Intravascular coagulation is aggravated by persistent hypovolemia, and treatment requires restoration of vascular volume, the adequacy of which can be monitored by urinary output and central venous pressure measurements. If the status of cardiovascular volume is uncertain, pulmonary artery wedge pressure monitoring with the Swan-Ganz catheter is used.

While bleeding from venous suture lines is relatively rare, associated bleeding from other lacerations or associated organ injuries may result in unsatisfactory hemostasis at the time of closure. When this is the case, reintervention is planned for 12 to 24 hours later, after anticoagulation defects have been corrected. This permits removal of blood clots, assessment of the status of vital organ perfusion, and assessment of the quality of venous repair.

After major venous injuries have been repaired, *thrombotic complications* are possible, and when major systemic veins such as iliac or cava have been repaired, extensive distal thrombosis is common. This can produce considerable morbidity, whereas clean ligation without thrombosis usually results in very little immediate and late morbidity. Therefore, when the iliac vein or vena cava is ligated, or when venous reconstruction has been performed, postoperative management should include an antithrombotic regimen when possible. This can consist of the administration of low molecular weight dextran, 10 cc/kg for the first 24 hours and 5 cc/kg in subsequent days, until normal activity is resumed. Elastic wraps and elevation of the extremities are essential to prevent morbidity, provided there has been no associated arterial injury. If prolonged immobility is anticipated, anticoagulation with warfarin sodium, keeping the prothrombin time elevated to twice normal, is used to prevent thromboembolic complications. With careful monitoring, bleeding complications can be minimized.

COMPLICATIONS

Complications of venous injury consist of those related to bleeding, thrombosis, and ischemia. These include transfusion reactions and bleeding problems as previously mentioned. Coagulation factors should be monitored, particularly if circulation to the liver has been temporarily interrupted. These consist of prothrombin time and partial thromboplastin time. Coagulation defects noted should be treated with fresh frozen plasma. *Disseminated intravascular coagulation* with a consumption coagulopathy is best treated by restoration and maintenance of normal volume and by reoperation if there is a question of intestinal or liver ischemia, so that ischemic tissue can be removed.

Thrombosis of venous repairs is a major problem. This is usually manifested by swelling distal to the injury. If extensive thrombosis occurs, the swelling can be massive. If a visceral vein is involved, ischemia of the GI tract or ascites may be the result. Renal infarction is a possibility following renal vein injury. The manifestation may be negligible if the clot is not firmly adherent to the vein wall, but this type of clot usually renders the patient vulnerable to pulmonary embolism seven to ten days post-injury, as he is being mobilized and/or venous pressure is raised by performance of a Valsalva maneuver. If there is no contraindication, major thrombosis or pulmonary embolism is most appropriately treated with heparin. The author utilizes 150 units/kg as an initial bolus in the average patient followed by approximately 25 units/kg/hr by continuous infusion for thrombosis. Pulmonary embolism is best treated by high doses of heparin consisting of a 300 unit/kg initial bolus followed by 40 units/kg/hr by continuous intravenous infusion. If anticoagulation is contraindicated because of associated injuries, ligation of the vena cava at the level of the renal veins is the treatment of choice.

Injuries to the portal venous system may result in bowel *ischemia* or in *portal* hypertension and ammonia intoxication if the portal vein was ligated or thrombosis of the repair occurs. If this is suspected in the immediate postoperative period, reoperation is indicated to evacuate clot from the portal or mesenteric vein and revise the repair. When this is accomplished, the risk of anticoagulation must be accepted to prevent recurrent thrombosis. Renal function should be monitored whenever the renal veins or suprarenal vena cava have been injured and repaired. Renal infarction may be relatively silent or associated with prostrating symptoms. In the latter instance, nephrectomy may be indicated.

REFERENCES

1. Ablaza SGG, Ghosh SC, Grana VP: Use of a ringed intraluminal graft in the surgical treatment of dissecting aneurysms of the thoracic aorta. J Thorac Cardiovasc Surg 76:390, 1978.
2. Albo D, Christensen C, Rasmussen BL, King TC: Massive liver trauma involving the suprarenal vena cava. Am J Surg 118:960-963, 1968.
3. Allen RE, Blaisdell FW: Injuries to the inferior vena cava. Surg Clin North Am 52:699, 1972.
4. Boyce FF, Lampert R, McFetridge EM: Occlusion of the portal vein. J Lab Clin Med 20:935, 1935.
5. Bricker BL, Morton JR, Okies JE, Beall AC: Surgical management of injury to the inferior vena cava: changing patterns of injury and newer techniques of repair. J Trauma 11:725, 1971
6. Brunschwig A, Bigelow R, Nichols B: Elective occlusion and excision of portal vein; an experimental study. Surg 17:781-785, 1945.
7. Buckberg G, Ono H, Tocornal J, et al.: Hypothermic assanguinous liver perfusion in dogs. Surg Forum 18:372-374, 1967.
8. Busuttil RQ, Kitahanea A, Cerise E, et al.: Management of blunt and penetrating injuries to the porta hepatis. Ann Surg 191:641-648, 1980.
9. Carrel A: La technique operatoire des anastomoses vasculaires et la transplantation des visceres. Lyon Med 98:859, 1902.
10. Chavez-Peon F, Gonzales E, Malt RA: Vena cava catheter for assanguinous liver resection. Surg 67:694-696, 1970.
11. Child CG III: The hepatic circulation and portal hypertension. W.B. Saunders, Philadelphia, 1954.
12. Colp R: Treatment of pylephlebitis of appendicular origin with report of three cases of ligation of portal vein. Surg Gynecol Obstet 43:627, 1926.
13. Conti SL: Gore-Tex grafts for vein replacement: effect of anti-platelet agents and volume expansion on patency. In press.
14. Dale WA: In discussion of Mattox et al., reference 23.
15. Duke JH Jr, Jones RC, Shires GT: Management of injuries to the inferior vena cava. Am Surg 110:759-763, 1965.
16. Feldman EA: Injury to the hepatic vein. Am J Surg 111:244-246, 1960.
17. Fish JC: Reconstruction of the portal vein: Case reports and literature review. Am Surg 32:472, 1966.
18. Gaspar MR, Treiman RL: The management of injuries to major veins. Am J Surg 100:171, 1960.
19. Haimovici H, Hoffert PW, Zimicola N, Steinman C: An experimental and clinical evaluation of grafts in the venous system. Surg Gynecol Obstet 131:1173, 1970.
20. Johnson CC, Baggenstross AH: Mesenteric vascular occlusion 1. Study of 99 cases of occlusion in veins. Proc Staff Meet Mayo Clinic 24:618, 1949.
21. Johnson V, Eiseman B: Evaluation of arteriovenous shunt to obtain patency of venous autograft. Am J Surg 118:915, 1969.
22. Kunlin J, Kunlin A: Experimental venous surgery. Major Prob Clin Surg 23:37-66, 1979.
23. Mattox K, Espada R, Beall AC: Traumatic injury to the portal vein. Ann Surg 181:519-522, 1975.
24. May R, De Weese JA: Surgery of the pelvic veins. WB Saunders, Philadelphia, 1979, p. 158.
25. Norton L, Eiseman B: Replacement of portal vein during pancreaticoduodenectomy for carcinoma. Surg 77:280-284, 1975.
26. Ochsner JL, Crawford ES, DeBakey ME: Injuries of the vena cava caused by external trauma. Surg 49:397-405, 1961.
27. Peterson SR, Sheldon GF, Lim RC: Management of portal vein injuries. J Trauma 19:616, 1979.
28. Quast DC, Shirkey AL, Fitzgerald JB, et al: Surgical correction of injuries of the vena cava: an analysis of sixty one cases. J Trauma 5:1-10, 1965.
29. Rabinowitz R, Golfarb D: Surgical treatment of axillo subclavian venous thrombosis: A case report. Surgery 70:703, 1971
30. Rich NM, Hobson RW II, Wright CB, Swan KG: Techniques of venous repair. In: Swan KG, et al (Eds), Venous Surgery in the Lower Extremities. Warren H. Green Publishers, St. Louis, 1975.
31. Rich NM, Hughes CW: Vietnam Vascular Registry, a preliminary report. Surg 65:218, 1969.
32. Rich NM, Hughes CW, Bough JG: Acute arterial injuries in Vietnam: 1000 cases. J Trauma 10:359, 1970.
33. Rich NM, Levin PM, Hutton JE: Effect of distal arteriovenous fistulas on venous graft patency. In: Swan KG, et al (Eds), Venous Surgery in the Lower extremities. Warren H. Green Publishers, St. Louis, 1975.
34. Rich NM, Spencer RC: Vascular Trauma. WB Saunders, Philadelphia, 1979.
35. Robson AWM: Case of perforating wound of abdomen. Br Med J 2:77, 1897 (Sept).
36. Scherck JP, Kerstein MD, Stansel HL: The current status of vena cava replacement. Surg 76:209-233 1974.
37. Schnug E: Ligation of the superior mesenteric vein. Surg 14:610-616, 1973.
38. Soyer T, Lempineur M, Cooper P, et al: A new venous prosthesis. Surg 72:864, 1972.
39. Schrock T, Blaisdell FW, Mathewson C: Management of blunt trauma to the liver and hepatic veins. Arch Surg 96:698-704, 1968.

40. Starzl TE, Broadaway RK, Dever RC, Reams GB: The management of penetrating wounds of the inferior vena cava. Am Surg 23:455-461, 1957.
41. Stone HH: In discussion of Busuttil et al., reference 8.
42. Taylor DC: Two cases of penetrating wounds of the abdomen involving the inferior vena cava. Lancet 2:60, 1916.
43. Timmis HH, Rosanova AR Jr, Larkin WB: Bloodless hepatic resection with an internal caval shunt. Surg 65:109-117, 1969.
44. Turpin I, State D, Schwartz A: Injuries to the inferior vena cava and their management. Am J Surg 134:25-32, 1977.
45. Yellin AE, Chaffer CB, Donovan AJ: Vascular isolation in treatment of juxta-hepatic venous injuries. Arch Surg 102:566-573, 1971.
46. Vaughn GD, Mattox KL, Feleciano DV, et al.: Surgical experience with expanded polytetrafluoroethylene (PTFE) as a replacement graft for traumatized vessels. J Trauma 19:403, 1979.
47. Waltuck TL, Crow RW, Humphrey LJ, Kaufman HM: Avulsion injuries of the vena cava following blunt abdomial trauma. Ann Surg 171:67-72, 1970.
48. Williams CD, Brenowitz JB: Sequential aortic and inferior vena caval clamping for control of suprarenal vena caval injuries: case report. J Trauma 17:164-167, 1977.
49. Wilms EF, *cited by* Harsha WN, Orr TG: Ligation of superior mesenteric vein. Am Surg 18:148-155, 1952.

Chapter Fourteen

RETROPERITONEAL HEMATOMA

KENNETH A. KUDSK AND GEORGE F. SHELDON

INTRODUCTION

Retroperitoneal hematoma (RH) continues to be a major cause of morbidity and mortality in patients with both blunt and penetrating injury (Table 14-1). The blood accumulating in the retroperitoneal space—after injury—has its origin in an organ or blood vessel posterior to the lining of the peritoneal cavity. The contribution of RH to ultimate morbidity or mortality depends on the source and quantity of blood loss.

Retroperitoneal hematomas generally center on one of three locations: upper abdominal (central), flank, or pelvic. A primary cause of morbidity or mortality, the central upper abdominal RH is usually caused by injury to the aorta, inferior vena cava, or the liver, pancreas, or duodenum.[2] Injury to these structures are difficult to diagnose and even more difficult to treat.

Flank retroperitoneal hematomas are of significance, primarily because they are associated with injury to the kidneys (see Chapter 11). The intraoperative decision-consists of whether to explore the hematoma or leave the hemorrhage contained.

By far, the most common cause of RH is fracture of the pelvis.[20] Hemorrhage secondary to pelvic fractures again poses a therapeutic dilemma—whether or not to explore. Blood loss is the major cause of morbidity and mortality from RH, regardless of exploration or management by leaving the peritoneum intact with the expectation that bleeding will be controlled by tamponade.

Table 14-1 RETROPERIOTNEAL HEMATOMA MORTALITY

	Percentage	Number of Patients
Baylis et al.[3]	18%	50
Allen et al.[1]	24%	75
Nick et al.[19]	31%	65

CLINICAL-ANATOMICAL CORRELATIONS

The retroperitoneal anatomy is shown in Figure 14-1. The retroperitoneum is the areolar space behind the posterior layer of the sack-like peritoneum which contains the viscera of the abdominal cavity and the vertebral column, diaphragm, back,

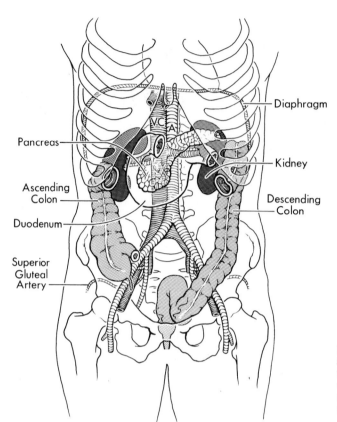

Pancreas—

Ascending
Colon

Duodenum—

Superior
Gluteal
Artery

—Diaphragm

—Kidney

Descending
Colon

Figure 14–1. Retroperitoneal
anatomy. Retroperitoneal hematomas originate from organs or
vasculature of the retroperitoneum in which bleeding is contained by the retroperitoneum.

and pelvic muscles. The posterior peritoneum covers the lower boundaries of the
diaphragmatic reflection and the aorta, vena cava, and their branches in the upper
abdomen. It descends over the duodenum, pancreas, and kidneys to reach the pelvis.
The retroperitoneum is an anatomic area into which hematomas dissect from posteriorly oriented structures such as the caudate lobe of the liver or other structures,
such as the right or left mesocolon in continuity with the retroperitoneum of the
upper and lower abdomen. Rupture, or injury of the supradiaphragmatic aorta may
dissect into the abdomen and present as an RH also.

The solid organs which lie completely inside the retroperitoneum include the
pancreas, adrenal glands, and kidneys. These structures are especially vulnerable
to blunt upper abdominal trauma. The hollow viscera, which lie entirely in the
retroperitoneum, are the third and fourth portion of the duodenum and the supra-
levator portion of the rectum. However, the posterior surface of the ascending,
transverse, and descending colon also form part of the anterior surface of the retroperitoneum. Injuries to the posterior aspect of these structures or their mesentery
may produce hematomas in the retroperitoneum. The cause can be penetrating injury
or crushing injury such as that in conjunction with a pelvic fracture. Operative
exposure of the duodenum and posterior portion of the colon or rectum, or other
retroperitoneal viscera is necessary to determine if injury has occurred.

The uterus and ovaries lie outside the retroperitoneum and rarely contribute to
a pelvic hematoma. Bladder and rectal injuries may contribute to the problem, but
for the most part pelvic hematomas are due to rupture of the vessels lining the

pelvis—most commonly, pelvic branches of the internal iliac vein, but also the internal iliac artery, and occasionally the common or external iliac artery and vein. Fractures to the pelvic ring with associated vascular injury will frequently result in extensive posterior dissection of blood, and may extend to the diaphragm and, on occasion, dissect above the peritoneum to the anterior abdominal wall. A pelvic fracture may also result in decompression of the RH through a peritoneal laceration with resultant bleeding into the peritoneal cavity. Open pelvic fractures, by definition, are uncontained sources of blood loss as the potential for tamponade of bleeding by the retroperitoneum is lost.

Peritoneal lavage, a common method for diagnosing intra-abdominal bleeding, will not necessarily detect bleeding or injury to the pancreas or other retroperitoneal structures.[14,21] However, pelvic retroperitoneal hematomas, secondary to fractures, commonly result in the oozing of small quantities of blood into the peritoneal cavity, producing a positive lavagate.

Because different problems are encountered when the hematoma presents in various portions of the retroperitoneum, the retroperitoneum has been arbitrarily classified into three areas (Figure 14-2). The first (Area 1) is the upper central area of the retroperitoneum. This corresponds to the area from the diaphragmatic hiatus of the aorta and esophagus, and extends to the sacral promentory. Principal structures in this area are the aorta, vena cava, proximal renal vessels, the portal vein, pancreas, and duodenum.

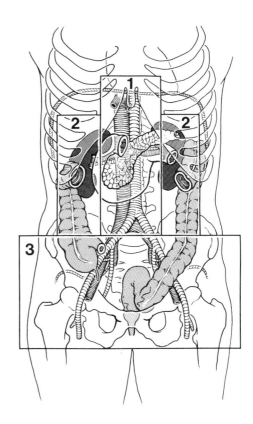

Figure 14–2. Relation of anatomic zones to indication for exploration of retroperitoneal hematomas, correlating the retroperitoneal anatomy with indications for operative management.

ZONE 1: *Central-medial retroperitoneal hematomas*

ZONE 2: *Flank retroperitoneal hematomas*

ZONE 3: *Pelvic retroperitoneal hematomas.*

Area 2 consists of the right and left flank. It contains the kidneys and suprapelvic ureters and the right and left mesocolon.

Area 3 consists of the pelvis and contains the rectum, posterior aspect of the bladder, and the distal or pelvic segment of the ureters.

ASSESSMENT

Retroperitoneal hematoma is usually a secondary diagnosis. Although RH is frequently associated with significant blood loss, initial assessment is directed to establishing a diagnosis of injury to a specific organ. Most significant RH (80 percent) are caused by blunt trauma, usually (50 percent) associated with pelvic fractures, but commonly resulting from injury to the kidney, pancreas, or liver.[9] Penetrating injuries of retroperitoneal structures from gunshot or stab wounds, or bone spicules from fractures, are the cause of 20 percent of RH. As with other injuries, the assessment begins in concert with resuscitation. The mechanism of injury and details of the accident may arouse suspicion of injury to retroperitoneal structures (Table 14-2). Steering wheel injuries, or injuries resulting in ejection of the patient from a moving vehicle, or injuries from the patient being thrown forward from an unprotected vehicle (e.g., a motorcycle), are common injuries which cause RH. Although initial emergency room assessment is usually targeted toward looking for injuries to primary organ systems, signs of retroperitoneal hemorrhage should be sought. However, the most common clue that RH is present is the clinical, or x-ray diagnosis of pelvic fracture. If physical examination identifies an exit wound, or if x-ray evidence of retroperitoneal penetration by gunshot or knife is present, an RH can be expected to be present. An uncommon physical finding is the so called Grey-Turner sign, classically associated with pancreatitis, but sometimes resulting from flank hematomas. It is not possible with a dissection into the flank, to differentiate a flank contusion from bleeding from a retroperitoneal organ.

As resuscitation and evaluation proceed, unexplained evidence of blood loss should raise suspicion that the source of blood loss is in the retroperitoneum. When blood loss from the chest has been excluded, and peritoneal lavage does not indicate gross intraperitoneal hemorrhage, retroperitoneal bleeding must be suspected as a cause of shock (Table 14-3).

Table 14–2   RETROPERITONEAL HEMATOMA, ETIOLOGY

	MVA	Pedestrian	Motorcycle	Fall	Other*
Retroperitoneal Hematoma					
Allen et al.[1]	31	28	–	12	4
Greico and Perry[9]	35	12	14	10	9
Pelvic Fracture					
Flint et al.[7]	10	19	9	–	2
(severe injuries)					
Hamilton[11]	31	–	–	9	–
Hawkins et al.[12]	16	16	2	1	–
Rothenberger et al.[24]	233	162	38	114	47
Trunkey et al.[26]	42	62	16	52	–

*Includes penetrating trauma

Table 14–3 PERCENTAGE OF PATIENTS HYPOTENSIVE ON ADMISSION
WITH DIAGNOSED RETROPERITONEAL HEMATOMA OR PELVIC FRACTURE

Allen et al.[1]	48%	(36/75)
Flint et al.[7]	62%	(31/50)
Hawkins et al.[12]	34.3%	(12/35)
Rothenberger et al.[24]	53%	(320/604)

Hemorrhage of unexplained origin—usually RH—is diagnosed by a serial fall of the hematocrit, in conjunction with hemodynamic instability. Another laboratory test of value consists of an amylase determination. An amylase elevation suggests the possibility of duodenal and/or pancreatic injury.[27]

Emergency room evaluation should proceed with a flat film of the abdomen and an x-ray of the pelvis. Abnormalities of the renal shadow or absence of the psoas muscle unilaterally suggest the probability of hemorrhage.[17] If a pelvic fracture is present, the urine should be examined, and if bloody, the patient should have a cystogram. If blood is present at the tip of the penis in a male patient, or if difficulty is encountered in passing a Foley catheter, the cystogram should be preceded by a urethrogram since there is high probability of urethral injury.

Retroperitoneal injury is often associated with hematuria. Microscopic hematuria may be caused by blunt trauma or deceleration injuries of minimal violence. If gross or microscopic hematuria is present, intravenous pyelograms should be obtained, although significant, penetrating, or blunt injury to the vascular pedicle of the kidneys can occur in the absence of hematuria. An intravenous pyelogram is of value to assess injury to the kidneys, ureteral displacement, and to confirm the presence of two functioning kidneys. If exploration of the retroperitoneum ultimately becomes necessary, and nephrectomy is required for exposure or therapy, pre-operative IVP evidence of good contra-lateral renal function is of great value.[5,18]

Arteriography is occasionally useful for assessing RH. An absolute indication for arteriography is the lack of visualization of a kidney or intravenous pyelogram. An arteriogram is done to determine if the kidney is present, and if the renal artery has been injured. A second indication for arteriography occurs when complex vascular injuries, usually secondary to penetrating injury, are suspected. Arteriograms, however, are practical only if the patient is hemodynamically stable. When complex retroperitoneal injury is suspected by the presence of abdominal bruits or hemodynamic and hematologic evidence of arteriovenous fistulae, localization of the area of vascular injury may be the key to salvaging the patient. Rarely, during operation, there may be evidence of vascular injury in a relatively inaccessible area in a hemodynamically stable patient. If such is the case, it may be advisable to close the abdomen, maintain anesthesia, move the patient to the angiography suite, and perform arteriography.

A third indication for angiography in the management of RH is for diagnosis and treatment of bleeding from pelvic fractures.[22] An expanding pelvic hematoma secondary to pelvic fracture is usually caused by disruption of the pelvic venous plexus.[23] Various methods of intra-operative management of expanding pelvic hematomas have been attempted but the results are often unsatisfactory. A small but significant number of pelvic hematomas secondary to pelvic fracture are due to arterial, not venous injuries. The most common arteries injured are the superior gluteal artery or greater sciatic artery and the obturator artery (Figure 14-3).

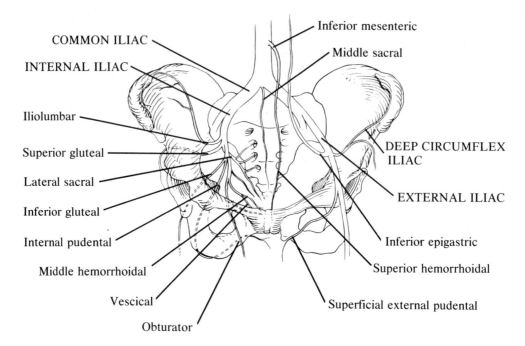

COMMON ILIAC
INTERNAL ILIAC
Iliolumbar
Superior gluteal
Lateral sacral
Inferior gluteal
Internal pudental
Middle hemorrhoidal
Vescical
Obturator

Inferior mesenteric
Middle sacral
DEEP CIRCUMFLEX ILIAC
EXTERNAL ILIAC
Inferior epigastric
Superior hemorrhoidal
Superficial external pudental

Figure 14–3. Arterial anatomy of the pelvis.

A complete assessment of the trauma patient with pelvic fracture includes rectal and stool examination for occult blood. In severe pelvic fractures, intraoperative determination of penetration of bone spicules into the retroperitoneal rectum is difficult. For that reason, preoperative proctoscopic examination is of value to ascertain if the lumen of the lower sigmoid colon or rectum contain blood. If the patient is hemodynamically stable, a water soluble contrast examination of the rectosigmoid colon should be done as well to determine if extravasation of contrast material, indicating rectal perforation, has occurred. Water soluble contrast material is preferred for this examination to avoid soiling the peritoneal cavity with barium if perforation of the rectum or sigmoid colon has occurred. If the diagnosis of rectal perforation in association with pelvic fracture or penetrating injury is established before operation, an operative consent to perform a diverting colostomy should be obtained.

Recently, it has become apparent that retroperitoneal hematomas can be directly documented by computerized tomography. The signs, symptoms, and other evaluation techniques continue to have value; however, plain abdominal radiographs may demonstrate lack of a psoas margin, which, with slight rotation or minimal spinal scoliosis, can cause a similar picture. Approximately 25 percent of normal individuals show unequal definition of psoas borders. Moreover, other indirect findings, e.g., intestinal ileus or soft tissue mass may be visible on contrast radiographs. Because sharp delineation of the retroperitoneal structures by surrounding extraperitoneal fat is seen in all but extremely malnourished patients, computed tomography can be an accurate, non-invasive method for evaluation of retroperitoneal hemorrhage. Published studies to date indicate that trauma is the most common cause of retroperitoneal hemorrhage that is detectable by computed tomography. Other causes less common than trauma, are hemorrhagic diathesis or abdominal aortic aneurysm rupture. The method appears to have the most value in the trauma patient by evaluating the presence of a retroperitoneal hematoma in a patient who has had a negative peritoneal dialysis as a possible explanation for blood loss. Moreover, the computed tomography may allow quantitation and following of the retroperitoneal hematoma. Computed tomography, of course, will not substitute for an arteriogram when non-visualization of an intravenous pyelogram has occurred. In that instance, damage to a renal artery is determined best by angiography.

INTRA-OPERATIVE EVALUATION

Retroperitoneal hematomas most commonly are first recognized during systematic exploration of the abdomen to determine sites of hemorrhage and injury to intra-abdominal organs. When the small intestine is eviscerated to allow evaluation, it is convenient to examine the root of the mesentery and determine the presence and amount of blood in the retroperitoneum with the intent to re-examine that area later in the operation and determine if the hematoma is increasing. Next, the cecum, ascending colon, transverse colon, descending colon, sigmoid colon, and rectum are evaluated. While the colon is examined, the root of the mesentery is palpated and visualized to determine if a hematoma is present on the right side of the retroperitoneum. If such is the case, or if a penetrating injury has occurred, the colon should be mobilized by severing its lateral attachments (See Chapter 9).[25] Both surfaces should be inspected with particular attention directed toward the-mesenteric border. As exploration proceeds, evisceration and/or elevation of the small bowel makes possible identification of central and flank RH. Upper abdominal central RH are easily identified when the esophagus and stomach are inspected and the lesser sac explored. They are usually visible through the gastrohepatic ligament. Hematomas in the pelvis are easily identified by visualization of the pelvic cavity. It is useful to palpate pelvic fractures by placing the examining hand within the pelvis and sweeping it over the bony surface to determine if sharp bony spicules from the fracture are present and if they have potential for penetrating the rectum or bladder.

If rectal injury is demonstrated by preoperative sigmoidoscopy and x-ray contrast studies, a proximal end colostomy with distal mucous fistula is performed. The defunctionalized rectum should be irrigated clean and antibiotic solution instilled. Open pelvic fractures with markedly contused rectum should also be treated by a defunctionalizing colostomy to avoid stool contamination of an open perineal wound. If the diagnosis is not established prior to operation, it is difficult to diagnose a damaged rectum intra-operatively, as mobilization of the rectosigmoid results in opening the RH, which is best avoided.

Although the intra-operative diagnosis of RH is not difficult, management of RH is often complex and remains controversial.[8] The need for exploration of RH depends upon the (1) wounding mechanism, blunt or penetrating; (2) the location of the hematoma; and (3) intra-operative increase in hematoma size.

Blunt trauma, as a general rule, is not associated with a high incidence of major vascular injury, and the decision whether or not to explore is determined by the region involved. In contrast, all penetrating injuries of the retroperitoneum should be explored and any repairable injuries of the retroperitoneal structures dealt with.[25]

The highest mortality is associated with hematomas in the upper part of Zone 1, which includes the superior, central RH.[2] This mortality is due to the high incidence of injuries to the aorta, coeliac axis, or vena cava, in the difficult-to-expose area below the diaphragm.[2,9,15] Blood may also be present in that area from hepatic vein injuries or to posterior injuries to the liver which dissect into the retroperitoneum. In two out of 100 cases in a recent series (Perry), central superior hematomas were caused by a transected thoracic aorta, which had dissected into the retroperitoneum below the diaphragm.[9] If a bruit is associated with a superior central hematoma which is not expanding, the patient's abdomen may be closed, and while maintaining anesthesia, an aortogram performed. Although this maneuver is useful in selected cases, hematomas in upper Zone 1 are usually associated with shock, which precludes delay of exploration for x-rays. When a central superior RH is explored, the aorta and vena cava may be exposed or controlled transthoracically as well as subdiaphragmatically, above the coeliac axis to allow rapid proximal control in anticipation of massive bleeding from significant injuries to the major vascular structures. Techniques for managing these major injuries was provided in Chapters 12 and 13.

Injuries to the pancreas are associated with Zone 1 retroperitoneal bleeding. When bleeding from the aorta or vena cava has been excluded, careful exploration of the pancreas is performed to identify organ damage and the source of bleeding (see Chapter 6). Portal vein injuries may also present as RH, and are frequently associated with injuries to the pancreas. Duodenal injuries, with or without associated pancreatic injuries, are another source of hemorrhage.[10,27] Assessment requires a generous Kocher maneuver, and often mobilization of the right colon and its mesentery, to facilitate exposure of the entire duodenum (see Chapter 6).

If a superior central hematoma has been excluded, and the hematoma is in the region of a kidney (Zone 2), several intra-operative considerations are of importance. The pre-operative intravenous pyelogram will provide information as to the (1) presence or absence of two kidneys; (2) extravasation of contrast material; and (3) altered or absent renal function. If the function of one kidney is absent or markedly altered, or if extravasation of contrast material has occurred, exploration of the kidney is mandatory (See Chapter 11). If the IVP has demonstrated loss of function and an arteriogram has delineated an injury to the renal artery or its tributaries, exploration and operative repair should be attempted. If pyelography is not obtained pre-operatively, this should be carried out on the operating table prior to entering the flank hematoma. In particular, the function of the opposite kidney should be verified (see Chapter 11). If the injury is from a penetrating wound, exploration of the kidney in conjunction with other retroperitoneal structures is performed.

Renal injury from blunt trauma as manifest by a flank RH usually does not require exploration. Even kidneys with IVP demonstrated stellate fractures will often appear normal when IVP is done several months after injury. The decision to explore the retroperitoneum and kidney following blunt trauma in the presence of a normal IVP is determined intra-operatively by the stability of the retroperitoneal hematoma.[4,13,16] If the RH does not increase in size during the operation, it usually does not require exploration.

Fracture of the pelvis is the most frequent injury which results in RH (Zone 3). Pelvic fractures are usually the result of crushing injuries such as those associated with motor vehicle accidents or those occurring when a pedestrian is struck by an automobile (Table 14-2). They can also be the result of motorcycle accidents or falls from heights. Regardless of the mechanism of injury, pelvic fractures occur when great mechanical force is transmitted to the bony pelvis. Evaluation and assessment of the patient with pelvic fractures includes bone x-rays, cystograms, and pelvic and rectal examinations. Attention to femoral artery pulses in the pre-operative evaluation is important as intimal disruption and subsequent dissection and thrombosis of the iliac artery may be associated with pelvic fracture.

Blood loss from pelvic fracture into the retroperitoneum is usually of considerable quantity and one of the reasons for the high morbidity and mortality of pelvic fractures. Blood transfusion is often required in quantities which can frequently approach the normal blood volume (Table 14-3).

The orthopedic evaluation and treatment is beyond the scope of this chapter, and was referred to in Chapter 4. The magnitude of the pelvic fracture associated RH is usually best appreciated at exploratory laparotomy. During exploration, the pelvis should be internally palpated for sharp bony spicules and evaluation for bladder, urethral, vascular, and rectal injuries performed.

When associated organ injuries are evaluated and treated, attention is directed to the retroperitoneal hematoma associated with the pelvic fracture. Because most bleeding associated with pelvic fractures is from the low pressure venous system, bleeding will usually tamponade if the retroperitoneum is intact and the pelvic fracture is a closed one. Because control of pelvic bones and venous plexus hemorrhage is virtually impossible by usual surgical techniques, open exploration of RH associated with pelvic fracture is avoided if possible.[23] The peritoneal convering, if intact, will contain and tamponade bleeding of potentially great magnitude. [25]

If the hematoma continues to expand, arterial bleeding is often the source. Several procedures can be employed in sequence, to control the bleeding. The first maneuver is to pack the pelvis as tightly as possible with laparotomy tapes. When ten to twenty minutes have elapsed, the packs are gently removed and the status of the hematoma reassessed. During the period of packing, platelet transfusion and fresh frozen plasma are administered to correct transfusion-related dilutional thrombocytopenia and other coagulopathies.

If the pelvic hematoma continues to expand after packing and transfusion therapy, the source of the hemorrhage should be considered to be arterial rather than venous. Because hypogastric artery ligation and other methods for controlling pelvic fracture bleeding have been unsatisfactory, our preference for treatment of the expanding pelvic hematoma is to repack the pelvis and perform arteriographic localization and embolization. Recent experience in several centers, including our own, suggests that an arterial origin of beeding from pelvic fractures may be more common than previously appreciated.[28] The arteries most commonly injured during pelvic fracture are the superior gluteal and greater sciatic artery, both originating from the hypogastric artery. Another artery that is injured frequently is the obturator artery. Because these arteries course deep through and exit from the bony pelvis, direct operative ligation is difficult. Moreover, ligation of the hypogastric arteries will not necessarily control hemorrhage, since the arterial collateral to the pelvis is so great. In addition, attempts to expose the pelvic arteries risk decompression and hemorrhage from associated venous injuries.

When hemorrhage from a distal branch of the hypogastric artery is identified by arteriography (Figure 14-4), treatment is by embolizing blood clot, muscle, absorbable gelatin sponge, or "biological glue" into the bleeding point (Figure 14-5). The success of arteriographic embolization is confirmed by repeating the angiogram after embolization has been completed.

If arteriographic embolization is unsuccessful in controlling hemorrhage, but the bleeding artery has been identified, the patient is returned to the operating room,

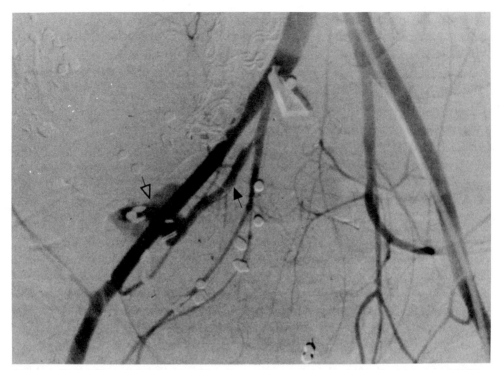

Figure 14–4. Distal aortogram (before balloon occlusion). Contrast has pooled (open arrow) after extravasation from the superior gluteal artery. (*From* Sheldon GF, Winestock DP: Hemorrhage from open pelvic fracture controlled intra-operatively with balloon catheter. J Trauma 18:68-70, 1978.)

where the ipsilateral (and, if necessary, the contralateral) hypogastric arteries are occluded in sequence with vascular clamps. Hemorrhage from distal branches of the hypogastric artery may be controlled by this maneuver. If bilateral hypogastric artery occlusion fails to control hemorrhage, the hypogastric artery feeding the bleeding branch is ligated at its junction with the common iliac artery. A Fogarty balloon catheter can be threaded into the hypogastric artery and passed into its distal branches.[6,28] Inflation of the balloon on the catheter will arrest hemorrhage in some instances (Figure 14-5). If all maneuvers fail to control hemorrhage, the surgeon's remaining choice is to tightly pack the pelvis, close the abdomen, transfuse with fresh blood, and plan to re-explore the patient 12 to 24 hours later, to remove the packs.

RETROPERITONEAL HEMATOMAS—THE TREATMENT CONTROVERSY

Because retroperitoneal hematoma is (1) a secondary diagnosis; (2) associated with considerable morbidity and mortality; (3) the source of considerable blood loss; and (4) treated with difficulty, opinions differ as to the optimal operative therapy.

Therapeutic controversy, to a large degree, is focused on the intra-operative decision to open the retroperitoneum. Advocates of routine exploration of all retroperitoneal hematomas maintain that exploration allows identification and control

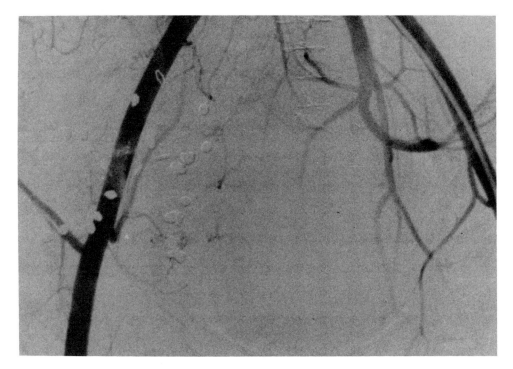

Figure 14–5. Distal aortogram (after balloon occlusion). The internal iliac artery and its branches have been occluded and do not opacify. There is no longer extravasation of contrast. (*From* Sheldon GF, Winestock DP: Hemorrhage from open pelvic fracture controlled intra-operatively with balloon catheter. J Trauma 18:68-70, 1978.)

of specific organ or vascular injury, and direct control of bleeding. Authors favoring non-exploration of RH point out that venous bleeding will eventually be controlled if the posterior peritoneum is left intact to contain the bleeding.[20] Moreover, urologists have contended that precipitous exploration of RH often results in uncontrollable bleeding from a kidney which might be salvaged, were the bleeding allowed to tamponade.[13,18]

A sequential approach to the management of RH reconciles both points of view. The decision to explore or leave intact the retroperitoneum is based on the following principles, which take into consideration the mechanism and location of the injury and the stability of the hematoma.

Because most penetrating injuries of the retroperitoneum are associated with a specific entrance and exit wound, and are amenable to operative management of the organ or vascular structure injured, exploration is routinely performed for penetrating injuries.[27] However, blunt injuries which result in RH require considerable intra-operative judgement. Retroperitoneal hematomas in Zone 1 (centro-medial hematomas), particularly if subdiaphragmatic, are associated with a 65 percent incidence of major vascular injury. All hematomas that are expanding in that region should be explored and operative repair of any vascular injury performed. An additional reason for exploring hematomas in that region is the inability to diagnose significant pancreatic or duodenal injuries without exploring the hematoma.[2]

Hematomas in Zone 2 usually do not require exploration as the presumed source is the kidney. The decision to explore or observe Zone 2 retroperitoneal hematomas is primarily based on the preoperative or operative evaluation of the kidney by x-ray contrast studies.[4,13] However, expanding hematomas in Zone 2 often require exploration to control bleeding and manage the renal injury. Non-expanding Zone 2 hematomas are not explored unless a specific urological indication for exploration is present.

Hematomas in Zone 3 are managed by avoiding retroperitoneal exploration if possible. Pelvic RH are explored only when rapid massive expansion of the hematoma occurs which cannot be controlled by arteriographic embolization and/or packing.

Although specific anatomic regions in which RH occur can be delineated which are best managed by exploration or observation, retroperitoneal bleeding usually dissects throughout the entire retroperitoneum. It is essential that the most likely anatomic zone in which the RH originates is identified prior to exploration, so that the proper management maneuvers can proceed in sequence.

POSTOPERATIVE CARE

The postoperative management of patients with RH is comparable to that required for all patients with critical injury. The availability of skilled intensive care unit personnel, in a unit familiar with the care of patients who are at risk for developing multiple sequential organ system failure, is essential. Specific details of special aspects of care required for the treatment of the various organs that are present in the retroperitoneum are included in the chapters dealing with those structures.

Pelvic fractures, the injury most commonly associated with RH, requires skilled management by a knowledgeable orthopedic surgeon (Table 14-4). Because pelvic fractures usually require a period of immobilization, pulmonary complications are common.

Perhaps the most unrecognized feature of postoperative management of RH is the failure to adequately replace blood volume during the initial 2 to 3 days after injury. If the RH is caused by a fracture, continued low volume bleeding may persist for several days, particularly if a pelvic fracture has not been stabilized. Unlike many injuries, patients with RH frequently require 5 to 10 additional units of blood transfusion during the immediate postoperative period.[9] Moreover, eventual resorption of large quantities of retroperitoneal blood may cause a transient increase in serum bilirubin values, which have to be differentiated from other causes of postoperative jaundice. When doubt about the status of a retroperitoneal hematoma exists the C.T. Scan has proven useful to diagnose and follow the status of the hematoma (Figures 14-6, 14-7).

Table 14–4   LOCATION OF RETROPERITONEAL HEMATOMAS

	Pelvic	Perirenal	Other*
Baylis et al.[3]	33	9	8
Greico and Perry[9]	23	36	21
Nick et al.[19]	22	39	41
	78 (33.6%)	84 (36.2%)	70 (30.1%)

*Primarily central

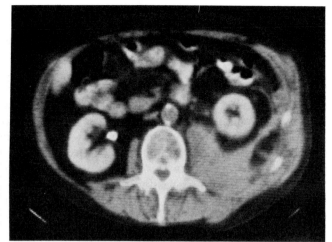

Figure 14–6. Large intraperitoneal hemorrhage primarily in posterior pararenal space and ileopsoas muscle which displaced the kidney forward. The above CT section was obtained in a patient with minor blunt trauma but who was anticoagulated.

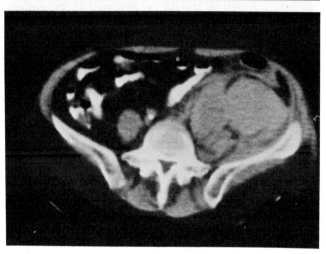

Figure 14–7. Large ileopsoas hemorrhage in a patient with intraabdominal injury.

The patient with the magnitude of injury which results in RH is subject to profound degradation of muscle protein. Early tube feeding or parenteral nutrition will sustain healing and metabolic function while recovery occurs.

Finally, when fractures are associated with RH, early aggressive physical therapy will shorten convalescence and hasten recovery.

COMPLICATIONS

The complications associated with retroperitoneal hematomas are in themselves relatively few, and relate primarily to the associated injuries. The primary complications relate to organ failure syndromes—the respiratory distress syndrome—and renal and hepatic failure. Prompt volume resuscitation with postoperative monitoring of vascular volume will accomplish the most toward preventing or modifying the severity of these complications.

Urine output should be monitored closely, and a fall in urine output should be assumed to relate to inadequate volume replacement. If doubt as to volume status exists, a Swan-Ganz catheter should be passed and fluid or cardiotonic agents administered, depending upon the filling pressures of the heart.

Arterial blood gases should be monitored frequently. A progressive fall in arterial PO2 or a PO2 below 70 in a patient receiving supplemental oxygen is an indication to carry out endotracheal intubation and mechanical ventilation.

Hematologic problems are often present. Platelet count and function should be monitored, as well as the prothrombin and partial thromboplastin times. Evidence of persistent bleeding is the indication to treat specific abnormalities noted, using platelet transfusions and/or fresh frozen plasma, as appropriate.

Immobilization increases the risk of thromboembolic problems. While anticoagulants are contraindicated in the immediate post-injury period, they should be utilized as appropriate if thrombotic complications become evident. Once the first three to four days have passed, unexplained cardiac arrhythmia or alteration in pulmonary function should be assumed to be embolic in nature and appropriate studies carried out to determine the cause.

REFERENCES

1. Allen RE, Eastman BA, Halter BL, Conolly WB: Retroperitoneal hemorrhage secondary to blunt trauma. Amer J Surg 118:558, 1969.
2. Attard J: Upper retroperitoneal injuries. Brit J Sur 58(1):55-60, 1971.
3. Baylis SM, Lansing EH, Glas WW: Traumatic retroperitoneal hematoma. Amer J Surg 103(4):477 480, 1962.
4. Cass AS, Ireland GW: Comparison of the conservative and surgical management of the more severe degrees of renal trauma in multiple injured patients. J Urol 109(1):810, 1973.
5. Dart CH, Braitman HE, Lanorb S: Management of renal arterial injuries secondary to penetrating abdominal trauma. J Urol 121:94-96, 1979.
6. Davidson AT: Direct intralumen balloon tamponade: A technique for the control of massive retroperitoneal hemorrhage. Amer J Surg 136:393-4, 1978.
7. Flint LM, Brown A, Richardson JD, Polk HC: Definitive control of bleeding from severe pelvic fractures. Ann Surg 189(6):709-716, 1979.
8. Gill W, Champion HR, Long WB, Austin EA, Cowley RA: Controversial aspects of abdominal trauma. J Royal College Surg 20:174-197, 1975.
9. Greico JG, Perry JF: Retroperitoneal hematoma following trauma: Its significance. J Trauma Aug.1980.
10. Gue S: Obstruction of second part of duodenum by retroperitoneal hematoma due to blunt abdominal trauma: A report of two cases. Injury 4(1):65-68, 1972.
11. Hamilton SG: Pelvic fractures and their complications. Proc Royal Soc Med 66:629-631, 1973.
12. Hawkins L, Pomerantz M, Eiseman B: Laparotomy at the time of pelvic fracture. J Trauma 10(8):619623, 1970.
13. Holcroft JW, Trunkey DD, Minagi H, Korobkin MT, Lim RC: Renal trauma and retroperitoneal hematomas: Indications for exploration. J Trauma 15(12):1045-1052, 1975.
14. Hubbard SG, Bivins BA, Sachatello·CR, Griffen WO: Diagnostic errors with peritoneal lavage in patients with pelvic fractures. Arch Surg 114:844846, 1979.
15. Killen DA: Injury of the superior mesenteric vessels secondary to nonpenetrating abdominal trauma. Am Surg 30(5):306-312, 1964.
16. Lucey DT, Smith MJV, Koontz WW: A plea for the conservative treatment of renal injuries. J Trauma 11(4):306-316, 1971.
17. McCort JJ: Plain film diagnosis of perirenal hemorrhage. Radiologia Clin 47:280-294, 1978.
18. Morrow JW, Mendey R: Renal trauma. J Urol 104:649-653, 1970.
19. Nick WV, Zollinger RW, Pace WG: Retroperitoneal hemorrhage after blunt abdominal trauma. J Trauma 7(5):652-659, 1967.
20. Orloff MJ, Charters AC: Injuries of the small bowel and mesentery and retroperitoneal hematoma. Surg Clin No Am 52(3):729-734, 1972.
21. Parvin S, Smith DG, Asher M, et al.: Effectiveness of diagnostic peritoneal lavage in blunt trauma. Ann Surg 181:255-261, 1975.

22. Paster SB, Van Houton F, Adams DF: Percutaneous balloon catheterization: A technique for the control of arterial hemorrhage caused by pelvic trauma. JAMA 230:573, 1974.

23. Ravitch MM: Retroperitoneal hemorrhage. Med Times 98(9):175-177, 1970.

24. Rotherberger DA, Fischer RP, Strate RG, Velasco R, Perry JF: The mortality associated with pelvic fractures. Surg 84(3):356-361, 1978.

25. Steichen FM, Dargan EL, Pearlman DM, Weil PH: The management of retroperitoneal hematoma secondary to penetrating injuries. Surg Gynecol Obstet 123(1):581-591, 1966.

26. Trunkey DD, Chapman MW, Lim RC, Dunphy JE: Management of pelvic fractures in blunt trauma injury. J Trauma 14(11):912-923, 1974.

27. Wilson TS, Castopoulos LB: Retroperitoneal injury to the duodenum by blunt abdominal trauma: Report of eight cases. Can J Surg 14:114-121, 1971.

28. Sheldon GF, Winestock DP: Hemorrhage from open pelvic fracture controlled intraoperatively with balloon catheter. J Trauma 18:68-70, 1978.

INDEX